Supportive Care
of Children
with Cancer

Supportive Care of Children with Cancer

CURRENT THERAPY AND GUIDELINES FROM THE CHILDREN'S CANCER GROUP

Second Edition

EDITED BY

Arthur R. Ablin, M.D.
Professor Emeritus of Clinical Pediatrics
Director Emeritus, Division of Pediatrics
   Clinical Oncology
Department of Pediatrics, School of Medicine
University of California, San Francisco

THE JOHNS HOPKINS UNIVERSITY PRESS
BALTIMORE AND LONDON

Drug dosage: The authors and publisher have exerted every effort to ensure that the selection and dosage of drugs discussed in this text accord with current recommendations and practice at the time of publication. However, in view of ongoing research, changes in governmental regulations, and the constant flow of information relating to drug therapy and drug reactions, the reader is urged to check the package insert of each drug for any change in indications and dosage and for warnings and precautions. This is particularly important when the recommended agent is a new and/or infrequently used drug.

© 1993, 1997 The Johns Hopkins University Press
All rights reserved. Published 1997
Printed in the United States of America on acid-free paper

9 8 7 6 5 4 3 2 1

The Johns Hopkins University Press
2715 North Charles Street
Baltimore, Maryland 21218-4319

The Johns Hopkins Press Ltd., London

Library of Congress Cataloging-in-Publication Data will be found at the end of this book.
A catalog record for this book is available from the British Library.

ISBN 0-8018-5726-0
ISBN 0-8018-5727-9 (pbk.)

Contents

Foreword:
Supportive Care Is
More Than Supportive

If children being treated for cancer today do as well as projected by national data, more than 85% will reach the plateau on the survival curve and presumably be cured of their malignant disease. If so, the overall prognosis for children with cancer in the United States will have turned a full 180°, from an 85% *mortality rate* for children and adolescents pre 1948 to an 85% *cure rate* at present! I believe the role of supportive care in this dramatic turnaround has been underestimated and certainly is underappreciated. Supportive care has become more than supportive in the role it has come to play in helping improve the survival of children and adolescents with cancer and in its critical importance in achieving the current successes of pediatric cancer therapy (Figure F.1). Although surgery, chemotherapy, and radiotherapy account for most of the 180° turn, advances in supportive care allowed the reversal to occur. Without supportive care there would have been little progress in the major therapeutic disciplines. Supportive care made it all possible.

Because six of every seven children and adolescents can now be cured, the quality of life during and after treatment is displacing cure as the paramount objective. Now, like the venerable Ford Motor Company slogan, "Quality is job #1." With this shift in emphasis, supportive care in pediatric cancer therapy is in the limelight and should be regarded as a primary modality, along with surgery, chemotherapy, and radiotherapy. In this book, now in its second edition, the discipline of supportive care in pediatric oncology is covered in depth by members of the Children's Cancer Group. This book continues to be unique: there is no other work of its kind. Although the editor was careful to describe the recommendations of the authors as "guidelines" rather than standards of care, most of the recommendations could be considered benchmarks of therapy, since they are current, tested by virtue of having been scrutinized during the first edition, and offered by experts in the field. Moreover, these guidelines may serve as the basis for critical pathways in pediatric cancer management and for the needs of our rapidly changing health care environment. The authors and editor provide this service and more. As the

Figure F.1.
The multiple modalities of supportive care interacting with care to achieve therapeutic goals.

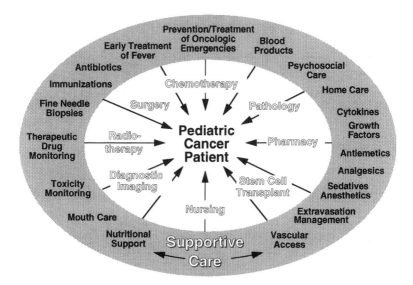

chair of the Children's Cancer Group, I am proud of my colleagues and what they have accomplished in the second edition. If you work in our field, you will benefit from this treatise.

W. Archie Bleyer, M.D.
Chair, Children's Cancer Group

Preface

The editor and contributors of the first edition of *Supportive Care of Children with Cancer* have been pleased with the reception this handbook has received by those directly responsible for providing patient care. The presence of dog-eared copies in hospital ward resident rooms, nursing stations, treatment rooms, and outpatient departments attests to its pertinence and usefulness.

Driven by innovative and ever-more-aggressive therapeutic approaches to children with cancer, their supportive care must constantly be intensified and improved. This new edition makes those changes and brings *Supportive Care of Children with Cancer* to the cutting-edge.

Five new chapters have been added, and very significant revisions have been made in each of the others. The new chapters are "Hemorrhagic and Thrombotic Complications in Children with Cancer," "Care of the Hematopoietic Stem Cell Transplant Patient after Leaving the Transplant Center," "Alternative Medicine in Pediatric Oncology," "Home Care for Children with Cancer," and "Terminal Care for Children with Cancer." These reflect, respectively, new ideas in the management of heretofore incompletely understood mechanisms of hemorrhage and thrombosis, the recognition of the increasing numbers of patients with various kinds of transplants and the more prominent role their long-term follow-up plays in pediatric oncology, the socioeconomically driven rapid changes in the practice and delivery of health care, and the deservedly increased attention to the child with terminal illness. The important changes in individual chapters are too numerous to mention, but it suffices to say that the reader will find many recommendations that continue to keep this bedside handbook current and representative of the "state of the art." Although there may be, and probably are, other approaches to the supportive care problems discussed, one may be confident that the recommendations made are up-to-date and reasonable.

Documenting the current state of supportive care of children with cancer does more than assist the bedside practitioner, the clinical nurse, and other health professionals with the details of treatment; it is also a mechanism for decreasing variables from creeping into clinical studies. Indeed, the influence of supportive care as a variable on clinical outcome could be as great as or greater than that of a specific therapeutic manipulation. This speaks for the adoption of some uniformity in supportive care measures in the conduct of cooperative clinical therapeutic studies.

This second attempt to document supportive care of children with cancer, like the first, will certainly not be the final one in this wonderful and constantly changing field of pediatric oncology. The contributors look forward to the readers' critical suggestions to help make this a living document, sensitive to change and ever improving, to better serve the children who so justly deserve our best efforts.

Abbreviations

ADH	antidiuretic hormone	CSA	cyclosporine
AIDS	acquired immuno-deficiency syndrome	CSF	colony-stimulating factor
ADH	antidiuretic hormone	CT	computed tomography
ALL	acute lymphoblastic leukemia	CTZ	chemoreceptor trigger zone
ALT	alanine aminotransferase	CVA	cerebrovascular accident
ANC	absolute neutrophil count	CVT	cerebral sinovenous thrombosis
ANLL	acute nonlymphoblastic leukemia	CVL	central venous line
APC	absolute phagocyte count	D5W	dextrose 5% in water
APTT	activated partial thromboplastin time	DIC	disseminated intravascular coagulation
AST	aspartame aminotransferase	DLCO	diffusion capacity of carbon monoxide
ATIII	antithrombin III	DT	diphtheria-tetanus
ATG	antithymocyte globulin	DTaP	diphtheria, tetanus, acellular pertussis
BCNU	bis chlorethyl nitrosourea (carmustine)	DVT	deep vein thrombosis
b.i.d.	twice daily	ECG	electrocardiogram
BUN	blood urea nitrogen	EEG	electroencephalogram
CBC	complete blood count	EBV	Epstein-Barr virus
CCNU	chlorethyl cyclohexyl nitrosouria (lomustine)	EPO	erythropoietin
		FAB	French-American-British
CDC	Centers for Disease Control and Prevention	FDA	Food and Drug Administration
cGy	centiGray	FS	fractional shortening
CHF	congestive heart failure	G-CSF	granulocyte-colony-stimulating factor
CMV	cytomegalovirus	GFR	glomerular filtration rate
CNS	central nervous system	GM-CSF	granulocyte-macrophage-colony-stimulating factor

GVHD	graft-versus-host disease
h	hour
HBIG	hepatitis B immune globulin
HBsAg	hepatitis B surface antigen
HBV	hepatitis B vaccine
Hct	hematocrit
Hgb	hemoglobin
HGF	hematopoietic growth factor
HIT	heparin-induced thrombocytopenia
HLA	human leukocyte antigen
HSTC	hematopoietic stem cell transplant
HSV	herpes simplex virus
HT3	serotonin
hu	human
HUS	hemolytic uremic syndrome
Ig	immunoglobin
IGIV	immune globulin intravenous
IL	interleukin
IM	intramuscular
INR	international normalized ratio
IPV	inactivated killed polio vaccine
IT	intrathecal
ITP	immune thrombocytopenic purpura
IV	intravenous
IVIgG	intravenous gamma-globulin
LDH	lactate dehydrogenase
LVEF	left ventricular ejection fraction
min	minute
MMR	measles, mumps, rubella

MRI	magnetic resonance imaging
NCI	National Cancer Institute
NHL	non-Hodgkin lymphoma
NPO	nothing by mouth
NSAID	nonsteroidal anti-inflamatory drug
OPV	oral polio vaccine
OTC	over-the-counter
pAO_2	partial pressure of arterial oxygen
pCO_2	partial pressure of carbon dioxide
PBSC	peripheral blood stem cells
PCA	patient-controlled analgesia
PCR	polymerase chain reaction
PE	pulmonary embolus
PFT	pulmonary function test
PICC	percutaneous intravenous central catheter
PLT	platelet
PO	by mouth
PR	by rectum
prn	as needed
PT	prothrombin time
PTT	partial thromboplastin time
q	each, every
q.i.d.	four times daily
r	recombinant
RBC	red blood cell (count)
RDA	Recommended Dietary Allowance
RNA	radionuclide cardiac cineangiography
RSV	respiratory syncytial virus
SC	subcutaneous

SGOT	aspartate amino-transferase
SIADH	syndrome of inappropriate antidiuretic hormone
SGPT	alanine aminotransferase
SMS	superior mediastinal syndrome
SMX	sulfamethoxazole
STI	systolic time interval
T_4	thyroxine
TBI	total body irridiation
TCT	thrombin clotting time
t.i.d.	three times daily
TMP	trimethoprim
TNF	tumor necrosis factor
TPN	total parenteral nutrition
TSH	thyroid-stimulating hormone
VIQ	ventilation perfusion scan
vWf	von Willebrand factor
VZIG	varicella-zoster immune globulin
VZV	varicella-zoster virus
WBC	white blood cell (count)
WK	week
WNL	within normal limits
ZIG	zoster immune globulin

Contributors

Consulting Editor: **Arnold J. Altman, M.D.,** Immediate Past Chair, Supportive Care Committee, Children's Cancer Group; Hartford Whalers' Professor of Childhood Cancer, Department of Pediatrics, University of Connecticut School of Medicine; and Head, Division of Pediatric Hematology/Oncology, Connecticut Children's Medical Center, Hartford, Connecticut

Consulting Editor: **James H. Feusner, M.D.,** Chair, Supportive Care Committee, Children's Cancer Group; and Adjunct Professor, Department of Pediatrics, University of California, San Francisco, California

Edythe A. Albano, M.D., Assistant Professor, Department of Pediatrics, University of Colorado School of Medicine, Denver, Colorado

Maureen E. Andrew, M.D., Professor, Department of Pediatrics, McMaster University, Hamilton, Ontario, Canada

Dorothy R. Barnard, M.D., Associate Professor, Department of Pediatrics, Dalhousie University, Halifax, Nova Scotia, Canada

Jean B. Belasco, M.D., Clinical Associate Professor, Department of Pediatrics, University of Pennsylvania School of Medicine, Philadelphia, Pennsylvania

Donna L. Betcher, R.N., M.S.N., P.N.P., Pediatric Oncology Nurse, Mayo Clinic, Rochester, Minnesota

Bruce R. Blazar, M.D., Professor, Department of Pediatric Hematology and Oncology, University of Minnesota, Minneapolis, Minnesota

Lu Ann Brooker, R.T., Research Assistant, Hamilton Civic Hospitals Research Center, Hamilton, Ontario, Canada

Gina Cavalieri, R.Pharm., Oncology Pharmacist, Children's Hospital of Philadelphia, Philadelphia, Pennsylvania

Pamelyn Close, M.D., M.P.H., Assistant Professor and Associate Chief, Division of Pediatric Hematology/Oncology, Harbor/UCLA Medical Center, University of California School of Medicine, Los Angeles, California

Ruth Daller, R.N., M.S., Pediatric Oncology Nurse, Children's Hospital of Philadelphia, Philadelphia, Pennsylvania

Patricia Danz, R.N., B.S.N., Supportive Care Coordinator, Children's Hospital Home Care, Children's Hospital of Philadelphia, Philadelphia, Pennsylvania

Kenneth De Santes, M.D., Assistant Professor, Division of Bone Marrow Transplantation, Department of Pediatrics, University of California, San Francisco, California

Peter W. Dillon, M.D., Professor and Chief, Division of Pediatric Surgery, Department of Surgery, College of Medicine, Pennsylvania State University, Hershey, Pennsylvania

Connie Goes, M.S.N., P.N.P., Oncology Nurse, Department of Oncology, Children's Hospital of Oakland, Oakland, California

Darryl C. Grendahl, B.Pharm., Oncology Pharmacist, Mayo Clinic, Rochester, Minnesota

Paula K. Groncy, M.D., Associate Clinical Professor, Department of Pediatrics, Harbor/UCLA School of Medicine, Torrance, California

Caroline Hastings, M.D., Assistant Clinical Professor, Department of Pediatrics, University of California, San Francisco, California

John J. Iacuone, M.D., Clinical Professor, Department of Pediatrics, Texas Tech University Health Sciences Center, Lubbock, Texas

F. Leonard Johnson, M.D., Robert C. Neerhout Professor, Department of Pediatrics, Oregon Health Sciences University, Portland, Oregon

Anne Kazak, Ph.D., Associate Professor, Division of Oncology, Department of Pediatrics, Children's Hospital of Philadelphia, Philadelphia, Pennsylvania

Sandra Luna-Fineman, M.D., Assistant Clinical Professor, Department of Pediatrics, University of California School of Medicine, San Francisco, California

M. Patricia Massicotte, M.D., Assistant Professor, Department of Pediatrics, The Hospital for Sick Children, University of Toronto, Toronto, Ontario, Canada

Rita S. Meek, M.D., Chief, Division of Hematology and Oncology, Alfred I. duPont Institute of the Nemours Foundation, Wilmington, Delaware; Associate Clinical Professor, Thomas Jefferson University, Philadelphia, Pennsylvania

John S. Murphy, B.Pharm., Senior Oncology Pharmacist, Pharmacy Department, Princess Margaret Hospital, Subiaco, Western Australia

Robert B. Noll, Ph.D., Professor, Division of Hematology/Oncology, Department of Pediatrics, Children's Hospital Medical Center, Cincinnati, Ohio

Melanie G. Oblender, M.D., Assistant Clinical Professor, Department of Pediatrics, Texas Tech University Health Sciences Center, Lubbock, Texas

Richard S. Pieters, M.D., Clinical Assistant Professor, Department of Radiology, Boston University School of Medicine, Boston, Mssachusetts

John J. Quinn, M.D., Professor, Department of Pediatrics, University of Connecticut School of Medicine, Hartford, Connecticut

Nancy Sacks, M.S., R.D., C.N.S.D., Pediatric Oncology Dietician, Department of Clinical Nutrition, Children's Hospital of Philadelphia, Philadelphia, Pennsylvania

Neil L. Schechter, M.D., Professor, Department of Pediatrics, University of Connecticut Health Center, Farmington, Connecticut

Susan F. Sencer, M.D., Clinical Instructor, Department of Pediatric Hematology-Oncology, University of Minnesota, Minneapolis, Minnesota

Kevin M. Shannon, M.D., Associate Professor, Division of Pediatric Hematology and Oncology, Department of Pediatrics, University of California, San Francisco, California

Laurel Steinherz, M.D., Associate Professor, Department of Pediatrics, Cornell University Medical Center, New York, New York

Richard D. Udin, D.D.S., Chair, Department of Pediatric Dentistry, University of Southern California, Los Angeles, California

Jean Wadman, R.N., M.S.N., C.R.N.P., Advanced Practice Nurse, Pediatric Hematology/Oncology, DuPont Hospital for Children, Wilmington, Delaware

Steven J. Weisman, M.D., Associate Professor, Department of Anesthesia, Yale University School of Medicine, New Haven, Connecticut

Eugene S. Wiener, M.D., Professor, Department of Surgery, University of Pittsburgh, Pittsburgh, Pennsylvania

Michael L. N. Willoughby, M.D., Oncologist Emeritus, Princess Margaret Hospital, Subiaco, Western Australia

Lawrence J. Wolff, M.D., Professor, Department of Pediatrics, Oregon Health Sciences University, Portland, Oregon

Supportive Care
of Children
with Cancer

1

The Prevention of Infection

Arnold J. Altman, M.D., and Lawrence J. Wolff, M.D.

Children receiving treatment for cancer are at increased risk of infection from bacterial, viral, protozoal, and fungal agents. Among the factors responsible are myelosuppression with decreased blood cell function, changes in humoral and cellular immunity, loss of integrity of physical defense barriers, hyponutrition, and changes in colonizing microflora. The following guidelines for care are considered to minimize the risk of infection and its associated morbidity and mortality in children with cancer who are undergoing treatment and to maintain the uniformity of care in a cooperative group study population to minimize treatment variables.

I. GENERAL MEASURES

A. Appropriate environment
1. Neutropenia alone is not a sufficient indication for hospitalization; the exposure to antibiotic-resistant nosocomial organisms would put the patient at additional risk. If the patient is afebrile and has no other evident medical problems, he or she should stay out of the hospital, but careful attention should be given to total body (especially oral) and environmental hygiene.
2. When hospitalization is necessary, place the patient in a private room or with another patient who has no active infection. The patient need not be restricted to the room, but must avoid contact with patients who have active infections.

3. Hospital staff, families, and visitors should wash their hands carefully before and after contact with the patient.

B. Hygiene
   1. Dietary precautions
      In view of the lack of evidence that dietary manipulation reduces the incidence of serious infection, the patient may eat a regular diet. The improvement in nutritional intake may compensate for any increased exposure to food-related organisms. Some prudent modifications to consider are:
      a. Have the patient avoid raw fruits and vegetables (especially salads).
      b. Have the patient avoid processed meats.
      c. Thoroughly wash the lids of canned foods and beverages with antiseptic soap and hot water before opening.
   2. Cleanliness
      a. Have the patient bathe and shampoo daily.
      b. Have the patient and all who come in contact with the patient wash their hands with antiseptic soap.
      c. Pay meticulous attention to skin, and practice asepsis with Betadine or a comparable agent before venipuncture or finger prick.
   3. Dental hygiene (see Chapter 14)
   4. Catheters (in blood vessels, urethra, nose, and elsewhere)
      a. Use catheters only when absolutely necessary.
      b. Use meticulous care during dressing changes, flushing, and connecting.
      c. Change peripheral intravenous (IV) lines at least every 4 days.

C. Activities
   The patient can attend school when the absolute neutrophil count (ANC) is > 200/μL and likely to increase.

D. Protection of the anal-rectal mucosa
   1. Prevent constipation with age-appropriate diet and, if necessary, a stool softener [(e.g., sodium docusate, 1–3 mg/kg/day PO)].
   2. Avoid rectal suppositories to minimize the chance of fissures and proctitis.
   3. Do not insert thermometers into the rectum.

II. PROPHYLAXIS AGAINST *PNEUMOCYSTIS CARINII*

A. Background
  1. Patients being treated for cancer have a higher incidence of *P. carinii* infection. This risk can effectively be reduced by administering trimethoprim/sulfamethoxazole (TMP/SMX).
  2. The low dosage suggested below does not appear to enhance bone marrow suppression from moderately aggressive programs of chemotherapy. However, this may not be true with more intensive cytotoxic regimens. When prolonged marrow suppression occurs in patients receiving TMP/SMX, consider withholding this agent rather than decreasing the dosage of chemotherapy and using pentamidine or dapsone.
  3. The incidence of pneumocystis infection varies from institution to institution and possibly from tumor to tumor and protocol to protocol, so the indications for prophylaxis may vary. However, in the interest of achieving uniformity of care, the use of TMP/SMX to prevent pneumocystis pneumonia is recommended for all patients on chemotherapy.

B. Dosage
  1. TMP 5 mg/kg/day (150 mg/m^2/day) and SMX 25 mg/kg/day (750 mg/m^2/day) are given in two divided doses 3 days a week.
  2. TMP/SMX therapy should start with the initiation of chemotherapy and continue for 8 to 12 weeks after chemotherapy is stopped.

C. Preparations
  1. Tablet: TMP 80 mg/SMX 400 mg
     Double-strength tablet: TMP 160 mg/SMX 800 mg
  2. Suspension: TMP 40 mg/SMX 200 mg/5 mL

D. Intolerance of or allergy to TMP/SMX
  For patients who are repeatedly unable to tolerate full doses of chemotherapy because of allergy or myelosuppression, omit TMP/SMX prophylaxis. Consider inhalation or intravenous pentamidine or dapsone where the possibility of pneumocystis infection is high.

1. The prophylactic regimen for dapsone is 2 mg/kg/day as a single dose. (It comes in 25 and 100 mg tablets.)
2. The prophylactic regimen for IV pentamidine is 4 mg/kg (diluted in 50–250 ml of dextrose 5% in water) infused over 60 minutes IV q4wk.
3. The prophylactic regimen for inhalation pentamidine is 8 mg/kg for children < 5 years old and 300 mg for children > 5 years old. It is administered q4wk via the Respirgard II nebulizer.

III. PROPHYLAXIS AGAINST BACTERIA

A. Trimethoprim/sulfamethoxazole
Some evidence indicates that children have fewer serious bacterial infections; deaths related to infection; and episodes of otitis media, upper respiratory infection, urinary tract infection, cellulitis, pneumonitis, and sinusitis when prophylactic TMP/SMX is given. The following recommendations are made to ensure uniformity in multi-institutional trials.
1. Patients on chemotherapy should receive prophylactic TMP/SMX *unless* they have
   a. Allergy to TMP or SMX
   b. Glucose-6-phosphate dehydrogenase deficiency
   c. Malabsorption
2. Schedule
   a. Patients should commence TMP/SMX prophylaxis at the time of the diagnosis whether or not systemic antibiotic therapy is also indicated.
   b. Patients on aggressive regimens for whom the ANC can be expected to be < 500/μL for more than 14 days should take TMP/SMX daily when starting the chemotherapy in the hopes of diminishing the occurrence of bacterial infection.
   c. Patients on nonaggressive regimens of chemotherapy or those receiving systemic antibiotic therapy should be given TMP/SMX 3 consecutive days each week.
   d. Patients should discontinue TMP/SMX 1 day before and for 4 days after infusion of high-dose methotrexate.
   e. Bone marrow transplant recipients should discontinue TMP/SMX 2 days before transplantation and then

restart it when the ANC is > 500/μL.
   3. Dosage (see Section IIB)
   4. Preparations (see Section IIC)

B. Other antimicrobial agents
   The quinolones ofloxacin, norfloxacin, and ciprofloxacin have shown promise in adult prophylactic studies. Ciprofloxacin appears to have the broadest antibacterial effect and should be considered as prophylaxis in the neutropenic young adult with cancer; however, ciprofloxacin is not approved by the Food and Drug Administration for use in children. The dosage usually used for ciprofloxacin is 500 mg b.i.d.

C. Prophylaxis against *Haemophilus influenzae* type b
   1. The use of *H. influenzae* vaccine for children older than 2 months is recommended; however, remember that patients who receive very intense chemotherapeutic regimens may not form or maintain antibodies to *H. influenzae.* (see ChII A-2)
   2. Patients who have contact within the household or who have prolonged exposure to individuals with severe *H. influenzae* infection should receive rifampin prophylaxis regardless of their age.
   3. Dosage: 20 mg/kg/day of rifampin: (maximum 600 mg) PO for 4 days
   4. Preparations
      a. Capsule: 150 or 300 mg. Powders can be preweighed by a pharmacist to give precise dosages.
      b. Rifampin suspension (1% in simple syrup) can be prepared by a pharmacist.

D. Intravenous immune globulin
   1. Determine the use of intravenous immune globulin for bacterial prophylaxis for each study. Specifically designate whether or not it is to be used.
   2. Dosage: 200–400 mg/kg once a month
   3. Preparations vary. Listed are several:
      a. 5% solution (Cutter): 10, 50, or 100 mL vials
      b. Lyophilized powder (Sandoz): 1, 3, or 6 g vials
         Reconstitution fluid is provided to prepare a 3, 6, 9, or 12% solution.
   4. Administer in a separate IV line starting at 0.5–1.0

mg/kg/min for 15 minutes, 3 mg/kg/min for 15 minutes, and then 4 mg/kg/min until completed.

5. Compatible with 0.9% saline
6. Give the IV preparation only intravenously; never use the intramuscular (IM) preparation intravenously.
7. Side effects
   a. Interstitial extravasation can result in local irritation, inflammation, and phlebitis secondary to the alkaline pH.
   b. Rapid intravenous infusion can result in reversible increases in serum creatinine concentrations.
   c. A small percentage of patients may experience nausea, vomiting, headache, diarrhea, and/or rash.
   d. Anaphylactoid reaction in agammaglobulinemic or IgA-deficient patients
   e. Inflammatory reactions: fever, fatigue, shivering, local pain
   f. Hypersensitivity reactions
   g. Headaches, aseptic meningitis syndrome

E. Splenectomized children
1. Splenectomized children are susceptible to overwhelming infections with encapsulated bacteria.
2. Penicillin, amoxicillin, or erythromycin may be used for antibiotic prophylaxis. Dosage recommendations are as follows:
   a. Penicillin
      > 14 years: 250–500 mg b.i.d.
      5–14 years: 250 mg b.i.d.
      1–5 years: 125 mg b.i.d.
   b. Amoxicillin
      > 14 years: 250–500 mg daily
      5–14 years: 125 mg daily
      1–5 years: 10 mg/kg/day
   c. Erythromycin (base)
      > 8 years: 250–500 mg daily
      2–8 years: 150 mg daily
      1–2 years: 125 mg daily
3. Vaccination (see II A–Z)
   a. Polyvalent pneumococcal vaccine: 0.5 mL IM for children ≥ 2 years old

b. *Haemophilus* type b conjugate vaccine: 0.5 mL IM for children ≥ 2 months old
See the manufacturer's recommendations for the number of injections required.
c. Quadrivalent meningococcal polysaccharide vaccine

IV. PROPHYLAXIS AGAINST FUNGI

Fungal infections are a significant cause of morbidity and mortality in immune-suppressed patients undergoing prolonged periods of antibiotic therapy for fever/neutropenia. The most common fungal infections in patients receiving intensive chemotherapy include candidiasis and aspergillosis.

A. Candidiasis
   1. Candidiasis is the most common fungal infection in children receiving anticancer therapy.
   2. For prevention of oral or esophageal candidiasis during treatment with steroids or with intensive chemotherapy, use either of the following regimens:
      a. Mycostatin oral swish and swallow (5–10 mL b.i.d.).
      b. Clotrimazole troche (1 b.i.d. suck for 20 minutes).

B. Aspergillosis
   1. Aspergillus is primarily an airborne organism. Sinopulmonary colonization is thought to precede infection.
   2. Aspergillus infection may be avoided as follows:
      a. Efforts to prevent aspergillus infection should include respiratory isolation, use of laminar flow rooms, and use of high-efficiency particulate air filters.
      b. If the patient is hospitalized at an institution where aspergillus infections are common, consider eliminating plants from the patient's room, monitoring and controlling nasal microbial flora, and scrutinizing construction work (which may be a source of airborne aspergillus spores).
      c. Low-dose amphotericin B (0.1–0.25 mg/kg/day IV) or the inhalant form of amphotericin B may reduce the incidence of invasive aspergillosis. Itraconazole and other agents need to be further evaluated.

V. PROPHYLAXIS AGAINST INFECTIOUS COMPLICATIONS IN PATIENTS WITH CENTRAL CATHETERS

A. Background
In-dwelling central catheters are common in children receiving chemotherapy. These children frequently require operations or other invasive procedures and, much as patients with congenital heart disease, are at risk for colonization of the catheter during episodes of transient bacteremia.

B. Recommendations
All patients with indwelling central catheters (of either the external catheter type or the subcutaneous reservoir type) should receive standard prophylaxis against subacute bacterial endocarditis, as recommended by the American Heart Association, during invasive procedures, including operations on the gastrointestinal or genitourinary tract, endotracheal intubation, and dental manipulation.
1. Standard regimen
Amoxicillin 50 mg/kg (maximum 2 g) PO 1 hour before the procedure.
2. Regimen for patients allergic to penicillin
Clindamycin 20 mg/kg (maximum 600 mg) PO 1 hour before the procedure
or
20 mg/kg (maximum 600 mg) IV within 30 minutes before the procedure.

VI. PROPHYLAXIS AGAINST VIRUSES

Common viral infections that are known to have increased virulence in immune-compromised children include varicella-zoster virus (VZV), herpes simplex virus (HSV), cytomegalovirus (CMV), Epstein-Barr virus (EBV), hepatitis types A and B, respiratory syncytial virus (RSV), and rubeola (measles). Infection with these viruses has resulted in prolonged virus excretion, increased morbidity, and death.

A. General preexposure measures
1. At the time of diagnosis of malignancy
a. Obtain a history of immunization and previous infection with VZV, HSV, EBV, RSV, and measles.

b. Obtain viral titers against VZV (preferably using immu-
nofluorescence antibody or a similarly sensitive technique), HSV, CMV, EBV, and, for infants < 2 years old, RSV.
2. Decrease exposure
a. Do not administer live attenuated oral polio vaccine to
the siblings of patients receiving chemotherapy. Killed
polio vaccine may be given.
b. Notify appropriate teachers, caregivers, and friends of
the risk to these children of infection with measles and
VZV.
c. Prevent in-hospital exposure by preadmission screening of other hospitalized children.
d. Avoid having caregivers with active viral infection come
into direct contact with immune-suppressed patients.

B. Prophylaxis against varicella-zoster virus
1. Indications for, and use of, varicella-zoster immune globulin are discussed in Chapter 2III-D.
2. The decision to hold chemotherapy during the incubation period for the development of varicella should
be based on the intensity of exposure, the general condition of the patient, and the intensity of the chemotherapy.
3. If varicella develops, stop chemotherapeutic agents and
start acyclovir (1500 mg/m2/day IV divided q8h) with adequate hydration.

C. Prophylaxis against herpes simplex virus
1. Patients with recurrent HSV infections are at increased
risk of developing significant HSV infections while receiving chemotherapy or during and after bone marrow transplantation. The administration of acyclovir prophylacti-
cally may prevent or decrease the severity of recurrent
HSV infection. Its use is recommended.
2. Acyclovir
a. Dosage: 200–600 mg/m^2/day PO divided into 3 to 6
doses or 250 mg/m^2 IV q8h during periods of marked
leukopenia.
b. Preparations
i. Vial: 500 mg for IV use
ii. Capsule: 200 mg
c. Acyclovir may be infused in 5% dextrose, 5% dex-

trose/0.9% saline, Ringer's lactate, or 0.9% saline. Ensure adequate hydration.

    d. Acyclovir should not be added to or infused in the same line with blood products, protein hydrolysates or amino acids, or fat emulsions.

    e. The clearance of acyclovir is markedly decreased in neonates. The clearance in infants aged 3 to 12 months is unknown; that of infants > 1 year old is the same as that for adults. Adjust the dosage if the patient has renal insufficiency (the drug is excreted by the kidneys). Table 1.1 shows the dosage adjustment for patients with renal impairment.

D. Prophylaxis against cytomegalovirus

    1. CMV-seronegative patients who are candidates for a bone marrow transplant should receive CMV-negative or leukocyte-depleted blood products.

    2. When CMV-seronegative blood is not available for CMV-negative patients, white cell filters must be used (see Chapter 4-I-B). Whenever possible, filtering of blood products should occur at the blood bank shortly after collection, rather than at the bedside.

E. Prophylaxis against Epstein-Barr virus

    1. The significance of EBV infection in patients with malignancies is unknown, although children in leukemic remission have died after a hemophagocytic infection associated with EBV.

    2. α-Interferon can prevent EBV infections in patients who have undergone renal transplantation.

TABLE 1.1.
Dosage Adjustment of Acyclovir for Patients with Renal Impairment

Creatinine Clearance Rate (mL/min/1.73 m²)	% Usual Individual Dose	Dosing Interval
> 50	100	q8h
25–50	100	q12h
10–25	100	q24h
< 10	50	q24h

*Higher peak and trough values have also been suggested

3. The prevention of EBV infections in patients receiving chemotherapy is not practical.

F. Prophylaxis against infectious hepatitis types A and B (see Chapter 2 III B&C)

G. Prophylaxis against respiratory syncytial virus
The risk of nosocomial infection with RSV can be significantly reduced with rapid laboratory diagnosis combined with cohort nursing and the wearing of gowns and gloves for all contacts with RSV-infected children.

H. Prophylaxis against rubeola (measles) (see Chapter 2 III-A)

Bibliography

Balfour HH: Varicella zoster virus infections in immunocompromised hosts: A review of the natural history and management. *Am J Med* 85:68–73, 1988 (suppl).

Brigden D, Whiteman P: The clinical pharmacology of acyclovir and its pro-drugs. *Scand J Infect Dis* 47:33–39, 1985 (suppl).

Dajani AS, Taubert KA, Wilson W, et al: Prevention of Bacterial Endocarditis: Recommendations by the American Heart Association. *Circulation* 96: 358-66, 1997.

Dekker AW, Rozenberg-Arska M, Verhoef J: Infection prophylaxis in acute leukemia; a comparison of ciprofloxacin with trimethoprim-sulfamethoxazole and colistin. *Ann Intern Med* 106:7–12, 1987.

Hathorn JW: Critical appraisal of antimicrobials for prevention of infections in immunocompromised hosts. *Hematol Oncol Clin North Am* 7:1051–99, 1993.

Hughes WT: Recent advances in the prevention of *pneumocystis carinii* pneumonia. *Adv Pediatr Infect Dis* 11:163–80, 1996.

Madge P, Paton JY, McColl JH, Mackie PL: Prospective controlled study of four infection control procedures to prevent nosocomial infection with respiratory syncytial virus. *Lancet* 340:1079–83, 1992.

Meunier F: Prevention of mycoses in immunocompromised patients. *Rev Infect Dis* 9:408–16, 1987.

Novell VM, Marshall WC, Yeo J, McKendrick GD: High-dose oral acyclovir for children at risk of disseminated herpes virus infections. *J Infect Dis* 151:372, 1985.

American Academy of Pediatrics. In: Peter G, ed. 1997 *Red Book: Report of the Committee on Infectious Diseases.* 24th ed. Elk Grove, IL: American Academy of Pediatrics; 1997.

Wolff LJ: Use of prophylactic antibiotics. *Am J Pediatr Hematol Oncol* 3:267–76, 1984.

Working Party of the British Committee for Standards in Hematology, Clinical Hematology Task Force: Guidelines for the prevention and treatment of infections in patients with an absent or dysfunctional spleen. *Br Med J* 312:430, 1996.

2

Immunization of the Child with Cancer

Caroline Hastings, M.D., Connie Goes, M.S.N., P.N.P.,
and Lawrence J. Wolff, M.D.

The aggressive therapies children with cancer receive result in profound immune suppression. Additionally, the specific underlying diagnosis is important to consider with regard to the timing of and response to immunization. The recommendations that follow are based on clinical studies evaluating immunizations in these distinct patient populations.

I. ACTIVE IMMUNIZATION OF CHILDREN ON CHEMOTHERAPY (TABLE 2.1)

    A. Bacterial immunization

        1. Diphtheria, tetanus, acellular pertussis (DTaP) immunizations

            a. Few infections with these organisms are seen, probably due to some protection from earlier immunizations and herd immunity.

            b. Several studies report adequate responses to primary and booster DTaP immunizations given during chemotherapy.

            c. Children receiving more aggressive therapies may be less likely to respond as well as those receiving standard therapies.

            d. Recommendations

                i. Children on maintenance therapy should be given DTaP immunizations at scheduled times.

TABLE 2.1.
Immunization of the Child with Cancer, on Chemotherapy

Immunization	Recommendation
DTaP	Recommended at appropriate age intervals in unimmunized children (routine boosters can be deferred)
Polio	OPV contraindicated IPV given in lieu of OPV at appropriate age
MMR	Contraindicated
Pneumococcus, meningococcus	Recommended at appropriate age, especially if asplenic
H. influenzae type b	Recommended at appropriate age in unimmunized children
HBV	Recommended at start of therapy, if titer negative (recommended with HBIG for exposures)
Influenza	Recommended seasonally
Varicella	Recommended for ALL, in maintenance. Consider in other "lower risk" diagnoses

ii. If therapy is short in duration or to be discontinued shortly after the DTaP is due, then delay immunization until therapy is completed.

iii. DTaP titers may fall during active therapy; therefore, a booster dose of DTaP for children ≤ 7 yrs and (*diphtheria tetanus (DT)* for children ≤ 7 yrs of age) is recommended at 1 year after the completion of therapy.

2. Polysaccharide vaccines: pneumococcus, meningococcus, and *Haemophilus influenzae* type b

Children receiving chemotherapy are at an increased risk of infection with polysaccharide-encapsulated pathogens, especially during the first 4 years of life. An increased incidence of pneumococcal and *H. influenzae* type b disease is seen in children with acute lymphoblastic leukemia (ALL) and in splenectomized patients with Hodgkin disease. Although less frequent, meningococcal disease has been reported in such patients.

a. Several studies have documented an adequate response to the pneumococcal polysaccharide and *H. influenzae* vaccines in patients with acute leukemia, Hodgkin disease, and solid tumors.

b. Fifty to 85% of children with leukemia and 45% of children with solid tumors have a significant antibody response after receiving *H. influenzae* type b diphtheria toxoid conjugate.

  i. The response is greatest in children immunized in the first 12 months of therapy for leukemia, with antibody levels declining during continued therapy.
  ii. In Hodgkin disease, the antibody response is only minimally impaired if the vaccine is given more than 10 days before the initiation of therapy or before splenectomy. Responses to polysaccharide vaccines may not be normal for as long as 4 years after treatment.

c. Recommendations

  i. The Centers for Disease Control and Prevention (CDC) recommends immunization with pneumococcal, meningococcal, and *H. influenzae* type b conjugate vaccines for all immune-compromised patients. However, few data support vaccination for pneumococcus and meningococcus in children receiving chemotherapy.
  ii. Unvaccinated children with ALL or solid tumors should be vaccinated during maintenance therapy, per recommendations for age.
  iii. Patients with Hodgkin disease undergoing splenectomy or splenic radiation should be immunized at least 7–10 days before therapy begins and be given booster doses of pneumococcal and *H. influenzae* type b vaccines 3–5 years after the completion of therapy.
  iv. Patients with surgical or functional asplenia (due to radiation of the spleen) should be given meningococcal vaccine in the pretreatment period and then a booster 2–3 years later. After this period of time, boosters for pneumococcus and meningococcus should be given every 5–6 years, as recommended for high-risk adults. For ALL and solid tumor patients receiving *H. influenzae* type b during therapy, a booster should be given 1 year after the completion of therapy.

B. Viral immunization

  1. Measles, mumps, rubella (MMR)

     a. The safety of this vaccine in immune-compromised hosts has been a concern since the death of a patient who received it during therapy over 30 years ago! A further attenuated measle vaccine has been studied in a small study of leukemic children after cessation of therapy and was found to be safe. Several small studies, however, have found that, although the measles vaccine is relatively safe, patients have a suboptimal and short-lasting antibody response.

b. Recommendation
MMR is contraindicated for any child with cancer currently undergoing therapy. Reimmunization of all patients with MMR is recommended at 1 year after the completion of therapy, then every 10 years.

2. Polio
a. Do not give oral polio vaccine (OPV) to immune-compromised patients or their siblings, due to their increased susceptibility to vaccine-associated polio.
b. Inactivated killed polio vaccine (IPV) is an alternative for immune-compromised patients, but may not be adequate for primary immunization during therapy.
c. Recommendations
i. IPV can be substituted for booster doses at appropriate times for patients previously partially immunized.
ii. For unimmunized children (or in areas in which polio is endemic), IPV can be given for primary immunization, but reimmunization with OPV 1 year after the cessation of therapy is recommended.
iii. Partially immunized children can receive either OPV or IPV 1 year after cessation of therapy.

3. Hepatitis B
a. Children with cancer are at risk for blood-borne infections due to numerous procedures requiring venous access and frequent transfusion of blood products. Additionally, children with cancer have an increased risk of becoming chronic hepatitis B surface antigen (HBsAg) carriers.
b. Children receiving chemotherapy have an impaired, yet adequate, serologic response to hepatitis B vaccine (HBV). The protective titer of antibody after three doses of vaccine is achieved in up to 67% of children receiving chemotherapy for solid tumors and hematologic malignancies, compared with 97% in children with benign conditions.

    c. Recommendation

    The administration of HBV at 0-, 1-, and 6-month intervals is recommended for previously unimmunized children on therapy. Obtain titers after immunization to ascertain an adequate response.

4. Influenza

    a. The safety of inactivated influenza vaccine in cancer patients is well established, yet efficacy data are minimal and controversial. Studies of vaccination in children with cancer on therapy found both a significant impairment of antibody response while some demonstrate a protective antibody titer.

    b. Recommendation

    The CDC recommends influenza vaccine for all children, on a yearly basis, during periods of active immune suppression (on therapy and up to 1 year after cessation of therapy). It is recognized that this is not the general practice due to incomplete data. For optimal immunogenicity, two doses should be given, 4 weeks apart. It is not necessary to interrupt chemotherapy. Influenza vaccine can safely be given to immune-compromised patients over the age of 6 months.

5. Varicella vaccine

    a. Although safe and effective, the varicella vaccine has not been licensed for use in children with malignancies, but may be used on a compassionate basis in children with leukemia. Eighty-five percent of children with ALL during maintenance therapy have serologic evidence of an immune response after receiving one dose, and more than 90% after two doses, independent of whether chemotherapy is withheld or not.

    b. Immune-compromised children have a higher incidence of vaccine-associated varicella than healthy children (up to 40% versus <5%); however, the attack rate is much lower than with exposure to wild-type varicella and the vaccine-associated illness usually has an extremely mild, often subclinical, course. Overall, the vaccine is felt to be more than 80% effective in preventing clinical varicella in children with leukemia and 100% effective in preventing severe varicella in this high-risk population. Current data indicate that this immunity does not wane significantly with time.

    c. Additionally, the vaccine provides a protective effect against zoster and, with a booster, reduces the risk from 15% to a 3% risk.

    d. Recommendations

       i. Varicella vaccine is recommended for all susceptible children with ALL during maintenance, 12 months after documented remission. A first dose confers immunity and a second dose given 3 months later boosts the antibody titer. Varicella titers should be checked several months after the second dose and then yearly to determine if a third dose is necessary.

      ii. Therapy should be interrupted for 1 week before and 1 week after the patient receives the first dose of the vaccine and timed such that it not be given within one week of the prednisone pulse. It is not necessary to interrupt therapy for the second injection.

     iii. The absolute lymphocyte count should be at least 700/µL at the time of vaccination.

     iv. Due to the possibility of rash-associated transmission of the virus to other immune-compromised children, vaccinated children should be examined to rule out vaccine associated varicella before they come to the oncology clinic for 4–5 weeks after the vaccine.

II. ACTIVE IMMUNIZATION OF CHILDREN OFF CHEMOTHERAPY

A. Overview

The duration and severity of immune dysfunction after the cessation of chemotherapy are not known. Preliminary studies suggest that immune recovery, both humoral and cellular, is slow and at variable rates depending on the underlying diagnosis and type of therapy. Abnormalities in children with ALL and Hodgkin disease may be more pronounced and longer lasting than in children with solid tumors. Some recovery is evident in the majority of children 3–12 months from the end of therapy.

B. Recommendations

    1. DTaP, OPV, MMR, *H. influenzae* type b, pneumococcal and meningococcal vaccines, varicella, and HBV require boosters.

    2. Killed vaccines (boosters) may be resumed 6–12 months

after the cessation of therapy and live virus vaccines at 1 year.

III. PASSIVE IMMUNIZATION (TABLE 2.2)

The use of passive immunization is well established for certain pathogens, including measles, hepatitis A, hepatitis B, and varicella. Due to possible loss of immunity while patients are receiving chemotherapy and the potential for exposure, it may be worthwhile to check yearly titers. Most of the recommendations that follow are from the American Academy of Pediatrics *Red Book*.

  A. Measles

      1. Immune-compromised patients who are exposed to measles should receive immune globulin prophylaxis, even if previously immunized. The efficacy of immune globulin within 6 days of exposure in preventing serious

Table 2.2.
Passive Immunization of the Child with Cancer, during Chemotherapy

Disease	Recommendation
Hepatitis A	Immune globulin 0.02 mL/kg IM (maximum dose 2 mL) Give within 14 days of exposure. Start HAV vaccine
Hepatitis B	Previously unvaccinated children HBIG 0.06 mL/kg IM (maximum dose 5 mL) Start the first of three HBV vaccine doses Previously vaccinated children Known nonresponder (or unknown status), 0.5 mL HBIG IM + vaccine: HBIG should be given within 24 hours, and vaccine series initiated within 7 days of exposure
Measles	Immune globulin 0.5 mL/kg IM (maximum dose 15 mL) Give within 6 days of exposure, regardless of previous immunization status
Varicella	VZIG 1 vial/10 kg IM (maximum 5 vials) Give within 48 hours of exposure for maximum effect, may be effective up to 96 hours after exposure
Tuberculosis	Isoniazid 10 mg/kg/day PO (maximum 300 mg/day for 12 months) If patient is noncompliant, can change dose to twice weekly Directly observed therapy (20–30 mg/kg/day to maximum of 900 mg/day, preferably after 1 month of daily therapy)

complications in patients with cancer is not clear, but it is likely to be beneficial.

2. Recommendations

a. Immune globulin 0.5 ml/kg intramuscular (IM) (maximum dose 15 mL) should be given within 6 days of exposure to measles. (Note that this dose is higher than that recommended for immune-competent individuals.)

b. Combined prophylaxis with a live virus vaccine is contraindicated in immune-compromised children, but recommended in immune-competent contacts (siblings, other family members).

B. Hepatitis B

1. Administration of hepatitis B immune globulin (HBIG) effectively prevents hepatitis B for patients with a percutaneous or mucosal exposure or for household contact with a chronic HBsAg carrier. Vaccination after exposure is highly effective when combined with passive immunization in the prevention of disease, especially if the vaccine series begins within 7 days of exposure.

2. Recommendations

a. Combined prophylaxis with HBIG and HBV is recommended for the unvaccinated child or for the child with a documented negative titer despite previous vaccination.

b. For unvaccinated children, the dose of HBIG is 0.06 mL/kg IM (maximum dose 5 mL), to be given within 24 hours of exposure.

c. For vaccinated children with either unknown or negative titers, the dose of HBIG is 0.5 mL IM. For the child with a documented positive titer, HBIG is not indicated.

C. Hepatitis A

1. Immune globulin can prevent clinical disease resulting from hepatitis A virus in exposed susceptible individuals when given within 14 days of exposure.

2. Recommendation

The dose of immune globulin is 0.02 mL/kg (maximum dose 5 mL) as soon as possible after exposure.

D. Varicella

1. Exposure to varicella is defined as a continuing household exposure to someone with active varicella or having been in the same room with an individual who is in the

contagious state (i.e., 1–2 days before and 5 days after the eruption of vesicles) for at least 1 hour.
2. Varicella-zoster immune globulin (VZIG) is highly effective in preventing primary varicella.
3. The incubation period is prolonged by 7 days when VZIG is administered, therefore the isolation period extends from day 10 to day 28 after exposure. No data are available on the possible role of acyclovir in the prevention of varicella after exposure.
4. Recommendation
Immune-compromised children who have been exposed to varicella and have documented negative titers should receive VZIG 1 vial/10 kg IM (maximum dose 5 vials) within 96 hours of exposure. Children who have been vaccinated and/or have positive titers do not need to receive VZIG with exposures.

E. Tuberculosis
1. Children who are exposed to a potentially infectious case of tuberculosis should undergo tuberculin skin testing (purified protein derivative, with appropriate controls) and a chest roentgenogram. However, they may be anergic, and negative skin test results do not indicate lack of disease.
2. Recommendation
Administer prophylactic isoniazid (10 mg/kg/day by mouth; maximum dose 300 mg/day) for 12 months to immune-compromised patients with a significant exposure to tuberculosis, irrespective of skin test results.

IV. IMMUNIZATIONS OF SIBLINGS OF CHILDREN WITH CANCER

In general, siblings should continue to receive all their immunizations as per the guidelines of the American Academy of Pediatrics, with the exception of the live polio vaccine. IPV should be given in lieu of OPV at the designated times. If the sibling received only IPV in the primary series, a booster with OPV is recommended when the patient completes therapy and felt to be at minimal, if any, risk i.e. 1 year off therapy.

Varicella vaccine is recommended for siblings over the age of 12 months. Transmission of vaccine-type varicella from healthy children to immune-compromised siblings has not been documented. Additionally, transmission of the virus has been known to occur only when the vaccine causes a rash (incubation time 1 month), which occurs in less than 5% of immune-competent children. The vaccine type infection is spread not via respiratory secretions but by direct contact with skin lesions, and the transmission rate is less than one-fourth that of the wild-type vaccine.

To reduce exposure to their siblings with cancer, this population should be targeted for immunization with the influenza vaccine.

V. IMMUNIZATION OF CHILDREN AFTER BONE MARROW TRANSPLANTATION

See Chapter 17.

Bibliography

Ambrosino DM, Molrine DC: Critical appraisal of immunization strategies for prevention of infection in the compromised host. *Hematol Oncol Clin N Am* 7:1027–50, 1993.

American Academy of Pediatrics: In: Peter G, ed 1997 *Red Book. The Report of the Committee on Infectious Diseases.* 24th ed. Elk Grove Village, IL: American Academy of Pediatrics; 1997.

Bernini JC, Mustafa MM, Winick NJ, et al.: Evaluation of attenuated live virus measles vaccine in children with cancer. [Abstr] *Proc of Am Soc Clin Oncol* 13:438, 1994.

Gershon AA: Varicella vaccine: Its past, present and future. *Pediatr Infect Dis J* 14:742–44, 1995.

Gershon AA, LaRussa P, Steinberg S, et al.: The protective effect of immunologic boosting against zoster: An analysis in leukemic children who were vaccinated against chickenpox. *J Infect Dis* 73:450–53, 1996.

Gross PA, Gould AL, Brown AE: Effect of cancer chemotherapy on the immune response to influenza virus vaccine. Review of published studies. *Rev Infect Dis* 7:613–18, 1985.

Hovi L, Valle M, Siimes M, et al.: Impaired response to hepatitis B vaccine in children receiving anticancer chemotherapy. *Pediatr Infect Dis J* 14:931–35, 1995.

Shenep JL, Feldman S, Gigliotti F, et al.: Response of immunocompromised children with solid tumors to a conjugate vaccine for *Haemophilus influenza* type b. *J Pediatr* 125:581–84, 1994.

3

The Management of Fever

Lawrence J. Wolff, M.D., Arthur R. Ablin, M.D., Arnold
J. Altman, M.D., and F. Leonard Johnson, M.D.

Fever is a common occurrence with multiple causes. However, in the febrile neutropenic child with cancer, a temperature of 38° C (100.4° F) or greater sustained for at least 1 hour indicates infection until proven otherwise. The usual signs and symptoms of infection are sometimes absent. A careful physical examination is important because untreated infection will rapidly spread. Start antibiotic therapy promptly, and consider all organisms potentially pathogenic. Choose antibiotics by the microbial prevalence and antibiotic sensitivity patterns at each institution. If these principles are kept in mind the morbidity and mortality associated with infection in neutropenic children with cancer will be reduced.

I. DEFINITIONS

A. Fever

Fever is one of the most common and obvious signs that allows the clinician to presume that the patient is sick. The measurement of temperature is an approximation and can be taken orally, axillary, or by tympanic measurement; however, fever is defined as a single *oral* temperature above 38.3° C (101° F) or a temperature of 38.0° C or greater taken on two occasions at least 1 hour apart. Do not take rectal temperatures in patients with neutropenia.

B. Neutropenia

Severe neutropenia is defined as ANC < 200/μL [total leuko-

cytes × (% neutrophils + % band cells)]; moderate neutropenia is 200–500/μL; mild neutropenia is 500–1000/μL. The risk
for a serious infection in a child being treated for cancer is
directly related to the degree and duration of neutropenia.
The risk for bacteremia/septicemia escalates when the
absolute neutrophil count (ANC) is < 200/μL, while the risk
for serious infections (including pneumonitis, cellulitis, and
abscess) begins to increase when the ANC falls below
500/μL. Those patients whose course of neutropenia is brief
(ANC ≥ 500/μL within 7 days after fever) have a better clinical
response than those who remain neutropenic (ANC ≤500/μL)
more than 7 days.

C. Indicators of marrow recovery
An increase in circulating monocytes, an increase in platelet
count, and the presence of young myeloid precursors, toxic
granules, and Döhle bodies may reflect marrow recovery.
Some use an absolute phagocyte count [total leukocytes ×
(% neutrophils + % bands + % monocytes)] as a predictor of
recovery.

II. EVALUATION OF THE FEBRILE NEUTROPENIC CHILD WITH CANCER

A. History and physical examination
The evaluation of the febrile child with cancer should be
thorough but expeditious. If the patient is neutropenic,
remember that sometimes only faint clues of the inflammatory process will be present, such as minimal discharge, faint
tenderness, or redness. Pay special attention to the skin,
nose, pharynx, and perineal and perirectal areas. Palpate
over sinuses and range of motions in all joints. The identification of an infection in specific areas, such as the perirectum,
skin, or mouth, narrows the spectrum of likely infecting
microorganisms.

B. Laboratory evaluation
Laboratory evaluation should include a complete blood
count, urinalysis, and generous amounts of blood drawn
from all venous access catheter ports and one or two peripheral sites for culture. A catheter site that is inflamed or drain-
ing should be cultured. Any suspicious skin lesion, watery
blister, or prominent erythema should be aspirated, stained,

and cultured. If periodontal infection is suspected, the patient should be examined by a pediatric dentist and appropriate radiographs and tissue samples obtained. Patients with tenderness over a sinus(es) should have diagnostic imaging studies. A febrile, neutropenic child with cancer who demonstrates mental confusion or central nervous system dysfunction should have a lumbar puncture.

Examine diarrheal stools for bacterial, protozoal, and viral agents and *Clostridium difficile* toxin. Culture urine if there are signs of urinary tract infection, the urinalysis is abnormal, or a urine catheter is in place. Chest radiographs are indicated if there are clinical symptoms or signs suggesting pulmonary disease.

C. Other studies (optional)
  1. Phase reactants
     Although available to some only as research tools, C-reactive protein, interleukin-6, and serum amyloid A acute inflammatory response indicators may give a rapid indication of bacteremia or bacterial infection.
  2. Radiolabeled imaging
     To help locate occult site of infection, indium-111–labeled donor granulocytes and indium-111–labeled immunoglobulin may be useful.
  3. Special studies
     The polymerase chain reaction (PCR) and enzyme-linked immunosorbent assay (ELISA) may be helpful in the early diagnosis of invasive bacterial or fungal disease. *Candida* enolase antigenemia can detect invasive fungal disease.

D. Follow-up monitoring
  Reexamine and reevaluate patients carefully at least once a day. Obtain blood cultures at least daily while the patient is febrile. Repeat urine, stool, tissue cultures, obtain diagnostic imaging, and consultation as clinically indicated.

III. MANAGEMENT OF FEVER WITH SEVERE NEUTROPENIA

A. At onset with unknown pathogen
  After diagnostic evaluation, promptly commence empiric broad-spectrum antibiotic coverage (see Section IV antibiotics). If a central venous catheter is in place, rotate antibiotic infusions to include all ports and lumens. Modifications of a "standard" selected regimen should be considered as follows:

1. If the patient has a history of allergy to penicillin, avoid semisynthetic penicillins and use an aminoglycoside, ceftazadime, or imipenem.
2. If a central venous catheter is suspected as the cause of fever, use vancomycin, not nafcillin, but discontinue its use after 72 hours if cultures are negative for *Staphylococcus epidermidis.*
3. If perianal tenderness is present, this suggests anaerobes. Add antianaerobic therapy.
4. If oral mucositis is severe, this suggests lower intestinal infection with anaerobes. Add anaerobic therapy and, if *Streptococcus viridans* is found, add vancomycin.
5. If peritonitis is possible, add vancomycin to cover *Clostridia* sp.
6. If pulmonary infiltrate is present and persists after 48 hours with continued fever, consider the merits of empiric therapy versus bronchial brushings or bronchoalveolar lavage; if this is not diagnostic, then consider needle or open lung biopsy.
   a. Begin empiric therapy for *Pneumocystis* with trimethoprim-sulfamethoxazole and for *Legionella* with erythromycin.
   b. If there is disease progression after 2 days of empiric therapy, then brushings, bronchoalveolar lavage, needle, or open lung biopsy is strongly indicated. If this is not possible, add antifungal therapy.

B. When a specific pathogen is not identified on culture
   1. Continue antibiotic coverage until the patient is afebrile for 24 hours, and there is evidence of marrow recovery (increases in absolute phagocyte or neutrophil count for 1 or more days).
   2. If fever and granulocytopenia persist for about 3 or more days, and all diagnostic procedures remain negative
      a. Continue broad-spectrum antibiotics and add antifungal therapy if not already included.
      b. Continue daily blood cultures, thorough physical examinations, and repeated histories for clues.
      c. Consider brain, perirenal, perianal, pelvic abscess, pseudomembranous colitis, viral etiology, and recurrent malignancy.
      d. Stop antibiotics after 14 days and repeat cultures daily and monitor the patient several times daily.

3. Recurrence of fever demands prompt rehospitalization, complete diagnostic evaluation, and aggressive antibiotic therapy.

C. When a specific pathogen is identified on culture
  1. Coagulase-negative and positive staphylococci and streptococci, including *S. viridans,* are the most frequent pathogens.
  2. Organisms seen less frequently in immune-compromised patients are: *Pseudomonas aeruginosa, Escherichia coli, Klebsiella* species, *Enterobacter* species, *Proteus* species, *Salmonella* species, *Haemophilus influenzae, Neisseria* species, *Enterococcus faecalis, Cornebacterium* species, *Bacillus* species, *Listeria monocytogenes,* and anaerobic cocci and bacilli as well. Fungal isolates include *Candida, Aspergillus, Cryptococcus, Histoplasma,* and *Mucor* species, among others.
  3. Make certain that the optimal agent or agents are being used for the isolated organism when cultures and sensitivity are known, but continue empiric broad-spectrum coverage until the patient is afebrile and there is evidence of marrow recovery (increases in absolute monocyte, absolute neutrophil, and platelet counts for 2 consecutive days). Then antibiotics may be tailored to the specific agent.
  4. Continue antibiotic therapy for a minimum of 10 days total (14 days if an indwelling catheter is present).

D. When a fungal infection is suspected or documented
  1. Presume fungal infection when fever and neutropenia persist after 3–7 days of empiric broad-spectrum antibiotics.
  2. Predisposing factors leading to fungal infections include prolonged hospitalization, prolonged granulocytopenia, prolonged use of broad-spectrum antibiotics, use of indwelling catheters, damaged mucosal barriers, and hyperalimentation.
  3. The most common pathogens are *Candida albicans, Candida tropicalis, Aspergillus fumigatus,* and *Aspergillus flavus.* Less frequently seen are *Cryptococcus neoformans, Histoplasma capsulatum,* and mucormycosis.
  4. Drugs of choice are shown in Table 3.1.
  5. Recommended doses of antifungal agents are shown in Table 3.2.

Table 3.1.
Drugs of Choice for Serious Fungal Infections

| Disease | Drug | |
	Preferred	Alternative
Candidiasis, systemic	Amphotericin*± flucytosine	Fluconazole
Aspergillosis	Amphotericin*± flucytosine	Itraconazole
Coccidiodomycosis	Amphotericin*	Itraconazole and fluconazole
Cryptococcosis	Amphotericin and Flucytosine	
Histoplasmosis	Amphotericin*	
Mucormycosis	Amphotericin*	

Source: Adapted from *1997 Red Book. The Report of the Committee on Infectious Diseases.* Elk Grove Village, IL: American Academy of Pediatrics; 1997.

*Liposomal amphotericin B for children is in current clinical trials to determine its efficacy and safety in comparison to nonliposomal drug.

Table 3.2.
Recommended Doses of Antifungal Drugs

Drug	Route	Dose
Amphotericin B	IV	Initial test dose 0–0.1 mg/kg. If tolerated, within 2 hours commence with 0.6–1.0 mg/kg/day in 1–4 hours. Increase to 1 mg/kg/day.
Amphotericin B lipid complex	IV	5 mg/kg/day single infusion at 2.5 mg/kg/day
Flucytosine	PO	50–150 mg/kg/day divided every 6 hours
Fluconazole	IV/PO	3–6 mg/kg/day,* single dose
Itraconazole	IV/PO	Not established, but in 3–16-year-old children experience at 100 mg/day

Source: Adapted from *1997 Red Book. The Report of the Committee on Infectious Diseases.* Elk Grove Village, IL: American Academy of Pediatrics; 1997.

*Not established for newborns

E. When a viral infection is suspected or documented
1. For documented infection with herpes simplex treat with acyclovir 750 mg/m^2/day divided q8h intravenous (IV).
2. For documented infection with varicella zoster treat with

acyclovir 1500 mg/m²/day divided q8h IV until no new lesions appear. Ensure adequate hydration.
3. For documented infection with cytomegalovirus (CMV) treat with ganciclovir 10 mg/kg/day divided q12h IV plus CMV immune globulin.

F. For documented or suspected infection with *Pneumocystis carinii*
1. Treat with trimethoprim-sulfamethoxazole (TMP/SMX): TMP 15–20 mg/kg/day and SMX 75–100 mg/kg/day divided q8–12h for at least 14 days PO or IV.
2. If TMP/SMX is not tolerated, treat with pentamidine 3–4 mg/kg/day IV or TMP 5 mg/kg PO q6h plus dapsone 100 mg/day PO for 21 days.

G. For documented toxoplasmosis
Treat with Pyrimethamine loading dose 1 mg/kg/twice daily PO for 1–3 days, then 1 mg/kg/day for 4 weeks plus either sulfadiazine or trisulfapyrimidines 100 mg/kg/day PO in three to four divided doses for 4 weeks.

IV. ANTIBIOTICS

A. The choice of antibiotics (antimicrobials) to be used at an institution should be determined by the needs of the patient and the local patterns of infection and resistance to antibiotics. The underlying disease, the chemotherapy being used, theprophylactic antimicrobials taken, and the prevalent microorganismsin the hospital, community, and geographical area are factors that affect the empirical choice of initial antimicrobials. The presence of a central venous access device, recent invasive procedures such as a bone marrow puncture, spinal tap, endoscopy, drug allergy, renal or hepatic dyfunction, and other drugs that may affect hearing and kidney or liver function will influence the choice of antimicrobial.

B. Many combinations of antimicrobials are effective. Prevailing community microorganisms and their antibiotic sensitivity will direct the choices and combinations of antibiotics. The patient with severe mucositis or the patient who has recently developed a neoplasm of the gastrointestinal or genitourinary tract should receive coverage for anaerobic bacteria. Various combinations that are used

Table 3.3.
Frequently Used Antibiotics for Fever and Neutropenia

Drug	Dose	Route	Schedule
Aminoglycosides			
Amikacin	15 mg/kg/day	IV	Divided q8h
Gentamicin	6.0–7.5 mg/kg/day	IV	Divided q8h
Tobramycin	6.0–7.5 mg/kg/day	IV	Divided q8h
β-Lactam drugs			
Antipseudomonal, semisynthetic penicillins			
Azlocillin	300 mg/kg/day (maximum 24 g/day)	IV	Divided q4–6h
Mezlocillin	300 mg/kg/day (maximum 24 g/day)	IV	Divided q4–6h
Piperacillin	300 mg/kg/day (maximum 24 g/day)	IV	Divided q4–6h
Ticarcillin	300 mg/kg/day (maximum 24 g/day)	IV	Divided q4–6h
Carbenicillin	500 mg/kg/day	IV	Divided q4–6h
Cephalosporins (third generation)			
Cefoperazone	100 mg/kg/day (maximum 12 g/day)	IV	Divided q8h
Ceftazidime	100–150 mg/kg/day (maximum 6 g/day)	IV	Divided q8h
Imipenem/cilastatin	50 mg/kg/day (maximum 4 g/day)	IV	Divided q6–8h
Penicillinase-resistant penicillin			
Nafcillin	100–200 mg/kg/day	IV	Divided q4–8h
Other			
Vancomycin	40 mg/kg/day (maximum 2 g/day)	IV	Divided q6-8h
Anaerobic coverage			
Clindamycin	40 mg/kg/day	IV	Divided q6–8h
Metronidazole	30 mg/kg/day (loading dose initially 15 mg/kg)	IV	Divided q6h

are listed below. For help in making a selection, remember that drug resistance is a major problem and refrain from using vancomycin initially unless the clinical situation mandates its use. (see Table 3.3)

1. Aminoglycoside plus an antipseudomonal β-lactam drug
   a. Advantages
      i. Good gram-negative coverage
      ii. Synergism against some gram-negative bacilli
      iii. Minimal emergence of resistance

     iv. Some anaerobic activity
   b. Disadvantages
     i. Lack of activity against some gram-positive bacteria
     ii. Nephrotoxic and ototoxic
     iii. Hypokalemia
     iv. Anaerobic coverage not optimal
     v. Necessity to monitor serum aminoglycoside levels

2. Combination of two β-lactam drugs
   a. Advantages
     i. Good gram-negative coverage
     ii. Synergism against some gram-negative bacteria
     iii. Low toxicity without need to monitor drug levels
   b. Disadvantages
     i. Possible antagonism with some combinations
     ii. Anaerobic coverage not optimal
     iii. Lack of activity against some gram-positive bacteria
     iv. High cost

3. Penicillinase-resistant penicillin or vancomycin plus aminoglycoside and β-lactam drug
   a. Advantages
     i. Broad gram-positive effectiveness
     ii. Good gram-negative coverage
     iii. Synergism against gram-negative bacteria
     iv. Minimal emergence of resistance
     v. Some anaerobic activity
   b. Disadvantages
     i. Combination without vancomycin has suboptimal effectiveness against *S. epidermidis.*
     ii. Nephrotoxic and ototoxic, especially with vancomycin
     iii. Hypokalemia
     iv. Anaerobic coverage not optimal
     v. Necessity to monitor serum aminoglycoside and vancomycin levels
     vi. High cost, especially with vancomycin

4. Monotherapy with third-generation cephalosporin or imipenem/cilastatin
   a. Advantages
     i. Less toxic than other combinations
     ii. Fairly-good broad-spectrum activity against gram-positive, gram-negative, and anaerobic bacteria (imipenem)

b. Disadvantages
   i. Insufficient gram-positive and anaerobic effective-
      ness (ceftazidime)
   ii. Potential for β-lactam resistance
   iii. Lack of synergistic activity
   iv. Anaerobic coverage not optimal
5. Third-generation cephalosporin plus penicillinase-resistant penicillin or vancomycin
   a. Advantage
      Wide antibacterial coverage, including gram-positive
      organisms
   b. Disadvantages
      i. Combination without vancomycin has suboptimal
         effectiveness against *S. epidermidis*
      ii. Lack of synergism against gram-negative bacteria
      iii. Necessity to monitor vancomycin levels
      iv. Nephrotoxic and ototoxic with vancomycin
      v. Expensive

V. MONITORING FOR TOXICITY TO ANTI-INFECTIVE AGENTS

A. Available monitors
   1. Complete blood count (CBC) with differential for hema-
      topoietic effect
   2. Serum chemistries for specific effects (e.g., electrolyte
      depletion, hepatic and renal toxicity)
   3. Serum levels for specific antibiotics
   4. Audiologic testing
   5. Urinalysis for glycosuria, albuminuria, and hematuria
   6. Quantitative urine samples for sodium and potassium
   7. Nucleotide glomerular filtration rate or creatinine clearance

B. Specific monitoring
   1. Gentamicin and tobramycin
      a. Check serum creatinine, blood urea nitrogen (BUN),
         and electrolytes every other day to monitor renal func-
         tion. When creatinine rises over baseline, monitor
         renal function daily.
      b. Check peak and trough serum levels of antibiotic after
         24 hours at a fixed dose.
      c. Modify the dosage or dosage interval according to the
         guidelines in Table 3.4.

Table 3.4.
Guidelines for the Desired Serum Concentrations of Gentamicin and Tobramycin

	Gentamicin	Tobramycin
Concentration	(µg/mL)	(µg/mL)
Peak (µg/mL)		
Serious infection	6–8	6–8
Life-threatening infection*	8–10	8–10
Trough (µg/mL)		
Serious infection	<1	<1
Life-threatening infection*	1–2	1–2

*Higher peak and trough values have also been suggested.

      d. See guidelines for desired serum concentrations in Table 3.4.
  2. Amphotericin B
      a. Monitor serum creatinine, BUN, serum electrolytes, particularly serum sodium, potassium, and magnesium (supplemental K^+ almost always necessary), at 1- to 3-day intervals.
      b. With significant persistent abnormality, adjust the frequency of administration to every other day or less frequently.
      c. Check creatinine clearance or nucleotide glomerular filtration rate as indicated.
  3. Vancomycin
      Monitor serum antibiotic levels. Aim for a peak level of 20–24 µg/mL and a trough level of 5–10 µg/mL.
  4. Nafcillin
      Monitor liver transaminases.

VI. MANAGEMENT OF FEVER WITH MODERATE NEUTROPENIA

    A. Studies show that more than 80% of children with cancer having fever (as earlier defined) and moderate neutropenia who are carefully chosen as defined below may be managed successfully either as outpatients or hospitalized briefly (12–48 hours) and then followed as outpatients. They should:
      1. Be older than 1 year of age.

2. Have no significant source of infection (e.g., perirectal abscess, central line tunnel cellulitis).
3. Have ANC ≥200/µL and anticipation that it will increase.
4. Be normotensive.
5. Have a remission status of their cancer.
6. Not be a bone marrow transplant recipient.
7. Not have recent surgery.
8. Have no moderate or severe mucositis.

B. Such patients can receive monotherapy such as ceftazidime or ceftriaxone or one of these agents combined with an aminoglycoside. However, they must be examined and evaluated daily by a physician experienced in caring for immune-compromised children.

VII. MANAGEMENT OF FEVER WITHOUT NEUTROPENIA

A. Evaluation
   1. Detailed history and physical examination
   2. Bacterial cultures
      a. Obtain blood cultures from a venipuncture site and, for patients with a central venous catheter, from each port of the catheter.
      b. Obtain cultures of urine and other potential sites of infection as indicated by history and physical examination (e.g., aspiration of cellulitis site or cerebrospinal fluid if meningitis is suspected).
   3. Radiographs as indicated by history and physical examination

B. Therapeutic measures
   1. When a central venous catheter is not present
      a. If a specific infection is not documented, continue to examine daily and monitor clinically with daily blood cultures and other relevant laboratory studies, but do not start antibiotics.
      b. If a specific pathogen is isolated, treat with specific antibiotics.
   2. When a central venous catheter is present
      a. If only an exit-site infection is suspected, obtain blood cultures from all ports of the catheter, one venipuncture site (if practical), and the exit site.

i. Begin antibiotic therapy with dicloxacillin 25 mg/kg/day PO divided q6h.

ii. Re-examine at 24–48 hours.

iii. If improved, finish 10-day course of antibiotic therapy.

iv. If not improved after 48 hours of dicloxacillin, commence therapy with vancomycin 40 mg/kg/day IV divided q8h (maximum 2 g/day) and tobramycin or gentamicin 6–7.5 mg/kg/day IV divided q8h.

v. If not improved after 72 hours of parenteral therapy, change antibiotics or consider removing the catheter.

b. If there is no evidence of local infection, obtain blood cultures from all catheter ports and one venipuncture site. Many physicians would choose to commence parenteral therapy with ceftriaxone 50 mg/kg IV q24h.

c. If the cultures are negative and the fever defervesces, stop antibiotic therapy after 48 hours.

d. If the cultures are positive, adjust antibiotic therapy appropriately to sensitivity of the organisms. If cultures remain positive despite 48 hours of appropriate antibiotic therapy, strongly consider removing the central venous line.

e. If the cultures become negative, complete a 10- to 14-day course of antibiotics and do not remove the catheter.

Bibliography

Bash RO, Katz JA, Cash JV: Safety and cost effectiveness of early hospital discharge of lower risk children with cancer admitted for fever and neutropenia. *Cancer* 74:189–96, 1994.

Cohen KL, Leamer K, Odom L, et al.: Cessation of antibiotics regardless of ANC is safe in children with febrile neutropenia. *J Pediatr Hematol Oncol* 17:325–30, 1995.

Freifeld AG, Pizzo PA: The outpatient management of febrile neutropenia in cancer patients. *Oncology* 10:599–612, 1996.

Hughes WT, Armstrong D, Bodey GP, et al.: Guidelines for the use of antimicrobial agents in neutropenic patients with unexplained fever. *J Infect Dis* 161:381–96, 1990.

Mustafa MM, Aquino VM, Pappo A, et al.: A pilot study of outpatient management of febrile neutropenic children with cancer at low risk of bacteremia. *J Pediatr* 128:847–49, 1996.

Pizzo PA: Granulocytopenia and cancer therapy: Past problems, current solutions, future challenges. *Cancer* 54:2649, 1984.

Sculier JP, Weerts D, Klastersky J: Causes of death in febrile granulocytopenic cancer patients receiving empiric antibiotic therapy. *Eur J Cancer Clin Oncol* 20:55, 1984.

Yu LC, Shanneyfelt T, Warrier R, Ode D: The efficacy of ticarcillin-clavulanate and gentamycin as empiric treatment for febrile neutropenic pediatric patients with cancer. *Pediatr Hematol Oncol* 11:181–87, 1994.

4

Blood Component Therapy

Dorothy R. Barnard, M.D., James H. Feusner, M.D., and Lawrence J. Wolff, M.D.

I. GENERAL RECOMMENDATIONS FOR BLOOD COMPONENT TRANSFUSION

A. General risks of transfusion
1. Blood component transfusions are costly in terms of both of the following.
   a. Costs related to the procurement/production of components
   b. Potential complications for patients receiving blood component transfusions
      i. Acute intravascular hemolysis, extravascular hemolysis, anaphylaxis, transfusion-related acute lung injury, and graft-versus-host disease are potentially life-threatening noninfectious complications of transfusion.
      ii. Other noninfectious complications resulting in morbidity include fluid overload, sodium overload, iron overload, febrile reactions, allergic reactions, and delayed hemolytic reactions.
      iii. With continuing improvements in screening, the incidence of transfusion-acquired infections is decreasing rapidly. However, as long as the blood components are derived from human blood donations, the risk of acquiring blood-borne pathogens will persist.

2. These risks must be balanced by consideration of the expected benefits each time a transfusion with blood-derived components is contemplated. For these reasons, obtain informed consent from patients/parents before nonemergency transfusions.

B. Prevention of transfusion-acquired cytomegalovirus (CMV)
Transfusion-acquired CMV can produce significant morbidity and mortality in immunosuppressed patients. Transfusion-acquired CMV may be prevented by
1. Providing CMV-seronegative blood products for CMV-negative patients, or
2. If CMV-seronegative blood products are not available, filtering blood components (red cell concentrates and platelet concentrates) with leukocyte-depleting filters capable of >3 log removal of white blood cells.

C. Prevention of graft-versus-host reaction
1. The incidence of transfusion-acquired graft-versus-host disease can be decreased by
a. Avoiding directed blood donations by close relatives (except when indicated for aggressive bone marrow rescue procedures), and
b. Irradiating all blood transfusion components with the potential to contain leukocytes (red cell concentrates, white cell concentrates, and platelet concentrates; the recommendation for irradiation of plasma has not been clearly substantiated). The generally recommended dose for irradiation of blood products is 1500–2500 cGy to the midplane with at least 1500 cGy in the field.
2. In addition, the use of a leukocyte-depleting filter where applicable will contribute to decreasing the risk of graft-versus-host disease.

D. Reduction of leukocyte sensitization
The use of leukocyte-depleted blood components can decrease the incidence of alloimmunization and platelet transfusion refractoriness.

E. Reduction of immunomodulation effects of transfusion
The immunomodulating effects of transfusion appear to be related to the presence of lymphocytes in blood compo-

nents. Removal of the transfused lymphocytes can decrease the immunosuppression secondary to transfusion. An additional postulated complication of the immunomodulation of transfusions is a decrease in the effectiveness of the individual's own natural immune mechanisms of cancer control.

F. Reduction in and treatment of febrile transfusion reactions
   1. Febrile transfusion reactions are associated with the presence of leukocytes in the transfused products as well as tumor necrosis factor, interleukin-1, -6, and -8, and other cytokines released by the leukocytes.
   2. Cytokines released into the plasma of blood components from the granulocytes increase with storage time.
   3. Prestorage filtration of cellular blood components appears to be the most effective method to decrease these reactions.
   4. Rule out serious red cell transfusion reaction in patients with febrile transfusion reactions.
   5. Treat febrile transfusion reactions in patients who are otherwise not at risk for sepsis with antipyretics and meperidine (0.5–1.0 mg/kg) for rigors. Some febrile transfusion reactions can be prevented with premedication with antipyretics and Benadryl.
   6. Take cultures from patients who have febrile reactions at the time of transfusion and are at risk for sepsis and treat patients with antibiotics if appropriate.
   7. Storage of platelets at room temperature increases the risk of sepsis as a complication of platelet transfusion.

G. Precautions to ensure that the correct product is given to the correct patient
   It is essential that the blood sample taken for type and screen and cross-match is clearly labeled and checked with the patient's identification. Before administering the blood product, check the physician order, patient identification, and blood product type and numbers. Clerical error and misidentification are major risks of transfusion. When error is suspected
   1. Stop transfusion.
   2. Inspect anticoagulated and centrifuged blood specimen from the patient for reddish discoloration of the plasma.
   3. Inspect urine for dark discoloration of hemoglobinuria.

II. RED CELL TRANSFUSION

A. Definition of anemia
Significant anemia results in decreased oxygen-carrying capacity of the blood and, thus, a reduction in the oxygen available to the tissues. The hemoglobin concentration is only a rough guide for an individual's adequate oxygen-carrying capacity.

B. Symptoms of anemia
When anemia develops gradually, there may be few symptoms or signs. Common symptoms of anemia include fatigue, dyspnea, inactivity, difficulty concentrating, anorexia, headache, syncope, vertigo, and palpitations. Signs can include pallor, tachycardia, tachypnea, ejection systolic murmur, and gallop rhythm.

C. Specific risks of red cell transfusion
Electrolyte imbalances of potassium or calcium, arrhythmias, post-transfusion purpura, hypothermia, and hemolytic transfusion reactions are more common with red cell transfusion than with other blood component transfusions.

D. Options for the correction/prevention of anemia
1. Packed red blood cells—AS-1 (Nutricel) or AS-3 (Adsol)—are used as additive solutions to the anticoagulant. Each packed red blood cell unit is approximately 350–380 mL with a hematocrit of 55–60%.
2. Recombinant erythropoietin has been used successfully in some children with leukemia or solid tumors, giving an increase in hemoglobin and decreasing red cell transfusion requirements. A decreased erythropoietin serum level *may* help to predict the response to recombinant erythropoietin therapy. This treatment is still experimental.
3. Consider hemodilution and other methods of decreasing surgical blood loss for children undergoing surgical procedures.
4. Autologous transfusion in children with solid tumors may be an option. Consult local protocols for autologous donation.
5. Discourage directed donations from first-degree relatives. Transfusion may sensitize the child and interfere with an allogeneic bone marrow transplant. It is mandatory if

directed donations from relatives are used that the blood is irradiated to prevent graft-versus-host disease.
6. Before deciding to transfuse with red cells, consider symptoms and signs of anemia, not only the hemoglobin level.

E. Indications for red cell transfusion
1. The optimal hemoglobin level for children cannot be precisely defined. The following are prudent guidelines.
    a. For a well child recovering from treatment-induced bone marrow suppression, transfusion is usually indicated if the hemoglobin level is 70–80 g/L and the reticulocyte count is low.
    b. For a child with symptoms and signs of anemia and a hemoglobin level < 100 g/L, a transfusion may be indicated.
    c. A child beginning a course of chemotherapy with a hemoglobin level < 80 g/L usually benefits from a transfusion.
    d. A child receiving radiation treatment *may* require a hemoglobin level maintained above 100 g/L.
    e. A child with acute blood loss of > 10% of blood volume, ongoing blood loss resulting in a loss of > 10% of blood volume, or bleeding with a hemoglobin level < 80 g/L usually benefits from a red cell transfusion.
    f. A child with respiratory insufficiency requiring supplemental oxygen *may* benefit from maintaining a hemoglobin level > 120 g/L.
    g. A child may require a higher hemoglobin level (> 70 g/L) if undergoing an anesthetic.
    h. For a child with a platelet count < 20,000 mL and a hemoglobin level < 8g/L, a red cell transfusion is usually indicated.

F. Dose of red cell transfusion
1. For a severely anemic child without hypovolemia, use small incremental transfusions of packed cells.
    a. For hemoglobin < 30 g/L, transfuse with 5 mL/kg over 4–6 hours.
    b. For hemoglobin 30–40 g/L, transfuse with 6 mL/kg over 4–6 hours.
    c. For hemoglobin 40–50 g/L, transfuse with 7 mL/kg over 4–6 hours.

d. For hemoglobin > 50 g/L, transfuse the required amount over 4 hours.

(*Note:* the length of time over which an individual unit of packed red blood cells can be infused is normally 4 hours. This can be extended to 6 hours under exceptional circumstances.)

e. Unless the child is actively bleeding or hypoxemic, correction of the hemoglobin level can be achieved over several days for severely anemic children.

2. For a child with a hemoglobin level of > 50 g/L to achieve an increase of 30 g/L, a red cell transfusion of 15–18 mL/kg is required if transfusing packed red cells with Adsol or Nuricel additive solution. The total volume required is usually infused over 4 hours.

3. Rarely, an exchange transfusion is required for a safe transfusion in a severely anemic, hypoxic, hypervolemic child with cardiovascular compromise due to congestive heart failure.

III. PLATELET TRANSFUSION

A. Definition of thrombocytopenia

Significant thrombocytopenia (platelet count <100,000/μL) results in an increased risk of mucosal, skin, and central nervous system bleeding. The risk of bleeding is increased with coincident coagulation factor deficiencies, platelet dysfunction, mucositis, high peripheral blood blast count, fever, recent surgery, sepsis, or other causes of increased platelet turnover.

B. Symptoms of thrombocytopenia

When thrombocytopenia develops gradually, there may be few symptoms or signs. Common symptoms of thrombocytopenia include petechiae, epistaxis, gastrointestinal bleeding, and other mucosal bleeding. More serious bleeding can occur in the central nervous system and can be indicated by retinal hemorrhages.

C. Specific risks of platelet transfusion

1. The major risks of repeated platelet transfusions are CMV infection, platelet alloimmunization, and sepsis.

2. Rarely, in very small patients, there is a risk of volume overload when platelet transfusions are infused over a

short period of time. The hemoglobin level after platelet transfusion is often lowered because of the fluid shifts. Volume reduction of platelet concentrates is not recommended, as such manipulation will adversely affect platelet function.

D. Options for the correction of thrombocytopenia
  1. Platelet concentrates—AS-1 (Nutricel) or AS-3 (Adsol)—are used as additive solutions to the anticoagulant. Each platelet concentrate unit is approximately 60 mL.
  2. Single-donor platelet apheresis packs are strongly recommended. One unit equals approximately 6 units of random-donor platelets. The units can be split for more efficient use of blood bank resources.
  3. Washed platelet concentrates are not recommended unless the patient has severe allergic reactions.
  4. Discourage directed donations from first-degree relatives. Transfusion may sensitize the child and interfere with an allogeneic bone marrow transplant. It is mandatory if directed donations from relatives are used that the blood be irradiated to prevent graft-versus-host disease.

E. Indications for platelet transfusion
  The determination of a thrombocytopenic patient's need for platelet transfusion includes, in addition to the current platelet count and the rate of decrease of the platelet count, an assessment of concomitant factors that may increase the patient's risk of bleeding (see Section IIIA). The threshold for platelet transfusion may be lower in patients with any of these factors. General guidelines for platelet transfusion are the following.
  1. Any child with a platelet count < 10,000/μL should be given a transfusion.
  2. Children with acute promyelocytic leukemia or acute monocytic leukemia during induction treatment should be given a transfusion to maintain the platelet count above 20,000/μL. Patients with acute lymphoblastic leukemia during induction should have their platelet count kept > 15,000/μL.
  3. Children with brain tumors should have their platelet count maintained > 30,000/μL during radiation therapy and the early phase of chemotherapy.
  4. A child requiring surgery should have a platelet count

> 50,000/µL but > 100,000/µL for surgery of the eye or brain.

5. Children requiring a lumbar puncture should have a platelet count > 30,000/µL.
6. A child requiring an intramuscular injection should have a platelet count > 20,000/µL.
7. Any child with bleeding, in spite of a normal prothrombin time, partial thromboplastin, and fibrinogen level, whose platelet count is < 60,000/µL should be given a transfusion.
8. These recommendations are clinically reasonable but not in every circumstance supported by data.

F. Dose of platelet transfusion
1. Four units of platelet concentrates/m² or 1 unit/7.5 kg should increase the platelet count by 50,000/µL by 60 minutes after transfusion.
2. In the actively bleeding patient, attempt to increase the platelet count by at least 40,000/µL.
3. It is preferable to use Rh-matched platelet units for females; ABO compatibility is recommended for all patients. If using single-donor apheresed platelets with an anti-A or anti-B titer > 1:64 for an A, B, or AB recipient, remove the plasma.

G. Platelet refractoriness
1. One definition of platelet refractoriness is a post-transfusion increment of < 5000/µL/unit of platelet concentrate/m² transfused when measured at 15–60 minutes after transfusion and recurring on more than one occasion.
2. Treatment options for platelet refractoriness
   a. Try treatment with platelet units stored for less than 24 hours.
   b. Try human leukocyte antigen (HLA)-matched single-donor platelets.
   c. Try cross-matching compatible platelets.
   d. Intravenous immunoglobulins are unlikely to be of benefit. If tried, the dose of intravenous immunoglobulin is 400 mg/kg/day before the platelet transfusion for up to 9 days. Transfuse the child with platelet concentrates daily until a safe platelet count is achieved.
   e. Consider massive transfusion with random-donor platelets (to adsorb the antibodies) if the patient is bleeding seriously and all other therapies have failed.

    f. Consider a trial of vinblastine-loaded platelets.

    g. Consider a trial of plasmapheresis with immunoadsorption onto staphylococcal protein A column.

IV. GRANULOCYTE TRANSFUSION

A. Definition of granulocytopenia
Significant granulocytopenia results in an increased risk of bacterial and fungal infection. The risk increases dramatically as the absolute granulocyte count decreases below $200/\mu L$.

B. Granulocyte preparations
Granulocytes collected by discontinuous- or continuous-flow centrifugation have better function (chemotaxis, phagocytosis, degranulation, killing, and migration to sites of infection) and fewer side effects (fever, chills, and hypotension) than white cells collected by filtration leukapheresis.

C. Specific risks of granulocyte transfusion
There are particular risks of CMV infection, graft-versus-host disease, respiratory distress with pulmonary infiltration, alloimmunization, and hemolytic reactions associated with granulocyte transfusion.

D. Options for the correction/prevention of granulocytopenia
  1. The use of granulocyte transfusion has not been proven of significant benefit except for patients with severe neutropenia and gram-negative septicemia or systemic fungal infection.
    a. Circulating granulocytes have a half-life of 6–10 hours;
    b. Granulocytes obtained from ABO/Rh-compatible, HLA-matched, lymphocytotoxicity-negative, neutrophil-antibody-nonreactive donors appear to be the most effective.
  2. The use of granulocyte-colony-stimulating factor or other cytokines has markedly decreased the use of granulocyte transfusion.

E. Dose of granulocyte transfusion
  1. The dose of granulocytes is generally $> 1 \times 10^{10}/m^2$ granulocytes.
  2. It is preferable to use Rh-matched granulocyte units for females; ABO compatibility is recommended for all

patients. If using single-donor apheresed granulocytes with an anti-A or anti-B titer > 1:64 for an A, B, or AB recipient, remove the plasma.

F. Indications for granulocyte transfusion. All of the following
1. Severe neutropenia [absolute neutrophil count (ANC) < 100/µL] *and* serious bacterial or fungal infection that is culture-positive or deep-seated and persists > 48 hours despite appropriate antibiotic coverage.
2. The ANC is not expected to increase to > 500/µL for several days *and* prolonged survival is expected if the infection is controlled.

G. Additional indications for granulocyte transfusion may include patients with severe granulocyte dysfunction (e.g., chronic granulomatous disease) with life-threatening infection.

H. Administration
1. Administer through a 170-µ filter at a rate of 150 mL/m²/h as soon after collection as possible.
2. If not used immediately, store at room temperature.
3. Do not administer with a leukocyte-depleting filter.

Bibliography

Bolonaki I, Stiakaki E, Lydaki E, et al.: Treatment with recombinant human erythropoietin in children with malignancies. *Pediatr Hematol Oncol* 13:111–21,1996.

Dzieczkowski JS, Barrett BB, Nester D, *et al.*: Characterization of reactions after exclusive transfusion of white cell-reduced cellular blood components. *Transfusion* 35:20–25,1995.

Jeter EK, Spivey MA: Noninfectious complications of blood transfusion. *Hematol Oncol Clin North Am* 9:187–204,1995.

Kaushansky K: The thrombocytopenia of cancer. Prospects for effective cytokine therapy. *Hematol Oncol Clin of North Am* 10:431–55,1996.

Manno CS: What's new in transfusion medicine? *Pediatr Clin of North Am* 43:793–808,1996.

Miller JP, Mintz PD: The use of leukocyte-reduced blood components. *Hematol Oncol Clin of North Am* 9:69–90,1995.

Slichter SJ: Principles of platelet transfusion therapy. In Hoffman, R. ed. *Hematology: Basic Principles and Practice.* 2nd ed., New York: Churchill Livingstone;1995. pp. 1987–2006.

Tamary H, Danon YL: Recombinant human erythropoietin in children with cancer. *Pediatr Hematol Oncol* 13:305–08,1996.

5

Hemorrhagic and Thrombotic Complications in Children with Cancer

M. Patricia Massicotte, M.D., Lu Ann Brooker, R.T.,
and Maureen E. Andrew, M.D.

Normal Hemostasis

I. The normal hemostatic process is a balance between maintaining blood in a fluid state under normal physiologic conditions, and the ability to react to vascular injury by forming a blood clot to stop blood loss.

A. Blood is maintained in the fluid phase by the presence of inhibitors of proteins activated in the clotting mechanism [antithrombin III (ATIII), protein C, and protein S]. A strong stimulus (e.g., sufficient vascular injury) will initiate the explosive clotting mechanism and override the action of the inhibitors, allowing the formation of a blood clot.

B. The formation of a thrombus occurs in three stages:

1. Formation of a platelet plug due to activation of platelets in response to vascular injury
2. Activation of the proteins of the coagulation mechanism, with the ultimate formation of a fibrin clot (with platelets mixed in) (Figure 5.1)
3. Clot lysis (fibrinolytic system) due to a protein activated

Figure 5.1.
A schema of the coagulation system.

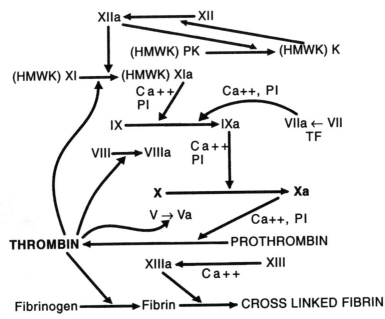

HMWK = High Molecular Weight Kininogen, K = Kallikrein, PK = Prekallikrein, Pl = Platelets, TF = Tissue Factor

at the initiation of the clotting cascade (plasminogen activated to plasmin) (Figure 5.2)

C. An abnormality in any part of the hemostatic system may
cause either abnormal bleeding or thrombosis.

II. TESTS MEASURING HEMOSTASIS

A. Platelets
1. Platelet count
2. Bleeding time
3. Platelet aggregation

B. Coagulation proteins and screening tests
1. International normalized ratio (INR)/prothrombin time
(PT)
2. Activated partial thromboplastin time (APTT)
3. Thrombin clotting time (TCT)
4. Fibrinogen level

Figure 5.2.
A schema of the fibrinolytic system.

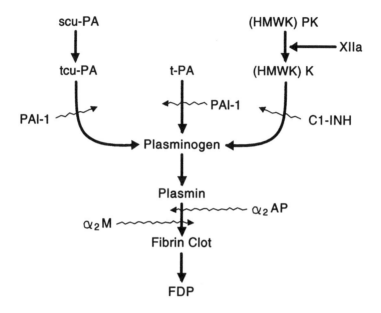

5. Functional and immunologic levels of inhibitors (ATIII, protein C, and protein S)

III. For many coagulation proteins, infants and children have different normal ranges from adults. Tests that measure hemostasis, therefore, also have age-dependent normal values. (Table 5.1).

A. Platelets
   1. Neonates have hyporeactive platelets due to an intrinsic defect but have shorter bleeding times than adults due to increased red blood cell size, high hematocrit, and increased levels of von Willebrand factor (vWf).
   2. Bleeding time has been shown to be longer in children than in healthy adults, with an unknown etiology or significance.

B. Mechanism of coagulation
   1. The vitamin K-dependent coagulation proteins (factors II or prothrombin, VII, IX, and X) are decreased in child-

Normal Values for Infants and Children for the Coagulation and Fibrinolytic System*

	Full-Term	Children Ages 6–10 Years	Adult
Fibrinogen (g/L)	2.83 (1.67–3.99)	2.79 (1.57–4.0)	2.78 (1.56–4.0)
II (U/mL)	0.48 (0.26–0.70)	0.88 ((0.67–1.07)	1.08 (0.70–1.46)
V (U/mL)	0.72 (0.34–1.08)	0.90 (0.63–1.16)	1.06 (0.62–1.50)
VII (U/mL)	0.66 (0.28–1.04)	0.85 (0.52–1.20)	1.05 (0.67–1.43)
VIII (U/mL)	1.00 (0.50–1.78)	0.95 (0.58–1.32)	0.99 (0.50–1.49)
vWf (U/mL)	1.53 (0.50–2.87)	0.95 (0.44–1.44)	0.92 (0.50–1.58)
IX (U/mL)	0.53 (0.15–0.91)	0.75 (0.63–0.89)	1.09 (0.55–1.63)
X (U/mL)	0.40 (0.12–0.68)	0.75 (0.55–1.01)	1.06 (0.70–1.52)
XI (U/mL)	0.38 (0.10–0.66)	0.86 (0.52–1.20)	0.97 (0.67–1.27)
XII (U/mL)	0.53 (0.13–0.93)	0.92 (0.60–1.40)	1.08 (0.52–1.64)
PK (U/mL)	0.37 (0.18–0.69)	0.99 (0.66–1.31)	1.12 (0.62–1.62)
HMWK (U/mL)	0.54 (0.06–1.02)	0.93 (0.60–1.30)	0.92 (0.50–1.36)
XIII_a (U/mL)	0.79 (0.27–1.31)	1.09 (0.65–1.51)	0.05 (0.55–1.55)
XIII_b (U/mL)	0.76 (0.30–1.22)	1.16 (0.77–1.54)	0.97 (0.57–1.37)
AT (U/mL)	0.63 (0.39–0.87)	1.11 (0.90–1.31)	1.0 (0.74–1.26)
α_2M (U/mL)	1.39 (0.95–1.83)	1.69 (1.28–2.09)	0.86 (0.52–1.20)
C_1E-INH (U/mL)	0.72 (0.36–1.08)	1.14 (0.88–1.54)	1.0 (0.71–1.31)
α_1AT (U/mL)	0.93 (0.49–1.37)	1.00 (0.69–1.30)	0.93 (0.55–1.30)
HCII (U/mL)	0.43 (0.10–0.93)	0.86 (0.40–1.32)	1.08 (0.66–1.26)
Protein C (U/mL)	0.35 (0.17–0.53)	0.69 (0.45–0.93)	0.96 (0.64–1.28)
Protein S (U/mL)			
Total	0.36 (0.12–0.60)	0.78 (0.41–1.14)	0.81 (0.60–1.13)
Free	0.42 (0.22–0.62)	0.45 (0.27–0.61)	
Plasminogen (U/mL)	0.54 (0.35–0.74)	0.92 (0.75–1.08)	0.99 (0.77–1.22)
TPA (ng/mL)	9.6 (5.0–18.9)	2.42 (1.0–5.0)	4.90 (1.40–8.40)
α_2AP (U/mL)	0.85 (0.55–1.15)	0.99 (0.89–1.10)	1.02 (0.68–1.36)
PAI (U/mL)	6.4 (2.0–15.1)	6.79 (2.0–12.0)	3.60 (0–11.0)

*All factors, except fibrinogen, are expressed as units per milliliter (U/mL), where pooled plasma contains 1.0 U/mL. All values are expressed as the mean, followed by the lower and upper boundary encompassing 95% of the population in parentheses. Between 40 and 77 samples were assayed for each value for the newborn. Some measurements were skewed due to a disproportionate number of high values. The lower limit, which excludes the lower 2.5% of the population, has been given.

Abbreviations: α_2AP, α_1AT, α1-antitrypsin; α_2M, $\alpha_2$macroglobulin; AT, antithrombin; C_1E-INH = C_1-esterase inhibitor; HCII, heparin cofactor II; HMWK, high-molecular-weight kininogen, PAI, plasminogen activator inhibitor; PK, prekallikrein, TPA, tissue plasminogen activator; vWf, von Willebrand factor.

hood compared with adult levels. Blood clots in neonates and children, therefore, have less thrombin incorporated into them due to decreased prothrombin levels. Optimal anticoagulant therapy of clots involves inactivating clot-bound thrombin and may be different in children from that in adults for this reason.

C. Inhibitors of coagulation
1. Protein C levels (both functional and antigenic) are lower than adult levels throughout childhood until puberty. Neonates can have levels as low as 20%. To rule out a deficiency, measure both functional and antigenic levels.
2. ATIII is 50% of adult levels until 3 months of age.
3. α_2-Macroglobulin levels are increased compared with adult values.
4. Protein S exists in both free and bound forms. Under normal conditions, approximately 60% of the total protein S in plasma is complexed to C4b-binding protein (a component of complement). Only the free protein S (40%) is functionally active as a cofactor with protein C to inhibit activated factors V and VIII. To rule out a deficiency, measure the total, free, and bound protein S (antigen) and functional protein S.

D. Fibrinolytic system
1. The fibrinolytic system is relatively downregulated in childhood.
2. Plasminogen is 50% of adult levels at birth.

Bleeding Disorders in Children with Cancer

I. ETIOLOGY (see Table 5.2.)

II. DIAGNOSIS

A. Assess bleeding by laboratory tests (initial).
1. Perform a complete blood count (CBC) including platelet count. If platelet count is $<100 \times 10^9$/L, check the smear to ensure there is no clumping (i.e., pseudothrombocytopenia).
2. Perform an APTT. If prolonged, consider a 1:1 mix with normal plasma and repeat the APTT. If the APTT is now normal, an acquired factor deficiency is likely, due to either decreased production or increased consumption (disseminated intravascular coagulation, DIC). Ensure

Table 5.2.
Bleeding in Children with Cancer

Malignancy or Clinical Disorder	Mechanism	Abnormal Hemostatic Tests*
Acute lymphoblastic leukemia	↓Platelet count	↓Platelet count
Acute myelogenous leukemia FAB M3	DIC/factor consumption	↑INR/PT ↑APTT ↑TCT ↓Fibrinogen Special tests: ↓factors V and VIII, ↑fibrinogen split products and fibrin split products
Metastases to liver or liver damage due to chemotherapy	↓Factor production (factors II, V, VII, IX, X, XI, XIII, fibrinogen)	↑INR/PT ↑TCT Special tests: ↓factors IX, and V
Antibiotic therapy, ↓oral intake in chronic illness and diarrhea	↓Vitamin K availability or absorption	↑INR/PT Special tests: ↓factors VII, IX, normal factors VIII and V
Neuroblastoma Wilms tumor	↓platelets Inhibitor to vWf	↓Platelet number ↑APTT special tests: ↓factor VIII, ↓vWf antigen, ↓vWf ristocetin cofactor, ↓vWf multimers

* Fragment 1.2 (F 1.2) and thrombin-antithrombin complex (TAT) are measurable markers of the degree of thrombin activation and thus activation of the coagulation pathway. D-dimer is a marker of activation of the fibrinolytic pathway and is a product of cross-linked fibrin degradation. F 1.2, TATs, and D-dimer may be increased in coagulopathies associated with malignancy (Andrew et al., 1990, 1992).

that the sample for APTT was not contaminated with heparin, as contamination will cause the APTT to be prolonged. This usually occurs if the blood sample was taken from a central line (especially arterial) that had not been adequately cleared of heparin before obtaining blood. If the 1:1 mix does not have a corrected normal value APTT in the absence of heparin, an antibody to a component in the coagulation mechanism is present (inhibitor).

3. Perform a PT or INR. If this is prolonged, consider deficiencies of factors II, V, VII, IX, X, or fibrinogen due to decreased production of functional coagulation factor (liver disease or vitamin K deficiency).
4. Perform a two-unit TCT. If abnormal, consider contamination of the sample with standard heparin or hypofibrinogenemia.
5. Perform a fibrinogen level if the TCT is abnormal. If DIC is a possibility, determine the fibrinogen level by a clottable (Claus) assay, as the nephelometric method based on particle light scatter may result in a falsely high value due to the presence of fibrinogen/fibrin split products.

III. RECOMMENDATIONS FOR TREATMENT

A. Assess the bleeding patient and institute emergency measures if necessary, including oxygen therapy (by nasal prongs, mask, or endotracheal tube) and intravenous fluids. Cross-match the patient for blood. If bleeding is life threatening, administer packed red cells (see Chapter 4).

B. Start an intravenous line. If it is a major bleeding episode, use as large a bore as possible (21 gauge for infants and children and 19 gauge for adolescents).

C. If the hemoglobin level is <70 g/L, consider red cell transfusion (see Chapter 4).

D. If there is a true thrombocytopenia and the platelet count is <20 × 10^9/L, consider platelet transfusion (see Chapter 4). If DIC is present (↓platelet count, ↑APTT, ↑TCT, and ↓fibrinogen), consider platelet transfusion, but treatment of the underlying cause (malignancy, sepsis) is the accepted method of therapy to eradicate the DIC.

E. If the APTT is prolonged (see Table 5.1) and is due to liver damage or DIC, consider plasma transfusion (see Section IID3). If there is liver damage with a resultant decrease in factor production causing the increased PT/INR, plasma transfusion is indicated (see Section IID3). Repeat the INR after the infusion of plasma. If the INR is prolonged (INR <4.5) but there is no bleeding, repeat the INR every 3–7 days but do not administer plasma.

F. If the PT/INR is prolonged (see Table 5.1) and vitamin K deficiency is present, administer vitamin K subcutaneously, intravenously, or orally (see Section IID6). If the patient is bleeding, consider a plasma transfusion. If the vitamin K deficiency is severe, the amount of plasma needed for total correction is so large that it may result in volume overload. If the bleeding is life threatening or is originating from an intracranial hemorrhage, consider using prothrombin complex (see Section IID3) as well as vitamin K. If the bleeding is not life threatening, repeat the PT/INR in 24 hours to confirm the correction of the deficiency. If the INR is still prolonged, repeat the vitamin K dose.

G. If the TCT is prolonged (without heparin contamination of the sample), this is most likely due to hypofibrinogenemia. Measure a fibrinogen level (see above). If the fibrinogen level is <75 mg/dL, infusion of cryoprecipitate may be necessary, especially if major bleeding is present.

H. Acquired von Willebrand disease is rare but has been reported with Wilms tumor. If the diagnosis is confirmed, the use of desmopressin can be tried; if unsuccessful, administer cryoprecipitate, a specific vWf concentrate, immunoglobulinG, or platelet transfusions.

IV. SPECIFIC THERAPY

    A. Red cell transfusion (see Chapter 4)

    B. Platelet transfusion (see Chapter 4)

    C. Plasma transfusion:
      1. Fresh-frozen plasma
        a. Plasma is frozen within 6 hours of collection.
        b. All coagulation factors are present in 1 U/mL concentration
        c. Indications are vitamin K deficiency, DIC, severe deficiencies of ATIII, protein C, or protein S with acute venous thrombosis.
        d. Dosage:10–20 mL/kg intravenous (IV) 8–12hs
        e. The risk of viral transmission per unit of properly screened fresh-frozen plasma is: human immunodeficiency virus, 1/500,000; hepatitis C, 1/100,000; human T-cell lymphotrophic virus 1 and 2, 1/500,000; hepatitis B, 1/50,000.
        f. Use of virally inactivated products
          These products, specifically solvent detergent inactivated fresh-frozen plasma, have been used in clinical

trials. Once approved, these products may become the main products used for therapy due to the decreased risk of viral transmission.

D. Cryoprecipitate
1. Cryoprecipitate is the cold-insoluble portion of plasma that remains after fresh-frozen plasma has been thawed under controlled conditions. One bag of cryoprecipitate has about 15–20 mL of fluid.
2. The main components are factor VIII, fibrinogen (250 mg/bag), vWf, and factor XIII.
3. Indications for use are fibrinogen <75 mg/dL or acquired von Willebrand disease.
4. Dosage: 1 bag/5 kg IV; continue until fibrinogen >75 mg/dL
5. The risk of viral transmission per bag of cryoprecipitate is the same as for fresh frozen plasma (see Section IIB3f).

E. Prothrombin complex
1. Prothrombin complex concentrates contain factors II, IX, and X with variable amounts of factor VII.
2. Patients with a life-threatening hemorrhage or an intracranial hemorrhage due to vitamin K deficiency could benefit from prothrombin complex concentrates.
3. Dosage: 50 U/kg

F. Vitamin K
1. Vitamin K preparations are usually synthetic derivatives of vitamin K_1 and K_2 as well as the synthetic water-soluble forms (e.g., vitamin K_3).
2. Subcutaneous vitamin K is the preferred route of administration due to reported anaphylaxis with intravenous preparation. Hypersensitivity reactions have been reported with subcutaneous administration in the form of peri-injection redness and pruritus with occasional development of skin necrosis. If this occurs, do not use the subcutaneous (sc) route.
3. Vitamin K can be administered orally using the intravenous preparation (vitamin K_1).
4. The indications for use is vitamin K deficiency.
5. Dosage: 2–20 mg SC
6. Infant formula contains an average of 83 mg/100 mL. This must be taken into consideration for infants receiving coumadin therapy.

Thrombosis in Children with Cancer

I. ETIOLOGY

A. Background
Thrombotic events in most children have been associated with at least two of the following factors.
1. Thrombophilic condition
2. Malignancy
3. Presence of a central venous line (CVL)
4. Total parenteral nutrition (TPN)
5. Immobility

B. Children with cancer
Many children with cancer already have two factors associated with increased thrombosis shortly after their diagnosis (i.e., malignancy and the placement of a CVL).

C. Thrombophilic condition
1. For a child with a confirmed thrombosis and a family history of thrombosis, consider the following conditions that have been shown to place a patient at increased risk of thrombosis: ATIII deficiency, protein C deficiency, protein S deficiency, nonspecific inhibitor, and anticardiolipin antibody.
2. The presence of activated protein C cofactor resistance or factor V Leiden mutation may increase the risk of thrombosis.

D. Malignancy
1. Certain malignancies have been associated with thrombosis due to the secretion of a thromboplastin-like material activating the coagulation pathway.
2. Acute promyelocytic leukemia [French-American-British (FAB) classification M3] and other malignancies have been associated with the development of DIC. Microthrombi at the level of the capillary bed are well recognized. Occasionally, this condition progresses to such an extent that thrombosis of extremities occurs.

E. Central venous lines
Prospective screening of patients with CVLs for thrombosis associated with the CVL has shown the incidence to be as high as 35%.

F. Total parenteral nutrition
   Endothelial cell damage has been shown in vitro with the use
   of TPN, and it has been postulated that the high osmolarity is
   the cause.

G. Immobility
   In adults, immobility has been shown to be a risk factor for
   thrombosis.

II. DIAGNOSIS

A. Clinical
   1. A swollen arm or leg suggests the presence of a deep
      venous thrombosis (DVT). Consider superficial venous
      dilatation on the arm or chest of a patient who has had a
      CVL in the upper venous system to be evidence of throm-
      bosis until proven otherwise (Figure 5.3).
   2. Acute-onset pleuritic chest pain, unexplained shortness
      of breath, and decreased oxygen saturation suggest the
      presence of a pulmonary embolism (especially if the DVT
      is in an arm or leg or if a CVL is in place). *Pulmonary*

Figure 5.3.
**A child with superficial venous dilation (and a central venous line) on
the left upper chest.**

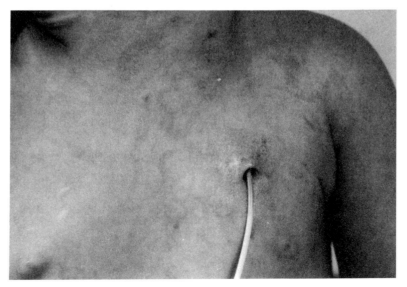

embolism can be a life-threatening emergency. If this diagnosis is a possibility and the patient is extremely symptomatic (tachycardia, hypotension, and hypoxia), initiate treatment immediately (see below).

3. Unremitting headache, seizures, and change in level of consciousness suggest the presence of a cerebral sinovenous thrombosis (CVT).

B. Deep vein thrombosis
   1. The gold standard for the diagnosis of an arm or leg thrombosis is a venogram. The contrast dye is injected in the hand of the affected arm or the foot of the affected leg. If there is a filling defect in more than two views of the limb, this is diagnostic for DVT (Figures 5.4, IIA and B).
   2. Ultrasound (either Doppler or compression) in the leg has been validated in adults to be as sensitive and specific as venography. There has been no validation of ultrasound to diagnose DVT in the arm.
   3. Recommendations
      a. If DVT suspected, perform venography on the affected limb if possible. If venography is not available, ultrasound of the leg may be used.
      b. Ultrasound of the upper venous system may be very inaccurate and may miss a DVT.
      c. If a DVT/pulmonary embolism is identified, treat the patient with anticoagulants (see Section IIIC).

C. Pulmonary embolus
   1. The gold standard for the diagnosis of a pulmonary embolus (PE) is a pulmonary angiogram. The test used most often is a ventilation perfusion (V/Q) scan. The presence of one segmental mismatch or two or more subsegmental mismatches define a scan as high probability for PE. All other V/Q scans are non high or normal.
   2. Recommendation
      When PE is suspected in children, perform a V/Q scan. If the V/Q scan is not high or normal and there is no alternative diagnosis for the respiratory symptoms, perform venography or ultrasound of the legs (a potential source of PE), or if an upper venous system CVL is present, a venogram of the arm with the CVL. If results are negative and respiratory symptoms persist, consider performing a pulmonary angiogram if the patient's condition is stable.

Figure 5.4.
A, normal venous system bilateral arm venogram; B, abnormal upper
venous system bilateral arm venogram. Complete loss of normal
venous system due to thrombus in deep vessels of the chest is seen.
Collateral vessels are responsible for blood return to the heart.

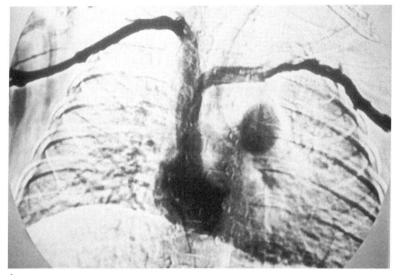

A

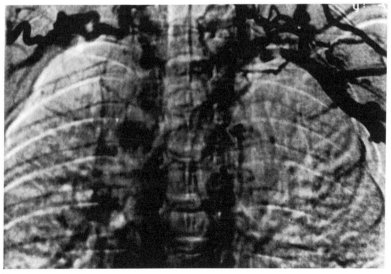

B

D. Cerebral venous thrombosis
1. A computed tomographic scan is not sensitive for the diagnosis of CVT.
2. Recommendation
   If CVT is suspected, use traditional angiography or magnetic resonance imaging angiography.

III. RECOMMENDATIONS FOR TREATMENT

A. Heparin
1. Treatment of children with confirmed DVT/PE:
   a. Loading dose: heparin 75 U/kg IV over 10 minutes
   b. Initial maintenance dose: 28 U/kg/h for infants <1 year, 20 U/kg/h for children >1 year
   c. Adjust heparin to maintain APTT of 60–85 seconds (assuming this reflects an antifactor Xa level of 0.30–0.70) (Table 5.3).
   d. Obtain blood for APTT 4 hours after administering the heparin loading dose and 4 hours after every change in the infusion rate.
   e. When APTT values are therapeutic, perform a daily CBC and APTT.
2. Reversal of heparin therapy
   a. If there is bleeding due to heparin that is clinically significant, the anticoagulant effect of heparin may be reversed with protamine sulfate according to dosages in Table 5.4 (maximum dose 50 mg).
   b. The infusion rate of a 10 mg/mL solution should not exceed 5 mg/min.
   c. Hypersensitivity reactions to protamine sulfate may occur in patients with known hypersensitivity reactions to fish or those previously exposed to protamine therapy or protamine-containing insulin.

B. Low-molecular-weight heparin
1. The following are guidelines for initiating and monitoring enoxaparin therapy. Modifications for individual clinical circumstances may be necessary. The only low-molecular-weight heparin that has been studied in children is enoxaparin (Lovenox, Rhone-Poulenc). Therefore, these dosage guidelines apply to this product *only* and cannot be directly extrapolated to other low-molecular-weight heparins. The treatment and prophylactic dose of enoxa-

Table 5.3.
Heparin Adjustments during Maintenance

APTT (s)	Bolus (U/kg)	Hold (min)	%Rate Change	Repeat APTT
<50	50	0	+10	4 h
50–59	0	0	+10	4 h
60–85*	0	0	0	Next day
86–95	0	0	-10	4 h
96–120	0	30	-10	4 h
>120	0	60	-15	4 h

*This therapeutic range must be established with the APTT reagent and instrument used in each particular laboratory. The range should correspond to a heparin level by protamine sulfate titration of 0.2–0.4 U/mL or an antifactor Xa level of 0.35–0.70 U/mL.

Table 5.4.
Heparin Reversal

Time Since Last Heparin Dose (min)	Protamine Dose
<3	1.0 mg/100 U heparin received
30–60	0.5–0.75 mg/100 U heparin received
60–120	0.375–0.5 mg/100 U heparin received
>120	0.25–0.375 mg/100 U heparin received

parin in children are extrapolated from adult clinical trials and a cohort study in children.

2. Consider the use of low-molecular-weight heparins for neonates, any patient requiring anticoagulation and deemed to be at increased risk of hemorrhage, and

3. Patients for whom venous access for administering and monitoring of standard heparin therapy is difficult.

4.. Dosage: enoxaparin (Lovenox has 110 antifactor Xa U/mg). (Table 5.5).

5. Avoid aspirin or other antiplatelet drugs during heparin therapy, if possible. If analgesia is required, prescribe acetaminophen.

6. Avoid intramuscular injections and arterial punctures during anticoagulation.

7. Measure platelet counts daily. If the platelet count drops below 100×10^9/L, on day 5 or later of initial heparin therapy or any day of heparin therapy if the patient received heparin therapy in the last 3 months, perform a heparin-induced

Table 5.5.
Dosage of Enoxaparin*

	Age <2 months	Age >2 months–18 years
Treatment dose	1.5 mg/kg/dose SC 12 h	1.0 mg/kg/dose SC 12 h
Prophylactic dose	0.75 mg/kg/dose SC 12 h	0.5 mg/kg/dose SC 12 h

*Maximum dose is 2.0 mg/kg/dose SC b.i.d.

thrombocytopenia (HIT) screen. In adults, the risk of HIT is greater after 5 days of treatment on the first exposure and anytime if the patient has been treated with heparin in the past. The epidemiology of HIT in children has not as yet been established. If a decrease in platelet count occurs and the total count is <100 × 10^9/L, consider performing a HIT screen.

C. Monitoring low-molecular-weight heparin
1. In treating a CVL-related thrombosis after the initial 3 months to 1 year of anticoagulant therapy, consider long-term low-dose anticoagulation as thromboprophylaxis if a functional CVL is in place.
2. On day 1 and/or day 2, draw a blood sample 4 hours after the subcutaneous administration of enoxaparin. If therapeutic, a weekly check on the antifactor Xa level is sufficient (Table 5.6.)
3. The therapeutic antifactor Xa level for treatment dose therapy is 0.5–1.0 U/mL. The target antifactor Xa level for prophylactic dose therapy is 0.2–0.4 U/mL.
4. For patients receiving long-term enoxaparin therapy (>3 months), consider bone densitometry studies at baseline and then every 6 months to assess for possible osteoporosis.
5. If an *antidote* for enoxaparin is needed, consider the following.
    a. If anticoagulation with enoxaparin needs to be discontinued for clinical reasons, termination of the subcutaneous injection will usually suffice. If an immediate effect is required, protamine sulfate has not been shown to completely reverse enoxaparin. Equimolar concentrations of protamine sulfate neutralize the antifactor IIa activity but result in only partial neutralization of the antifactor Xa activity.

Table 5.6.
Nomogram for Enoxaparin Treatment

Antifactor Xa Level	Hold Next Dose	Repeat Antifactor Xa Dose Change	Level
<0.35 U/mL	No	Increase by 25%	4 h after next dose
0.35–0.49 U/mL	No	increase by 10%	4 h after next dose
0.5–1.0 U/mL	No	0	and 1 × per week at 4 h after dose
1.1–1.5 U/mL	No	Decrease by 20%	4 h after next dose
1.6–2.0 U/mL	No	Decrease by 30%	4 h after next dose
>2.0 U/mL	For these patients, hold all further doses and measure the antifactor Xa level SC 12 hours until the level is <0.5 U/mL. Enoxaparin can then be restarted at a dose 40% less than was originally prescribed.		

    b. However, studies in experimental animal models indicate that increased microvascular bleeding produced by very high concentrations of enoxaparin is neutralized by protamine sulfate. The dose of protamine sulfate depends on the dose of enoxaparin used and the time of administration. If protamine is given within 3–4 hours of the enoxaparin, then a maximal neutralizing dose is 1 mg of protamine per 100 U (1 mg) of enoxaparin given in the last dose.

    c. The protamine should be administered intravenously and over a 10-minute period, as rapid infusion can cause hypotension.

D. Duration of heparin or low-molecular-weight heparin therapy

    1. The duration of heparin therapy depends on the primary problem. For DVT in children, heparin is usually administered for a minimum of 7 days. Maintenance coumadin should be instituted on day 1 or 2 of heparin therapy.

    2. If the thrombus is extensive or massive PE is present, administer heparin for 7–14 days and begin coumadin therapy on day 5.

    3. Continue heparin or low-molecular-weight heparin simultaneously with coumadin until the INR PT is therapeutic for a minimum of 2 days. Then, discontinue heparin or low-molecular-weight heparin and continue coumadin (see Section IIIB5).

4. Newborns may be treated for 10–14 days without the addition of coumadin.
5. Based on adult data, a first DVT or PE is treated with anticoagulants for 3 months to 1 year, depending on the extent of thrombosis. If an underlying thrombophilic condition is diagnosed, consider long-term anticoagulation.

E. Coumadin
Coumadin is an oral anticoagulant used for long-term anticoagulation for some children after heparin or low-molecular-weight heparin is discontinued (see Section IIIB4).
1. Loading dose
   a. Day 1: if the baseline INR is 1.0–1.3 U/mL, the dose is 0.2 mg/kg PO
   b. Days 2–4 (see Table 5.7).
2. Maintenance oral anticoagulation dose guidelines (see Table 5.8).

F. Thrombolytic therapy
1. Blocked catheters may be made patent with thrombolytic therapy (Table 5.9).
2. If local thrombolytic therapy for a blocked catheter fails, recommend diagnostic test to rule out CVL-related thrombosis (venography of upper system or ultrasound of lower venous system). If a CVL-related thrombus is confirmed, commence anticoagulation therapy. Consider systemic thrombolytic therapy with anticoagulation (Table 5.10).

G. Thromboprophylaxis for central venous lines
1. The reported incidence of CVL-related DVT is highly variable, reflecting a spectrum of diagnostic tools (clinical to

Table 5.7.
Adjusting Coumadin on Days 2 to 4 of Loading Dose

INR	Action
1.1–1.4	Repeat loading dose
1.5–1.9	50% of loading dose
2.0–3.0	50% of loading dose
3.0–3.5	25% of loading dose
>3.5	Hold until INR <3.5, then restart at 50% less than the previous dose

Table 5.8.
Guidelines for Maintenance Dosing

INR	Action
1.1–1.4	Increase by 20% of previous dose
1.5–1.9	Increase by 10% of previous dose
2.0–3.0	No change
3.1–3.5	Decrease by 20% of previous dose
>3.5	Hold dose, check INR daily until INR <3.5, then restart at 20% less than the previous dose

Table 5.9.
Low Dose for Blocked Catheters

	Regimen	Monitoring
Instillation	Urokinase (5000 U/mL) 1.5–3 mL/lumen for 2–4 h	None
Infusion	Urokinase (150 U/kg/h) per lumen for 12–48 h	Fibrinogen, TCT, PT, APTT

Table 5.10.
Systemic Thrombolytic Therapy*

Drug	Load	Maintenance	Monitoring
Urokinase	4400 U/kg for 6–12 h	4400 U/kg/h	Fibrinogen, TCT, PT, APTT
Streptokinase	2000 U/kg for 6–12 h	2000 U/kg/h	Same
Tissue plasminogen activator	None for 6 h	0.1–0.6 mg/kg/h	Same

*Start heparin therapy either during or immediately on completion of thrombolytic therapy. A loading dose of heparin may be omitted. The length of time for optimal maintenance is uncertain. Values provided are starting suggestions; some patients may respond to longer or shorter courses of therapy.

venography). When objective tests, such as venography, are used, the incidence ranges from 35 to 45%.

2. In adults, two studies [Bern et al. (1990) used low-dose coumadin and Monreal et al. (1995) used the low-molecular-weight heparin, Fragmin] demonstrated that prophylaxis of CVLs significantly decreases the incidence of thrombosis.

3. Side effects of thrombosis in a limb are the following.
   a. Postphlebitic syndrome, consisting of pain, swelling, and ultimately skin breakdown
   b. Mortality
      The Canadian Registry of Pediatric Thrombosis reported 2% mortality associated with thrombosis, usually in the form of PE.

4. Prophylaxis of CVLs in children is not recommended at this time due to the lack of prospective randomized controlled trials demonstrating safety and efficacy of anticoagulation prophylaxis.

5. If DVT associated with the placement of a CVL is objectively diagnosed, treatment with anticoagulation is recommended.

H. Cerebral venous thrombosis
   1. Therapy is controversial, but based on an adult study (Einhaupl et al., 1991) anticoagulation for 3 months should be considered.
   2. *Note:* Carry out thrombophilic blood studies on all children with thrombosis. If abnormal, offer screening of the family for the same abnormality. If the abnormality is confirmed, offer high-risk counseling.
      Questions on hemostasis may be directed to 1-800-NO-CLOTS or to Dr. Patti Massicotte or Dr. Maureen Andrew.

Acknowledgments

This work was supported by Project 7, from the Medical Research Council of Canada. Dr. M. Andrew is a Career Investigator of the Heart and Stroke Foundation of Canada.

Bibliography

Andrew M: Acquired disorders of hemostasis. In Nathan DG, Oski FA, eds. *Hematology of Infancy and Childhood.* 5th ed. Philadelphia: WB Saunders; in press.

Andrew M, Paes B, Johnson M: Development of the hemostasis system in the neonate and young infant. *Am J Pediatr Hematol Oncol* 12:95–104, 1990.

Andrew M, Vegh P, Johnson M, Bowker J, Ofosu F, Mitchell L: Maturation of the hemostatic system during childhood. *Blood* 80:1998–2005, 1992.

Andrew M, Adams M, Ali K, et al.:Venous thromboembolic complications (VTE) in children: First analysis of the Canadian Registry of VTE. *Blood* 83:1251, 1994.

Bern MM, Lokich JJ, Wallach SR, et al.: Very low doses of warfarin can prevent thrombosis in central venous catheters: A randomized prospective trial. *Ann Intern Med* 112:423, 1990.

Einhaupl KM, Villringer A, Meister W, et al.: Heparin treatment in sinus venous thrombosis. *Lancet* 338:597, 1991.

Leaker M, Massicotte MP, Brooker L, Andrew M: Thrombolytic therapy in pediatric patients: A comprehensive review of the literature. *Thromb Haemost* 76:132, 1996.

Lensing AWA, Prins MH, Davidson BL, Hirsh J, Academic Medical Centre: Treatment of deep venous thrombosis with low molecular weight heparins: A meta-analysis. *Arch Intern Med* 155:601–07, 1995.

Massicotte MP, Adams M, the Directors of the Canadian Children's Thrombophilia Program: Central venous line (CVL) related thromboembolic events (CVLT) in children with cancer. Proceedings of the 4th International Conference on the Longterm Complications of Treatment of Children and Adolescents for Cancer, Buffalo, NY, June 14–15, 1996.

Massicotte MP, Adams M, Marzinotto V, Brooker L, Andrew M: Low molecular weight heparin in pediatric patients with thrombotic disease: A dose finding study. *J Pediatr* 128:313–18, 1996.

Michelson AD, Bovill E, Andrew M: Antithrombotic therapy in children. *Chest* 108:506S, 1995.

Monreal M, Alastrue A, Rull M, et al.: Upper extremity deep venous thrombosis in cancer patients with venous access devices: Prophylaxis with a low molecular weight heparin (Fragmin). *Thromb Haemost* 75:251, 1996.

Schreiber GB, Busch MP, Kleinman SH, Korelitz JJ, for the Retrovirus Epidemiology Donor Study: The risk of transfusion-related viral infections: The Retrovirus Epidemiology Donor Study. *N Engl J Med* 334:1734–35, 1996.

6

The Use of Hematopoietic Growth Factors in Children with Cancer

Sandra Luna-Fineman, M.D., Kevin M. Shannon, M.D., and Bruce R. Blazar, M.D.

Several hematopoietic growth factors (HGFs) have recently been molecularly cloned, and recombinant (r) human (h) products are available for clinical use. Three products have been approved for clinical use. Granulocyte-colony-stimulating factor (rhG-CSF, filgrastim [Neupogen]) and granulocyte-macrophage-colony-stimulating factor (rhGM-CSF, sargramostim [Leukine]) stimulate, respectively, the proliferation, maturation, and function of granulocytes, and that of granulocytes, macrophages, and possibly megakaryocytes. Erythropoietin (rhEPO, epoetin alfa [Epogen, Procrit]) stimulates the proliferation and differentiation of committed erythroid progenitors, including burst-forming unit-erythroid cells and colony-forming unit-erythroid cells.

Even though HGFs are approved for use in children, both the indication for the administration of HGFs and their doses for children are largely unsettled. Although the absolute neutrophil count (ANC) may fall as low with these HGFs as without them, the duration of neutropenia is typically shorter. The intensification of some chemotherapeutic regimens might not be feasible without the use of rhG-CSF or rhGM-CSF for the faster recovery of granulocytes and macrophages. Little information exists for the use of rhEPO in children. However, there are unique situations in which the use of rhEPO is reasonable, such as for patients who will not accept blood transfusions for religious reasons.

These guidelines should be considered as a framework that will be refined with time. When no specific recommendation for the use of rhG-CSF, rhGM-CSF, or rhEPO is made in a study protocol or the patient is not in a study, the following guidelines will prove useful.

Recombinant Human Granulocyte-Colony-Stimulating Factor (rhG-CSF)

I. INDICATIONS AND CONTRAINDICATIONS

A. Proven indications
1. When the planned chemotherapy for a nonmyeloid malignancy is likely to result in an ANC < 500 cells/μL for 7 or more days
2. To accelerate myeloid recovery after chemotherapy in patients with myeloid malignancy and expected ANC < 500 cells/μL for 7 or more days
3. To accelerate myeloid recovery in patients who have undergone bone marrow transplantation after conditioning drugs have been given
4. To mobilize peripheral blood stem cells for autologous bone marrow transplantation

B. Controversial indications
1. When a prior cycle of the anticipated chemotherapy has been associated with at least one episode of fever and neutropenia
2. When an ANC of < 500 cells/μL for 7 days or more is anticipated, secondary to noncytotoxic myelosuppressive agents (e.g., ganciclovir, zidovudine)
3. To increase the granulocyte count in patients with aplastic anemia.
4. To treat myelodysplastic syndromes associated with an ANC <500 cells/μL.
5. To treat fever and neutropenia (ANC <500 cells/μL) in patients not yet receiving rhG-CSF. This might be especially important if the patient has signs of sepsis.

C. Inappropriate indications
  1. Neutropenia secondary to chemotherapy likely to result in an ANC < 500 cells/μL for < 7 days
  2. Infection without neutropenia (ANC > 1000 cells/μL).
  3. Neutropenia (ANC < 1000 cells/mm^3) secondary to radiation therapy
  4. To mature or cycle myeloid blasts for better chemotherapeutic response to therapy

D. Contraindication
  History of hypersensitivity to rhG-CSF or *Escherichia coli*-derived proteins.

II. ADMINISTRATION (rhG-CSF, filgrastim, Neupogen)

A. Dosage
  1. Starting dose: 5 μg/kg/d SC or IV over 30 minutes
  2. Based on limited information in adults, an improved response may be obtained with 10 μg/kg/d when there was a suboptimal response at 5 μg/kg/d. No studies in children have demonstrated significant increases in neutrophil count with doses > 5 μg/kg/d

B. Duration
  1. Start rhG-CSF 24 hours after the last chemotherapeutic agent and continue until the ANC is ≥ 10,000 cells/μL after the expected chemotherapy-induced nadir, but for a maximum of 14 days. However, a shorter duration of administration that is sufficient to achieve clinically adequate neutrophil recovery is reasonable. A lower ANC value can be used to stop rhG-CSF.
  2. Do not administer rhG-CSF within 24 hours of the administration of chemotherapy.
  3. Occasionally, the ANC will increase transiently 2 days after the initiation of rhG-CSF. Avoid premature discontinuation before the expected ANC nadir.

C. Monitoring
  1. Monitor complete blood clot (CBC), differential, and platelet counts before starting rhG-CSF and at least twice

weekly, past the neutrophil nadir until the ANC is $\geq 10,000$ cells/mm^3.
2. More frequent monitoring of WBC might be needed to avoid excessive leukocytosis.

D. Formulation and preparation
  1. rhG-CSF is supplied as single-dose, preservative-free vials containing 300 μg (1 mL at 300 μg/mL) or 480 μg (1.6 mL at 300 μg/mL) of rhG-CSF-injectable solution.
  2. Each 1 mL contains 300 μg of rhG-CSF in a solution containing 10 mM sodium acetate buffer at pH 4.0, with 5% mannitol and 0.004% Tween 80 and 0.035 mg sodium in 1 mL of water.
  3. Vials are single dose and should not be reentered for later administration, since rhG-CSF is supplied as a preservative-free solution.

E. Dilution
  1. Dilute rhG-CSF only in dextrose 5% in water (D5W). Avoid shaking. Do not dilute in saline.
  2. If the concentration of the diluted rhG-CSF is < 15 μg/mL, add albumin to the D5W to make a 0.2% albumin solution before adding the rhG-CSF.

F. Storage
  1. Store rhG-CSF at 2–8° C. Do not freeze. Vials are stable for a maximum of 24 hours at room temperature.
  2. After dilution in D5W, the solution is stable in the refrigerator or room temperature for 7 days. Since the solution is preservative-free, practice caution to maintain sterility.

III. ADVERSE EFFECTS

A. Common
Bone pain elevation of uric acid, lactate dehydrogenase (LDH), and alkaline phosphatase

B. Occasional
Fever, nausea and vomiting, rash, diarrhea, splenomegaly, exacerbation of psoriasis, and erythema at the injection site

Recombinant Human Granulocyte-Macrophage-Colony-Stimulating Factor (rhGM-CSF)

I. INDICATIONS AND CONTRAINDICATIONS

A. Proven indications

1. To accelerate myeloid recovery in patients who have just received an autologous bone marrow transplant secondary to non-Hodgkin lymphoma, Hodgkin disease, or acute lymphoblastic leukemia after conditioning drugs have been given

2. To accelerate myeloid recovery when delayed or failure of engraftment after autologous or allogeneic bone marrow transplant

3. To accelerate myeloid recovery after peripheral blood stem cell transplantation

B. Controversial indications

1. To accelerate myeloid recovery in patients who have undergone allogeneic bone marrow transplantation for any malignancy and in patients with myeloid malignancy undergoing autologous bone marrow transplantation

2. When the planned chemotherapy for a nonmyeloid malignancy is likely to result in an ANC < 500 cells/μL for 7 or more days

3. To treat myelodysplastic syndrome

C. Inappropriate indications

To mature or cycle myeloid blasts for better chemotherapeutic response to therapy.

D. Contraindications

1. Excessive myeloid blasts ($\geq$ 10%) in bone marrow or peripheral blood

2. Juvenile chronic myeloid leukemia or monosomy 7 syndrome.

3. History of hypersensitivity to rhGM-CSF or yeast-derived proteins

II. ADMINISTRATION (rhGM-CSF, sargamostim, Leukine)

A. Dosage
1. Starting dose is 250 µg/m²/day IV over 2–4 hours for both the prevention and the treatment of engraftment delay. rhGM-CSF can be administered subcutaneously if indicated.
2. If a severe adverse reaction occurs, reduce or discontinue the dose.

B. Duration
1. When given to prevent engraftment delay, the first dose should be given within 2–4 hours after the bone marrow transplant, then once a day for 21 days or until the ANC > 10,000 cells/µL .
2. rhGM-CSF should not be given within 24 hours of last chemotherapy or within 12 hours of last dose of radiation therapy.
3. In case of engraftment delay or failure of bone marrow transplant, 14 or more days of treatment may be necessary.

C. Monitoring
1. CBC with differential and platelet counts shuld be monitored at least twice weekly and rhGM-CSF should be discontinued when ANC >10,000 cells/µL; avoid white blood cell count (WBC) >50,000 cells/µL.
2. More frequent monitoring of WBC might be needed to avoid excessive leukocytosis.
3. If blasts appear or disease progresses, discontinue rhGM-CSF.
4. Monitor renal and hepatic function twice a week and more often for patients with organ dysfunction.
5. Due to possible fluid retention syndrome, monitor patients for weight gain, respiratory distress, and pleural or pericardial effusions.

D. Formulation and preparation
1. Sterile, white, preservative-free, lyophilized powder in vials containing 250 or 500 µg of rhGM-CSF with 40 mg of mannitol, 10 mg of sucrose, and 1.2 mg of tromethamine in 1 mL of water

     a. Reconstitute rhGM-CSF in 1 mL of sterile or bacterio-static water. Avoid shaking.

     b. Administer product reconstituted with sterile water within 6 hours of preparation; product reconstituted with bacteriostatic water may be stored for up to 20 days at 2–8° C.

  2. Sterile, preserved (1.1% benzyl alcohol), injectable solution in multiple-dose vials containing 500 µg of rhGM-CSF with 40 mg of mannitol, 10 mg of sucrose, and 1.2 mg of tromethamine in 1 mL of water

    Since this product is preserved, once the vial is entered, the drug may be stored for up to 20 days at 2–8° C. Discard any remaining solution after 20 days.

E. Dilution

  1. Dilute with 0.9% NaCl and administer as a 2 to 4 hour infusion.

  2. If the concentration of rhGM-CSF is <1 0 µg/mL, to prevent absorption to the drug delivery system, add albumin to the saline to make a 0.1% albumin solution before adding rhGM-CSF.

F. Storage

  1. Store all preparations at 2–8° C. Do not freeze.

  2. Prepared or diluted rhGM-CSF is stable for 6 hours after reconstitution. Since the diluted solution is preservative-free, practice caution to maintain sterility.

III. ADVERSE EFFECTS

A. Occasional

Bone pain, leukocytosis, diarrhea, asthenia, rash, malaise, headache, fever, chills, arthralgias, chest pain, thrombocytopenia, dyspnea, and thrombophlebitis

B. Uncommon

Fluid retention: peripheral edema, pleural effusion, pericardial effusion, dyspnea, respiratory distress syndrome, weight gain, renal failure, thrombosis of vena cava, hypotension, facial flushing, bundle branch block, supraventricular arrhythmias, and elevation of LDH, alkaline phosphatase, and liver function tests

Recombinant Human Erythropoietin

Three points must be emphasized if the use of rhEPO is being considered: 1) disproportional anemia compared with neutropenia and thrombocytopenia suggests other causes of low hemoglobin/hematocrit (iron deficiency, bleeding, or hemolysis) that will not be resolved with rhEPO; 2) not all patients will respond to rhEPO due to "end-organ" problems (myelodysplastic syndrome and, some anemias of chronic disease); and 3) some patients receiving cisplatin-containing regimens (due to renal damage) might respond better to rhEPO.

I. INDICATIONS AND CONTRAINDICATIONS

A. Proven indications
There are no proven indications in pediatric oncology.

B. Controversial indications
1. Anemia of chronic disease or secondary to chemotherapy to decrease the need of blood transfusions
2. Anemia associated with radiation therapy
3. Anemia secondary to myelodysplastic syndrome, when baseline serum EPO is low
4. Anemia after allogeneic bone marrow transplantation

C. Inappropriate indications
Anemia associated with cancer or myelodysplastic syndrome when the serum EPO is > 500 U/L

D. Contraindications
1. Anemia secondary to nutritional deficiencies (iron, folic acid, or vitamin B_{12}), bleeding, or hemolytic anemia
2. Uncontrollable hypertension
3. Hypersensitivity to mammalian cell-derived products
4. Hypersensitivity to human albumin

II. ADMINISTRATION (rhEPO, epoetin alfa, Epogen, Procrit)

A. Baseline laboratory tests
1. Before starting rhEPO therapy, all patients should have a baseline serum EPO and ferritin measurement.
2. If ferritin is less than 100 µ/L, prescribe iron supplementation (ferrous sulfate).

B. Dosage (Table 6.1)
1. Starting dose: 150 U/kg/day SC 3 times a week
2. If there is no response within 2 to 4 weeks, the dose can be increased to 300 U/kg/day SC 3 times a week.
3. If the hematocrit (Hct) reaches 40%, stop the rhEPO dose until the Hct is 36%; restart at a 25% dose. Titration might be necessary.
4. If the Hct increases very rapidly (> 4 percentage points in 2 weeks), reduce the rhEPO dose by 25%.

C. Duration
1. Continue rhEPO until the patient is considered not to need red blood cell support.
2. rhEPO can be given concurrently with chemotherapy treatment.

D. Monitoring
1. Measure baseline serum EPO level before starting rhEPO (Table 6.1).
2. Perform a baseline CBC with platelet count and reticulocyte count. Thereafter, monitor the hematocrit and hemoglobin weekly until the Hct becomes stable.

Table 6.1.
Dosage Guidelines for Recombinant Human Erythropoietin

Baseline Serum Erythropoietin (U/L)	rhEPO Dose

< 100	Start 150 U/kg/day 3 times a week
	Dose adjustment:
	    If Hct > 40%, hold EPO until Hct is 36% and restart at a 25% dose reduction
	    If rapid increase in Hct, (> 4 percent points in 2 weeks) reduce Epo 25%
	    If no response* in 2 to 4 weeks, increase dose to 300 U/kg/day 3 times a week

>100 and < 500	Start 150 U/kg/day 3 times a week
	Dose adjustment:
	    If no response in 4 weeks, increase dose to 300 U/kg/day 3 times a week
	    If no response after 8 weeks of dose escalation, stop rhEPO

>500	Do not use rhEPO

*Response: increase of Hct by 6 percentage points in 2–4 weeks. No blood transfusions given. Check ferritin if no response or response poor.

    3. Monitor blood urea nitrogen, creatinine, and potassium every 2 weeks for the 1st month and once a month thereafter.

    4. Monitor ferritin once a month.

E. Formulation and preparation

    1. Single-dose, preservative-free 1 mL vial containing rhEPO: 2000, 3000, 4000, or 10,000 U/mL of injectable solution.

    Each 1 mL of preservative-free solution contains the above amounts of rhEPO with 2.5 mg of albumin (human), 5.8 mg of sodium citrate, 5.8 mg of sodium chloride, and 0.06 mg of citric acid in water.

    2. Multiple-dose, preserved 2 mL vial containing rhEPO: 10,000 U/mL.

    Each 1 mL of preserved solution contains 10,000 U of rhEPO, 2.5 mg of albumin (human), 1.3 mg of sodium citrate, 8.2 mg of sodium chloride, 0.11 mg of citric acid, and 1% benzyl alcohol as preservative in water.

F. Dilution

Do not dilute rhEPO or give with other drugs. However, before subcutaneous injection, it can be mixed in bacteriostatic 0.9% sodium chloride with benzyl alcohol 0.9% at 1:1. The benzyl alcohol acts as a local anesthetic.

G. Storage

Store at 2–8° C. Do not freeze or shake.

III. ADVERSE EFFECTS

A. Common

Hypertension, local pain at site of injection, headache, fever, and diarrhea

B. Occasional

Nausea, flu-like symptoms, thrombosis of vascular access devices, and seizures

Bibliography

American Society of Clinical Oncology: Update of recommendations for the use of hematopoietic colony-stimulating factors: Evidence-based clinical practice guidelines. *J Clin Oncol* 14:1957–60, 1996.

Case DC: Recombinant human erythropoietin therapy for anemic cancer patients on combination chemotherapy. *J Natl Can Inst* 85:801–6, 1993.

Henry DH: Clinical application of recombinant erythropoietin in anemic cancer patients. *Hematol Oncol Clin North Am* 8:961–73, 1994.

Ludwig H, et al.: Prediction of response to erythropoietin treatment in chronic anemia of cancer. *Blood* 84:1056–63, 1994.

Ludwig H, et al.: Recombinant human erythropoietin for the correction of cancer associated anemia with and without concomitant cytotoxic chemotherapy. *Cancer* 76:2319–29, 1995.

Nemunaitis J: Growth factors of the future. *Leuk Lymphoma* 9:329–36, 1993.

Ozer H: American Society of Clinical Oncology Guidelines for the Clinical Use of Hematopoietic Colony-Stimulating Factors. *Curr Opin Hematol* 3:3–10, 1996.

Vose JM, Armitage JO: Clinical applications of hematopoietic growth factors. *J Clin Oncol* 13:1023–35, 1995.

Welte K et al.: Filgrastim (r-metHuG-CSF): The first 10 years. *Blood* 88:1907–29, 1996.

7

Modifications for Toxicity

John J. Iacuone, M.D., Laurel Steinherz, M.D.,
Melanie G. Oblender, M.D.,
Dorothy R. Barnard, M.D., and
Arthur R. Ablin, M.D.

Monitoring Patients Receiving Anthracyclines

I. BACKGROUND

A. The anthracycline antibiotics can cause both acute and long term cumulative cardiotoxic effects. Anatomic damage increases linearly with the cumulative dose, whereas clinical manifestations increase more logarithmically at higher doses.

B. The incidence of clinical cardiotoxicity can be anticipated to increase rapidly beyond a cumulative dose of about 450 mg/m^2 for both doxorubicin and daunorubicin and 125 mg/m^2 for idarubicin.

C. Individual patients may have a lower threshold and develop toxicity at significantly lower doses.

D. Mediastinal irradiation increases both anatomic and clinical toxicity at any cumulative dose.

E. Cardiac dysfunction may appear several months after anthracycline therapy, and cardiac status during the year after treatment predicts long-term effects. Therefore, continue monitoring after drug discontinuation.

F. In calculating the maximum allowable dose of anthracy-clines, consider the possibility of the future administration of other cardiotoxic drugs (e.g., high-dose cyclophosphamide), mediastinal radiation, or bone marrow transplantation.

II. MONITORING TECHNIQUES

A. Electrocardiographic changes are too nonspecific and occur too late to be reliably predictive of myocardial damage and changes in cardiac function.

B. Serial echocardiography
   1. Serial two-dimensional or M-mode echocardiograms in children may permit successful dose modification and reduce the incidence of congestive heart failure.
   2. The parameter to follow is the fractional shortening (FS), which is normally $\geq 29\%$.
   3. Other parameters that can be followed are end-diastolic internal diameter and volume, systolic time intervals, end-systolic wall stress compared with velocity of circum-ferential fiber shortening, parameters of diastolic func-tion, and increase of contractility with exercise or chemi-cally induced stress.
   4. Echocardiograms are a suitable modality for children because of their relatively thin chest and noncalcified ribs. Sedation is usually not required.

C. Radionuclide cardiac cineangiography
   1. Radionuclide cardiac cineangiography (RNA, also known as MUGA or RNCA) can be used in children and adults, with the advantage of providing a three-dimensional mea-surement of cardiac volume rather than the one- or two-dimensional measurements echocardiography provides.
   2. The results of RNA are more independent of thoracic pathologic conditions than are echocardiogram measure-ments.
   3. The disadvantages are possible obscuring of the image by "poor tag" of radionuclide or competitive uptake, less well-defined "areas of interest" compared with echocar-diograms in children, and the need for the patient to be motionless during the scan.
   4. Normal systolic function is defined by a left ventricular ejection fraction (LVEF) $\geq 55\%$. Normal stress response is

defined as an increase in the LVEF by at least 5 percentile points.

D. Myocardial biopsy
1. Myocardial biopsy is a measure of anatomic abnormality that may occur before clinical abnormality is detected.
2. It is used to determine the risk of additional anthracyclines when top recommended doses have been given or to clarify the role of chemotherapy in producing myocardial dysfunction and congestive heart failure.

III. TESTING FOR CARDIOTOXICITY

A. The probability of abnormal cardiac function is increased when both the echocardiogram and the RNA are abnormal, rather than when just one of the two is abnormal.

B. One modality, either echocardiogram or RNA, should be the consistent method of testing at every evaluation, with the other added when confirmatory testing is required.

C. Perform studies before anthracycline treatment as a baseline and then preferably 2–3 weeks from the preceding dose and early enough to allow the reporting of accurate calculations before the next dose. Also obtain an electrocardiogram (ECG) as a baseline for comparison with later ECGs, which may show changes in conduction and arrhythmias.

D. The patient should be normothermic and have a hemoglobin ≥ 9 g/dL at the time of the testing.

E. Frequency of testing (Figure 7.1)
1. Perform an echocardiogram (or RNA) before every other subsequent course of doxorubicin and/or daunorubicin when the total cumulative dose is < 300 mg/m^2.
2. Perform an echocardiogram (or RNA) before each subsequent course of doxorubicin and/or daunorubicin > 300 mg/m^2.
3. Perform an RNA (or echocardiogram) in addition to the consistent test modality as an optional confirmatory test, when a total dose of > 300 mg/m^2 of doxorubicin or daunorubicin plus mediastinal radiation above 1000 cGy are given.
4. Perform an RNA (or echocardiogram) in addition to the consistent test modality as an optional confirmatory

Figure 7.1.
The frequency of testing cardiac function for the anthracyclines, daunorubicin, and doxorubicin.

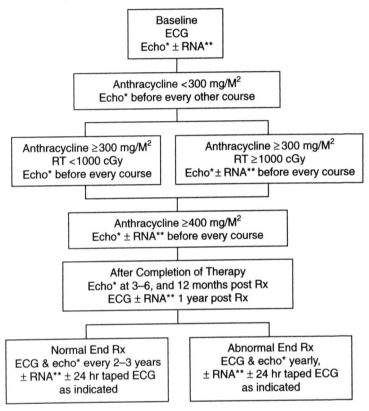

* Echocardiography (Echo) is the "first" testing modality to be used consistently for evaluation.
** RNA is the "second" testing modality to be used if indicated for better imaging and confirmation. Alternatively, RNA could be used as the "first" consistent modality and echocardiography could be used as the confirmatory modality. The second confirmatory modality is suggested at doses above 400 mg/m² or 300 mg/m² with radiotherapy (RT) because treatment in excess of these limits represents significantly higher risk of cardiotoxicity.
Source: Modified from Steinherz et al., 1992, p. 946.

test, when a total dose of > 400 mg/m² of doxorubicin or daunorubicin is given with or without mediastinal radiation.

5. For new cardiotoxic agents under investigation, perform an echocardiogram and RNA, if possible, before each course.

6. The current recommendation for idarubicin is to begin more frequent monitoring at a total cumulative dose of 75 mg/m². Confirmatory testing is suggested at 75 mg/m² if there is mediastinal radiation and at a total dose of 100 mg/m² of idarubicin with or without mediastinal radiotherapy.
7. Follow-up after cessation of therapy is advisable.
   a. Obtain an echocardiogram (or RNA) at 3–6 and 12 months after therapy and repeat the ECG at 12 months after therapy.
   b. RNA (or echocardiogram) may be added as a confirmatory test at 12 months after therapy, especially if there is difficulty with imaging with the primary modality.
   c. If cardiac function is normal (by criteria of Section IV) during the first year after therapy, then do the following.
      i. Obtain an echocardiogram (or RNA) and 12-lead electrocardiogram every 2 to 3 years.
      ii. Because of a high incidence of arrhythmias noted on late follow-up examination of patients after anthracycline therapy, a 24-hour ECG is recommended as indicated by symptoms or abnormalities of the other tests.
      iii. RNA (or echocardiogram) may be added as a confirmatory test less frequently, especially if there is difficulty imaging with the first testing modality.
   d. If cardiac function is abnormal during the first year after therapy, plan cardiac evaluation that includes an ECG and echocardiogram and, as indicated, RNA and 24-hour ECG, yearly or more often if required by symptoms.

IV. CRITERIA FOR DETERIORATING CARDIAC FUNCTION

A. A decrease in the FS by an absolute value of 10 percentile points from the previous test (e.g., from 41% to 31%)

B. A FS < 29%

C. A decrease in the RNA LVEF by an absolute value of 10 percentile points from the previous test (e.g., from 67% to 57%)

D. A RNA LVEF <55%

E. A decrease in the RNA LVEF with stress

V. MODIFICATION OF ANTHRACYCLINE THERAPY

A. Discontinuation

If both the echocardiogram FS and the RNA LVEF are abnormal by the criteria in Section IV, stop anthracycline therapy unless:

1. Myocardial biopsy (optional) shows no anatomic evidence of anthracycline toxicity.
2. There is a recovery of echocardiogram FS and RNA LVEF to normal on two serial tests taken 1 month apart.

B. Temporary cessation

If only one test modality was used and it was abnormal by the criteria in Section IV, confirm with the other modality. If either the echocardiogram FS or the RNA LVEF is abnormal while the other is normal, stop anthracyclines temporarily. Wait 1 month and repeat both tests. If one remains normal and the other becomes normal or does not deteriorate further, resume therapy. Stop therapy if further deterioration occurs in either test.

VI. CARDIOPROTECTIVE AGENTS AND ADMINISTRATION METHOD MINIMIZING CARDIOTOXICITY

A. There is evidence in the literature that both short- and long-term cardiotoxicity is related to the peak dose of exposure to the heart.

1. Decreasing the peak circulating dose by using split/lower weekly doses or continuous infusion has resulted in decreased clinical and pathologic cardiotoxicity for any cumulative dose.
2. The shortest infusion that has been reported to show benefit is 6 hours, with increasing benefit when the delivery time is prolonged to 72 hours.

B. The chelator ICRF-187 (Zinecard) has been shown, in adults, to decrease clinical and pathologic cardiotoxicity when given immediately before the administration of doxorubicin. Smaller studies reported this for daunorubicin and epirubicin as well.

1. These studies have used ICRF-187 in conjunction with delivery of the anthracycline by "push" rather than continuous infusion.

2. ICRF-187 is currently officially approved for adults who have already received 300 mg/m^2 of doxorubicin; it is not yet approved for routine use in children.
3. It is given as a rapid infusion in a dose that is 10 times the doxorubicin dose, minutes before each dose of doxorubicin.
4. There have been two promising reports of pediatric use, and larger pediatric studies are planned.

Prevention and Treatment of Urinary Tract Toxicity

I. ASSESSMENT OF RENAL FUNCTION

Assessment of renal function can provide information for early detection and monitoring of nephrotoxic treatments. Measurements of renal function that can provide information related to the etiology, site of injury, current activity, extent, and potential reversibility of nephrotoxicity are needed. Traditional screening tests of renal function (blood urea nitrogen, serum creatinine, and urine output) are inadequate.

As always in pediatric patients, carefully consider the importance of age-related reference values and physiologic developmental variations. Although rarely applicable in oncology clinical trials, the dynamic early postnatal renal changes can complicate treatment with potentially nephrotoxic medications.

A. Radioisotopic techniques
^{99}Tc-diethylene pentacetic combines low patient radiation dosimetry (40 mrad/mCi) and good correlation with inulin clearance. Using a compartmental analysis model, calculate glomerular filtration rate (GFR) after a single bolus injection of radioisotope. The two-compartment model has an error of approximately 3–4 mL/min when compared with inulin clearance. Errors in measurement can be introduced by edema, intravascular volume contraction or expansion, or severe renal failure. A correction factor for volume of distribution can be used.

B. Electrolytes
Screening for renal tubular dysfunction should include

serum potassium, sodium, chloride, glucose, magnesium, phosphate, alkaline phosphatase, bicarbonate, and pH. To aid interpretation of these values, corresponding evaluation of urine lytes is required. Screening for distal renal tubular function should include osmolality and pH of an early morning urine sample. Proximal tubular damage is associated with aminoaciduria and glucosuria.

II. RENAL TOXICITY TO BE EXPECTED WITH SPECIFIC CHEMOTHERAPEUTIC AGENTS

A. Toxicity
1. 5-Azacytidine
   5-Azacytidine can produce proximal tubular dysfunction with acidosis, hypokalemia, and hypophosphatemia.
2. Diaziquone (AZQ)
   AZQ given in high doses commonly leads to proteinuria and renal tubular dysfunction.
3. Carmustine (BCNU)/ Lomustine (CCNU)
   BCNU/CCNU, along with other nitrosoureas, can cause a progressive chronic nephropathy. The renal tubular disease frequently occurs after the completion of chemotherapy and can be irreversible.
4. Busulfan/melphalan
   Busulfan and melphalan have been associated with hemorrhagic cystitis and can increase the risk of hemorrhagic cystitis in patients who receive cyclophosphamide.
5. Carboplatin
   a. The nephrotoxic potential of carboplatin appears to be less than that of cisplatin.
   b. Hyponatremia secondary to increased urinary loss can occur but is reported rarely.
   c. Renal tubular damage has followed treatment with carboplatin.
   d. Carboplatin has not resulted in proteinuria.
6. Cisplatin
   Proximal and distal renal tubular damage, hemolytic uremic syndrome, and decreased GFR (acute and chronic) have been associated with cisplatin.
   a. Hypomagnesemia, hyponatremia, and hypocalcemia due to renal tubular damage have been documented.

b. Renal tubular damage is exacerbated by coincident hyperuricemia, hypoalbuminemia, amphotericin B, iodinated intravenous contrast dyes, abdominal radiation, and, perhaps, aminoglycoside therapy.

c. Cisplatin can increase nephrotoxicity related to ifosfamide or methotrexate.

d. The extent of GFR or renal tubular damage recovery after the completion of cisplatin is uncertain. In some patients, deterioration of renal function continues after the completion of treatment.

7. Cyclophosphamide

a. Hemorrhagic cystitis (microscopic to gross, life-threatening) is frequently associated with cyclophosphamide therapy.

i. The cystitis is accompanied by irritative voiding complaints. It can be diminished or prevented with vigorous hydration.

ii. Radiation to the bladder can increase the risk of hemorrhagic cystitis. Vesicoureteral reflux and hydronephrosis have also been reported.

iii. Symptoms frequently recur, with and without further exposure to cyclophosphamide or related compounds, radiation, or other radiomimetic therapy. The risk of recurrence is higher and the symptoms more severe with additional bladder-toxic treatments.

b. Transient dilutional hyponatremia and oliguria can occur 8–12 hours after moderate- to high-dose cyclophosphamide treatment.

8. Ifosfamide

a. Ifosfamide has been associated with proximal renal tubular dysfunction (impaired reabsorption of glucose, amino acids, sodium, and inorganic phosphate).

b. Nephrotoxic effects on the proximal tubule appear to be more severe in younger children, particularly increased urinary excretion of phosphate and glucose.

c. Distal renal tubular dysfunction is less common, and glomerular toxicity has not been reported without associated severe tubular dysfunction.

d. Fanconi syndrome (glucosuria, aminoaciduria, low fractional excretion of phosphate, and elevated fractional excretion of sodium bicarbonate) secondary to ifosfamide therapy has been reported. High urinary excretion of sodium in the presence of impaired concentrating ability can lead to significant dehydration.

e. Although the acute effects of each treatment are generally partially to completely reversible between courses of treatment, there is evidence that the capacity to recover from acute tubular damage is increasingly impaired after each course of therapy. Tubular damage, once established, may persist long term. Progression of renal toxicity can continue after the completion of treatment.

f. The incidence of ifosfamide-related nephrotoxicity increases with increasing cumulative doses.

g. The nephrotoxicity of ifosfamide and cisplatin may be additive. Ifosfamide nephrotoxicity is increased after abdominal irradiation or nephrectomy.

h. The onset of laboratory and clinical nephrotoxicity may occur during or years after the completion of treatment.

i. Hematuria resulting from bladder wall damage is common without the use of the uroprotective agent Mesna.

   i. The use of Mesna gives a false-positive result for ketones on urine dipstick measurements.

   ii. Mesna does not prevent nephrotoxicity.

j. Rarely, renal toxicity has led to a syndrome resembling that of inappropriate antidiuretic hormone, clinical nephrogenic diabetes insipidus, hypophosphatemic rickets, or renal tubular acidosis.

k. One study found decreased bone mineral density in 20% of children receiving ifosfamide.

9. Methotrexate

a. Precipitation of methotrexate in renal tubules or collecting ducts, direct biochemical damage of renal tubules, or a pharmacologic effect on proliferating cells resulting in renal failure can occur with high-dose methotrexate, especially in patients with acidic urine.

b. In general, renal failure secondary to methotrexate resolves within 14–21 days. Proteinuria and enzymuria frequently have resulted from treatment with methotrexate. These laboratory changes are usually clinically insignificant.

c. Systemic complications of methotrexate are increased in the presence of a decreased GFR. Patients with ileal conduits are at increased risk of methotrexate-induced renal complications. Patients receiving both methotrexate and cisplatin are at increased risk of nephrotoxicity.

10. Aminoglycosides
   a. Aminoglycosides can induce renal tubular dysfunction, decreased GFR, proteinuria, and urinary renal casts.
   b. Most patients with aminoglycoside nephrotoxicity develop nonoliguric azotemia.
   c. An occasional patient develops Fanconi renal syndrome or electrolyte wasting of calcium, magnesium, and potassium.
   d. Aminoglycosides may potentiate the renal damage of other nephrotoxic treatments.
   e. Usually, the renal effects of aminoglycosides reverse after the discontinuation of the drug. There is a range in the degree of renal toxicity caused by aminoglycosides.
   f. Gentamicin is associated with the greatest renal toxicity.

11. Amphotericin B
   a. Nephrotoxicity occurs to some degree in 80% of patients receiving amphotericin B.
   b. Amphotericin B decreases GFR through toxic effects on the renal vasculature.
   c. Decreases in GFR and renal plasma flow occur almost universally.
   d. These changes may be mediated by sodium status and intrarenal glomerulotubular feedback. Adequate hydration and sodium loading can decrease nephrotoxicity.
   e. Damage to proximal and distal renal tubules by amphotericin B frequently results in excess loss of potassium, magnesium, and protein.
   f. Renal tubular acidosis without systemic acidosis can develop.
   g. Patients receiving amphotericin B are predisposed to nephrocalcinosis.
   h. Alkalinization of the urine can decrease the risk of nephrocalcinosis and permanent renal damage.
   i. Hyposthenuria can precede azotemia

      j. Nephrotoxicity is increased in the presence of base-line renal dysfunction, hypovolemia, and the use of diuretics and concomitant nephrotoxic medications.

      k. The nephrotoxic effects of amphotericin B usually resolve over several months after the drug is discontinued.

B. Symptoms
1. Hypocalcemia
   Symptoms associated with hypocalcemia include vomiting, muscle weakness, irritability, tetany, ECG changes (prolonged QT interval), and seizures. Long-term consequences include ricketic changes.
2. Hypokalemia
   Symptoms associated with hypokalemia include fatigue, neuromuscular disturbances (weakness, hyporeflexia, paresthesia, cramps, restless legs, rhabdomyolysis, paralysis), gastrointestinal disorders (constipation and ileus), cardiovascular abnormalities (orthostatic hypotension, worsening of hypertension, and arrhythmias), ECG changes (T wave flattening, prominent U waves, and ST segment depression), and renal abnormalities (metabolic alkalosis, polyuria, polydipsia, and glucose intolerance).
3. Hypomagnesemia
   Symptoms related to hypomagnesemia include lethargy, confusion, tremor, fasciculations, ataxia, nystagmus, tetany, seizures, and ECG changes (prolonged PR and QT intervals, and arrhythmias). Hypomagnesemia can cause hypokalemia or hypocalcemia.
4. Hyponatremia
   Symptoms may occur if hyponatremia develops rapidly. These signs/symptoms can include lethargy, muscle cramps, anorexia, nausea and vomiting, agitation, disorientation, hypothermia, and seizures. The manifestations of hyponatremia depend on whether the hyponatremia results from water overload or sodium deficiency.
5. Hypophosphatemia
   a. Etiology of hypophosphatemia can be related to:
      i. Inadequate input (i.e., starvation, continuous vomiting, or impaired absorption)
      ii. Excessive losses (tubular reabsorptive defect, acidosis, massive diuresis, glycosuria, ketonuria, and catabolic states).

    iii. Acute volume expansion (syndrome of inappropriate antidiuretic hormone).

    iv. Redistribution (respiratory alkalosis, metabolic alkalosis, carbohydrate load, corticosteroids, and insulin). Hypophosphatemia can be exaggerated by hypomagnesemia.

  b. Symptoms associated with hypophosphatemia result from decreased availability of phosphate for synthesis of adenosine triphosphate and 2,3-diphosphoglycerol. Superimposition of an acute shortage of inorganic phosphate on cells with disturbed energy metabolism may result in clinical symptoms. Hypophosphatemia can lead to osteomalacia, paresthesia, paralysis, irritability, malaise, seizures, coma, myalgias, bone pain, increased oxygen binding by hemoglobin, dysfunctional granulocytes, increased platelet aggregation, hypercalcuria, anorexia, cardiac arrhythmias, metabolic acidosis, and poor diaphragmatic function.

  6. Metabolic acidosis (secondary to urinary bicarbonate losses)

Symptoms/signs of metabolic acidosis include tachypnea, hyperventilation, abdominal pain, vomiting, fever, and lethargy.

C. Grading of renal, genitourinary, and other toxicities

Grading toxicities caused by therapeutic interventions allows an assessment of an individual patient's response and comparison of complications of one treatment program with another (Table 7.1).

III. MONITORING STUDIES TO BE PERFORMED

  A. Baseline historical information necessary for monitoring for possible renal complications for all patients receiving cancer treatment

    1. Current nephrotoxic medications and medications that alter renal perfusion include diuretics, acetylcholinesterase inhibitors, nonsteroidal anti-inflammatory drugs, β-blockers, steroids, and contrast media.

    2. Hydration status during nephrotoxic cancer treatments

    3. Nutritional status, including serum albumin

    4. Urinary tract infections; coincident episodes of sepsis while receiving nephrotoxic treatments

Table 7.1.
Criteria for Toxicity and Complications

Site	Measure	0/WNL	1 (Mild)	2 (Moderate)	3 (Severe)	4 (Unacceptable)
					Grade	
Blood	WBC/uL	≥4.0	3.0–3.9	2.0–2.9	1.0–1.9	<1.0
	ANC/uL	≥2.0	1.5–1.9	1.0–1.4	0.5–0.9	<0.5
	PLT/uL	WNL	75.0–normal	50.0–74.9	25.0–49.9	<25.0
	Hgb, g/dl	WNL	10.0–normal	8.0–10.0	6.5–7.9	<6.5
	Lymphocytes/uL	≥2.0	1.5–1.9	1.0–1.4	0.5–0.9	<0.5
Marrow	cellularity	Normal	Mildly hypoplastic 25%↓	Moderate hypoplastic 50%↓	Marked hypoplastic 75%↓ >3 weeks to recovery	Aplastic 3 weeks to recovery
Liver	SGOT	WNL	≤2.5 × N	2.6–5.0 × N	5.1–20.0 × N	>20.0 × N
	SGPT	WNL	≤2.5 × N	2.6–5.0 × N	5.1–20.0 × N	>20.0 × N
	Alkaline phosphatase	WNL	≤2.5 × N	2.6–5.0 × N	5.1–20.0 × N	>20.0 × N
	Total bilirubin	WNL		<1.5 × N	1.5–3.0 × N	>3.0 × N
	Liver-clin.	WNL			Precoma	Hepatic coma
Pancreas	Amylase/creatinine clearance	WNL	<1.5 × N	1.5–2.0 × N	2.1–5.0 × N	>5.0 × N
	Amylase	WNL	<1.5 × N	1.5–2.0 × N	2.1–5.0 × N	>5.0 × N
	Glucose, mg/dL	WNL	55–64/116–160	40–54/161–250	30–39/251–500	<30/>500/ketoacid
	Ultrasound size	Normal	Normal	Increased	Increased	Pseudocyst
	and sonolucency	Normal	Increased	Increase localized	Increase generalized	Hemorrhagic
Renal and genitourinary	BUN	<20	20–39	40–59	60–79	≥80
	Creatinine	WNL	<1.5 × N	1.5–3.0 × N	3.1–6.0 × N	>6.0 × N
	Creatinine clearance	WNL	75%	50–74%	25–49%	<25%

Category	Parameter	0	1	2	3	4
	Blood pressure					
	Systolic	Baseline	±10%	±20%	±30%	±40%
	Diastolic	Baseline	±5%	±10%	±15%	±20%
	Proteinuria	Negative	1+/or <3 g/l	2-3+/or 3-10 g/L	4+/or >10 g/L	Nephrotic syndrome
	Hematuria	Negative	Micro only	Gross, no clots	Gross and clots	Transfusion required
	Bladder—frequency and dysuria	None	Slight	Moderate, responds to treatment	Severe, no response to treatment	Incapacitating, with severe hemorrhage
Gastrointestinal	Stomatitis	None	Erythema or Mild soreness	Painful/edema can eat	Cannot eat or drink	Requires parenteral or enteral support
	Abdominal pain					
	Severity	None	Mild	Moderate	Moderate-severe	Severe
	Treatment	None	Not required	Required—helps	Required—no help	Hospitalization, heavy sedation
	Constipation	No change	Mild ileus	Moderate ileus	Severe ileus	Ileus >96 hours
	Diarrhea	None	↑2-3 stools/day	↑4-6 stools/day or moderate cramps	↑7-9 stools/day or Severe cramps	↑≥10 stools/day, bloody, parenteral support required
	Nausea	None	Reasonable intake	Decreased intake	No significant intake	
	Vomiting	None	1x/day	2-5x/day	6-10x/day	>10x/day or IV required
Pulmonary	Vital capacity	WNL	10-20%↓	21-35%↓	36-50%↓	>51%
	pAO_2	>90	80-89	65-79	50-64	<49
	Functional	Normal	Tachypnea	Dyspnea	O_2 required	Assist ventilation
	DLCO	100-75%	74-65%	64-55%	54-40%	<40%
	Clinical	No change	Abnormal PFTs/ asymptomatic	Dyspnea on significant exertion	Dyspnea at normal activity	Dyspnea at rest
Cardiac	Cardiac rhythm	WNL	Asymptomatic/ transient No treatment required	Recurrent/ persistent	Requires treatment	Hypotension/ V tach/ fibrillation

Table 7.1.
Criteria for Toxicity and Complications (Continued)

Site	Measure	0/WNL	1 (Mild)	2 (Moderate)	3 (Severe)	4 (Unacceptable)
					Grade	
	Echo					
	%FS	>30	24–30	20–24	<20	
	%STI	<0.35		<0.40	>0.40	
	Ischemia	None	Nonspecific T-wave flattening	Asymptomatic/ECG change suggests ischemia	Angina/without evidence of infarction	Acute myocardial infarction
	Pericardial effusion	None	Asymptomatic effusion; no treatment required	Pericarditis	Drainage required	Tamponade; drainage urgently required
	Cardiac function	WNL	Asymptomatic	Asymptomatic	Mild CHF/responds to treatment	Severe or refractory CHF
	Hypertension	No change	Asymptomatic/transient ↑20%, no treatment required	Recurrent/persistent ↑20%, no treatment required	Requires treatment	Hypertensive crisis
	Hypotension	No change	No treatment required	Treatment but no hospitalization	Treatment and hospitalization <48 hours after stop agent	Treatment and hospitalization >48 hours after stop agent
Nervous system	Peripheral Sensory	No change	Mild paresthesias, loss of tendon reflex	Moderate sensory loss, moderate paresthesias	Interferes with function	
	Motor	No change	Subjective weakness/no objective findings	Mild objective weakness/no significant impairment	Objective weakness/impaired function	Paralysis weakness/impaired

	No change				
Central					
Cerebellar	No change	Slight incoordination/dysdiadokinesis	Intention tremor/dysmetria/slurred speech/nystagmus	Locomotor ataxia	Cerebellar necrosis
CNS					
General	No change	Drowsy/nervous	Confused	Seizures/psychosis	Comatose
Headache	No change	Mild	Transient/moderate/severe	Severe, unrelenting	
Cortical	No change	Mild somnolence/agitation	Moderate somnolence/agitation	Severe somnolence/agitation confusion/hallucination	Coma/seizures/toxic psychosis
Skin					
Skin	No change or WNL	Scattered eruption or erythema, asymptomatic	Urticaria/scattered eruption, symptomatic	Generalized eruption, treatment required	Exfoliation/ulcerative dermatitis
Alopecia	No loss	Mild hair loss	Marked/total hair loss		
Allergy	None	Transient rash	Mild bronchospasm	Moderate bronchospasm, serum sickness	Hypotension, anaphylaxis
Coagulation					
Fibrinogen	WNL	$0.99-0.75 \times N$	$0.74-0.50 \times N$	$0.49-0.25 \times N$	$\leq 0.24 \times N$
PT	WNL	$1.01-1.25 \times N$	$1.26-1.50 \times N$	$1.51-2.00 \times N$	$>2.00 \times N$
PTT	WNL	$1.01-1.66 \times N$	$1.67-2.33 \times N$	$2.34-3.00 \times N$	$>3.00 \times N$
Hemorrhage (clinical)	None	Mild/no transfusion	Gross/1–2 transfusions/episode	Gross/3–4 transfusions/episode	Massive/>4 transfusions/episode
Hearing					
Objective	No change	20–40 dB loss >4 kHz	>40 dB loss >4 kHz	>40 dB loss 2 kHz	>40 dB loss <2 kHz
Subjective	No change	Loss on audiometry only	Tinnitus, soft speech	Loss correctable with hearing aid	Deafness not correctable

Table 7.1.
Criteria for Toxicity and Complications (Continued)

Site	Measure	0/WNL	1 (Mild)	2 (Moderate)	3 (Severe)	4 (Unacceptable)
					Grade	
Electrolytes	Na, mEq/L	WNL	↓130–134/↑146–149	125–129/150–155	116–124/156–164	<115/>165
	K, mEq/L	WNL	↓3.1–3.4/↑5.5–5.9	2.6–3.0/6.0–6.4	2.1–2.5/6.5–6.9	<2.0/>7.0
	Ca, mg/dL	WNL	8.4–7.8/10.6–11.5	7.7–7.0/11.6–12.5	6.9–6.1/12.6–13.5	≤6.1/≥13.5
	Mg, mEq/L	WNL	1.4–1.2	1.1–0.9	0.8–0.6	≤0.5
Infection		None	Mild	Moderate	Severe	Life threatening
Fever		<38° C	38°–40° C	>40° C <24 hours	>40° C >24 hours	
Local		None	Pain	Pain/swelling with inflammation/phlebitis	Ulceration	Plastic surgery indicated
Mood		No change	Mild anxiety or depression	Moderate anxiety or depression	Severe anxiety or depression	Suicidal ideation
Vision		No change			Subtotal vision loss	Blindness
Weight change		<5.0%	5.0–9.9%	10–19.9%	≥20%	
Performance (Karnofsky %)		Normal (90–100)	Mild restriction (70–<90)	Ambulatory up to 50% (50–<70)	Bed or wheelchair (30–<50)	No self-care (<30)

Source: Modified from the Children's Cancer Group from the National Cancer Institute Common Toxicity Criteria.

Abbreviations: ANC, absolute neutrophil count; BUN, blood urea nitrogen; CHF, congestive heart failure; CNS, central nervous system; DLCO, diffusion capacity of carbon monoxide; ECG, electrocardiogram; FS, fractional shortening; HgB, hemoglobin; pAO$_2$, partial pressure of arterial oxygen; PFTs, pulmonary function tests; PLT, platelets; PT, prothrombin time; PTT, partial thromboplastin time; SGOT, aspartate aminotransferase (AST); SGPT, alanine aminotransferase (ALT); STI, systolic time interval; V tach, ventricular tachycardia; WBC, white blood cell count.

5. Radiation received to kidney or bladder; presence of a single kidney
6. Presence of hydronephrosis or obstructive uropathy
7. Tumor lysis syndrome and degree of hyperuricemia during remission induction treatment.

B. Laboratory data to consider before each course of chemotherapy (see Sections IA and IAB)

IV. SUPPORTIVE CARE MEASURES TO AVOID/AMELIORATE TOXICITY

A. Children with a single kidney or hydronephrosis
1. Are ineligible to receive ifosfamide in rhabdomyosarcoma protocols. The use of ifosfamide is discouraged for all patients with a single kidney.
2. Have greater nephrotoxicity with cisplatin than those without hydronephrosis, in spite of adjustment of doses for decreased GFR..

B. Primary prevention of nephrotoxicity including adequate to increased hydration, maintenance of normal intravascular fluid status, and avoidance of intravascular volume depletion
1. Adequate intravascular hydration and diuresis can be enhanced by the use of 0.45% or 0.9% saline, mannitol, and diuretics.
2. Use mannitol and diuretics to increase diuresis only after determining adequate intravascular hydration.

C. Where possible, avoid:
1. Nephrotoxic antimicrobials and other renal-toxic medications.
2. The use of intravenous contrast dye for computed tomographic scanning during and after infusion of nephrotoxic chemotherapy.

D. Prevention of bladder toxicity
1. Provide hyperhydration to ensure increased urine output to dilute and decrease the bladder mucosal contact time of toxic oxazaphosphorine metabolites.
2. Strongly encourage ample oral intake for the 12–24 hours preceding cyclophosphamide or ifosfamide infusion.
3. Maintain a urine output of > 65 mL/m^2/h for at least 18 hours after cyclophosphamide or ifosfamide therapy.

4. Encourage the patient to void at least every 2 hours for the 24 hours after oxazaphosphorine treatment.

E. Specific measures to prevent renal toxicity from renal-toxic drugs
   1. Hydration
      a. Before infusion of high-dose methotrexate, moderate- to high-dose cyclophosphamide, cisplatin, or ifosfamide, give hydration at 125 mL/m^2/h (2× maintenance) for a minimum of 2 hours to increase urine output to >100 mL/m^2/h (> 3 mL/kg/h).
      b. Before the chemotherapy infusion, urine specific gravity should be ≤1.010.
      c. The hydration fluid most frequently used is 5% dextrose /0.45% NaCl + 10 mEq/L KCL.
      d. During infusion of these agents, in general, maintain hydration at >125 mL/m^2/h and urine output at >90 mL/m^2/h.
      e. After the infusion of nephrotoxic chemotherapy (including high-dose melphalan), maintain urine output at 65–100 mL/m^2/h (depending on agent and protocol) with oral/intravenous fluids to equal 90–125 mL/m^2/h.
      f. Where needed to maintain isovolemic fluid balance (avoidance of over- and underhydration), diuresis can be forced (in the presence of adequate hydration) through the use of mannitol 6 g/m^2 (200 mg/kg) in at least 25 mL of fluid over 15–60 minutes and/or furosemide 0.5–1 mg/kg push intravenous (IV).
   2. Alkalinization
      Before infusion of high-dose methotrexate, urine alkalinization of >pH 6.5 can be achieved with 40–60 mEq NaHCO$_3$/L added to the intravenous hydration fluid.
   3. Uroprotectant
      a. Mesna has been used as a uroprotectant with high-dose cyclophosphamide and ifosfamide (oxazaphosphorines). Mesna, which has a half-life of 90 minutes, binds the toxic oxazaphosphorine metabolite acrolein within the urinary collecting system to detoxify it. In adult patients, Mesna may not be more effective in preventing bladder toxicity than vigorous hydration.

    b. The dosage guidelines for Mesna vary. The majority of Children's Cancer Group protocols recommend a total Mesna dose equivalent to the total ifosfamide dose (i.e., 1 mg of Mesna /1 mg of ifosfamide) and a total Mesna dose of about 80% of the total cyclophosphamide dose.

    c. Studies have shown that lower doses of Mesna may be uroprotective.

4. Hypertonic saline

    a. The effectiveness of prevention of cisplatin nephrotoxicity by infusion in 3% saline is controversial.

    b. Prevention or diminution of nephrotoxicity associated with cisplatin is possible with hydration with normal saline, continuous infusion of cisplatin, and prophylactic supplementation with magnesium.

5. Magnesium

    a. During infusion of cisplatin, add mannitol in a dose of 15 g/m^2 (10–24 $g/m^2/L$) and $MgSO_4$ in a dose of 20 mEq/L to the hydrating solution to prevent hypomagnesemia.

    b. Continue postchemotherapy hydration with 5% dextrose/0.45% NaCl + 20 mEq/L KCl + 20 mEq/L $MgSO_4$ + mannitol 20 g/L.

    c. When chemotherapy includes cisplatin, routine magnesium supplementation with a minimum of 6 $mEq/m^2/day$ by mouth (PO) or IV is recommended.

6. Continuous versus intermittent infusion

For cisplatin or ifosfamide, there are insufficient data to determine if continuous versus intermittent infusion or dosing by pharmacokinetic measurement of area under the curve can decrease their nephrotoxicity.

7. Adjust the administered dose of chemotherapeutic agents according to the GFR (Table 7.2).

8. Limited total dose of agent

More than eight courses of ifosfamide (approximately 72 g/m^2) are not recommended, as the incidence of serious nephrotoxic complications increases markedly when this dose is exceeded.

F. Hematuria

1. Microscopic hematuria

    a. Transient microscopic hematuria (no more than 2 abnormal urinalyses on 2 separate days during a course

Table 7.2.
Suggested Percentage Dose of Chemotherapeutic Agents Adjusted for GlomeruLar Filtration Rate

>60 mL/min:	30–60 mL/min (50–75% baseline)*			10–30 mL/min (25–49% baseline)		<10 mL/min (<25% baseline)	
100% dose	75%	50%	Omit	75%	Omit	50%	Omit
Adriamycin†	Bleomycin‡	Cisplatin	Nitrosureas	Carboplatin§	Cisplatin	Cyclophosphamide	Cisplatin
Bleomycin		Methotrexate	Bleomycin*	Ifosfamide§	Methotrexate		Methotrexate
Cisplatin			Cisplatin	Nitrosureas	Nitrosureas		
Cyclophosphamide							
Cytarabine†							
5-fluorouracil†							
Ifosfamide							
Melphalan†							
Methotrexate							
Nitrosureas							
Vinblastine†							
Vincristine							

Source: Modified from Patterson (1992).

* Percentage of baseline may not be suitable if high urine output renal dysfunction present.

† No dose modification for decreased glomerular filtration rate.

‡ Recommendations vary per protocol.

§ Reduce by 50%.

of therapy); no modification of the oxazaphosphorine or Mesna
b. Persistent microscopic hematuria (>2 abnormal urinalyses during a course of therapy)
  i.   Do not modify the oxazaphosphorine dose.
  ii. Change the Mesna to a continuous infusion: 360 mg/m^2 during oxazaphosphorine, followed by 120 mg/m^2/h for 24 hours.
2. Gross hematuria
   Evaluate all episodes of gross hematuria by cystoscopy. Also consider further testing, such as urine culture, excretory urogram, and voiding cystogram, and perform as indicated.
   a. Transient gross hematuria during or after a course of therapy (only one episode, which clears to less than gross hematuria)
     i.   Do not modify the oxazaphosphorine dose.
     ii. Change the Mesna to a continuous infusion: 360 mg/m^2 during oxazaphosphorine, followed by 120 mg/m^2/h for 24 hours.
   b. Persistent gross hematuria after completion of a course of therapy
     i.   Hold subsequent oxazaphosphorine until the urine shows less than gross hematuria.
     ii. Reinstitute oxazaphosphorine at full dose, with the Mesna changed to a continuous infusion: 360 mg/m^2 during oxazaphosphorine, followed by 120 mg/m^2/h for 24 hours after each dose of oxazaphosphorine.
     iii. If gross hematuria does not resolve to microscopic hematuria or less, withhold further oxazaphosphorine therapy.
   c. Persistent gross hematuria occurring during a course of oxazaphosphorine
     i.   Interrupt the oxazaphosphorine.
     ii. Withhold further oxazaphosphorine until the next course of therapy.
     iii. If the gross hematuria resolves to microscopic hematuria or less, subsequent courses of oxazaphosphorine may be administered at full dose, with Mesna changed to a continuous infusion: 360 mg/m^2 during oxazaphosphorine, followed by 120 mg/m^2/h for 24 hours.

    d. Occurrence of a second episode of gross hematuria or persistence of microscopic hematuria on the continuous infusion regimen

      i. Continue the oxazaphosphorine when the urine shows less than gross hematuria.

      ii. Double the loading dose of Mesna to 720 mg/m^2 and the subsequent hourly dose to 240 mg/m^2/h.

      iii. Continue to give Mesna by continuous infusion for 48 hours after the last dose of oxazaphosphorine.

    e. Persistent gross hematuria in the face of the "double dose, continuous infusion" regimen

    Discontinue oxazaphosphorine.

G. Renal tubular dysfunction

If significant renal Fanconi syndrome (serum phosphate <3.5 mg/dL, potassium <3 mEq/L; 1+ glycosuria with serum glucose <150 mg/dL, bicarbonate <17 mEq/L, and ratio of urine protein/urine creatinine <0.2) develops while receiving ifosfamide, consider substituting cyclophosphamide.

IV. LONG TERM FOLLOW-UP/LATE EFFECTS

A. Cyclophosphamide and ifosfamide

Cyclophosphamide and ifosfamide can lead to vesicoureteral reflux, hydronephrosis, or contracted bladder, which may not become symptomatic for months to years after treatment. These complications are usually preceded by acute episodes of hemorrhagic cystitis and are increased in patients who have received pelvic radiation.

B. Ifosfamide and cisplatin

Both ifosfamide and cisplatin have caused persistent renal Fanconi syndrome, occasionally resulting in hypophosphatemic rickets, growth failure, and/or renal tubular acidosis.

1. The onset of renal tubular dysfunction can occur years after the completion of chemotherapy.

2. Ifosfamide has been associated with persistent nephrogenic diabetes insipidus.

Prevention and Treatment of Chemotherapy-Induced Liver Toxicity

The liver has a central role in the metabolism and detoxification of many chemotherapeutic agents and is therefore a target for drug toxicity. It is important to distinguish drug causes from viral hepatitis or tumor-related effects of hepatic abnormality. Furthermore, agents that depend on the liver for metabolism may have their organ-specific effects heightened in the face of abnormal liver metabolism. Thus, to reduce toxicity it becomes necessary to modify therapy with chemotherapeutic agents with liver-dependent metabolism. (See Table 7.1 to grade liver toxicity.)

I. MODIFICATION OF CHEMOTHERAPEUTIC AGENTS THAT PRODUCE LIVER TOXICITY

A. L-Asparaginase
   1. L-Asparaginase can result in fatty metamorphosis.
   2. Liver enzyme abnormalities may be reversible while continuing therapy.
   3. Stop therapy for grade 3 or greater liver toxicity; resume at grade 2.

B. 6-Mercaptopurine and 6-Thioguanine
   6-Mercaptopurine (6-MP) or 6-thioguanine (6-TG) can result in cholestasis.
   1. Stop if toxicity is grade 3 or greater.
   2. Rule out viral hepatitis, Gilbert disease, or tumor effect.
   3. If drugs are the cause of liver toxicity, restart at 50% dose when the toxicity decreases to grade 2.
   4. If grade 3 or greater toxicity persists, it may be necessary to perform a liver biopsy to determine the histologic extent of the disease and whether 6-MP/6-TG can be restarted.

C. Methotrexate
   Methotrexate can result in fibrosis and cirrhosis.
   1. There does not appear to be a need to modify the dosage in patients with preexisting liver damage, other than to consider whether the patient can tolerate the potential additional hepatic dysfunction induced by methotrexate.

   2. Stop if toxicity is grade 3 or greater.
   3. Rule out viral hepatitis, Gilbert disease, or drug effect.
   4. If the drug is the cause of liver toxicity, restart at 50% dose when toxicity decreases to grade 2.
   5. If grade 3 or greater toxicity persists, it may be necessary to perform a liver biopsy to determine the histologic extent of the disease and whether methotrexate can be restarted.

D. Carmustine and lomustine
BCNU and CCNU can result in increased liver enzymes.
   1. Stop if toxicity is grade 3 or greater.
   2. Rule out viral hepatitis or tumor effect.
   3. If drugs are the cause, restart at 50% dose when the toxicity decreases to grade 1.
   4. If grade 3 or greater toxicity persists, it may be necessary to perform a liver biopsy to determine the histologic extent of the disease and whether BCNU/CCNU can be restarted.

II. SPECIFIC MODIFICATIONS OF CHEMOTHERAPEUTIC AGENTS WITH LIVER-DEPENDENT METABOLISM

A. Vincristine, vinblastine, and VP-16 (etoposide)
   1. Bilirubin <1.5 mg/dL and aspartate aminotransferase (SGOT) <60 U/mL: give 100% dose.
   2. Bilirubin 1.5–3.0 mg/dL or SGOT 60–180 U/mL: give 50% dose.
   3. Bilirubin >3.1 mg/dL or SGOT >180 U/mL: hold dose.

B. Adriamycin, daunorubicin, idarubicin, and actinomycin-D
   1. Bilirubin <1.5 mg/dL and SGOT <60 U/mL: give 100% dose.
   2. Bilirubin 1.5–3.0 mg/dL or SGOT 60–180 U/mL: give 50% dose.
   3. Bilirubin 3.1–5.0 mg/dL or SGOT >180 U/mL: give 25% dose.
   4. Bilirubin >5.0 mg/dL: hold dose.

C. Methotrexate and cyclophosphamide
   1. Bilirubin <1.5 mg/dL and SGOT <60 U/mL: give 100% dose.
   2. Bilirubin 1.5–3.0 mg/dL or SGOT 60–180 U/mL: give 50% dose.
   3. Bilirubin 3.1–5.0 mg/dL or SGOT <180 U/mL: give 25% dose.

4. Bilirubin >5.0 mg/dL: hold dose.
5. Restart at 50% dose when bilirubin <1.5 mg/dL and SGOT <60 U/mL.

   D. Actinomycin-D
   1. Restart at 50% dose when the toxicity decreases to grade 0.
   2. Increase the dose by 25% increments if tolerated.

   E. Hold all the following drugs when bilirubin >5.0 mg/dL or SGOT >180 U/mL:
   1. CCNU
   2. BCNU
   3. 5-Fluorouracil
   4. Cytosine arabinoside
   5. Dacarbazine (DTIC)
   6. Procarbazine

Diagnosis and Treatment of Chemotherapy-Induced Pulmonary Toxicity

Pulmonary toxicity is a significant complication of bleomycin. Less frequently, methotrexate, busulfan, and CCNU have been incriminated in acute lung syndrome, which is believed to be idiosyncratic and not predictable. Radiation therapy to the lung parenchyma reduces pulmonary toxicity thresholds.

Pulmonary toxicity from radiation and chemotherapeutic agents may be partially reversible. Ultimately, enough damage to the parenchymal lung tissue could result in death. (See Table 7.1 to grade pulmonary toxicity.)

I. TOXICITY OF BLEOMYCIN

A. Diagnosis of bleomycin toxicity
1. Slow inspiratory vital capacity and pulmonary capillary blood volume appear to be the proper lung function assessments that specifically reflect alterations induced by bleomycin.
2. Diffusion capacity of carbon monoxide (DLCO) is not a suitable parameter to monitor pulmonary toxicity induced by bleomycin specifically when it is part of a multidrug regimen.

a. Investigators have found a poor correlation between DLCO and lung toxicity, and DLCO fails to predict the development of serious bleomycin lung toxicity in the majority of patients. When a low DLCO is encountered, look at other parameters as well (see b. below). The clinician should decide to continue bleomycin when it is in the best interest of patient care.

   i. Bleomycin may be stopped inappropriately after low DLCO measurement. DLCO <65% has a high false positive incidence when used as the standard for withholding chemotherapy.

   ii. When a low DLCO is encountered, examine and consider other parameters of lung function before discontinuing bleomycin.

b. It is important to monitor for respiratory system and chest x-ray abnormalities during bleomycin treatment, as these will be the earliest signs of lung toxicity in most patients.

   i. The combination of respiratory symptoms and an abnormal chest x-ray is the earliest manifestation in many patients.

   ii. Therefore, a careful history of respiratory symptoms and regular chest x-rays is more likely to detect clinically significant bleomycin lung toxicity than the DLCO.

   iii. Diffuse infiltration with tumor, interstitial pneumonias, generalized pulmonary infections such as pneumocystis pneumonia, and bleomycin nodularity may have similar signs and symptoms.

   iv. An aggressive approach is justifiable because the consequence of stopping bleomycin in a patient with a curable cancer may be as devastating as continuing bleomycin in one at risk of bleomycin lung damage.

B. Factors contributing to bleomycin toxicity
   1. Dose-related toxicity of bleomycin is shown in Table 7.3.
   2. The serum half-life of bleomycin can be increased in the presence of renal dysfunction such as that induced by cisplatin. Monitor renal function closely when patients are receiving both bleomycin and nephrotoxic chemotherapeutic agents.

Table 7.3.
Dose-related Pulmonary Toxicity of Bleomycin

Bleomycin Total Dose (U)	% Individuals Demonstrating Clinical Toxicity
0–49	2.7
5–149	3.9
150–249	4.4
250–349	4.9
350–449	5.5
450–549	12.5
> 550	17.2

3. The administration of oxygen in high concentrations, (e.g., during general anesthesia) may cause fulminate respiratory failure in patients previously treated with bleomycin.

C. Modifications for pulmonary toxicity
Bleomycin lung toxicity remains an unpredictable side effect by comparison with the toxicities of many other anticancer drugs. Therefore, it would be advisable to avoid bleomycin in situations in which other drugs can be substituted without compromising results.

D. Late effects
Bleomycin pulmonary toxicity may be reversible. A decreased force vital capacity and DLCO in the first 15 months after treatment, in terms of long-term follow-up, did not predict outcome.

Recognition and Management of Chemotherapy-Induced Neurotoxicity

I. BACKGROUND

A. Signs and symptoms may be difficult to recognize because they are woven into a background of underlying disease, metabolic abnormalities, psychologic responses, and the effects of other medications.

B. Neurologic toxicity may occur with the first course of treatment or with subsequent courses.

C. Neurotoxicity generally occurs with high-dose therapy and when the cumulative dose is high.

D. Neurotoxicity may be seen months or years after the completion of chemotherapy.

II. TOXICITY

Table 7.1 serves as a guide to determining the grade of toxicity. It provides a way to assess an individual patient's response to therapy. In addition, it provides the investigator with standard criteria to compare the toxicity and complications of one treatment program with another.

III. MONITORING FOR NEUROTOXICITY

A. History
1. Question the patient and family about numbness, tingling, vertigo, or visual disturbances.
2. Question the patient's family about changes in personality, affect, or lethargy.
3. Inquire about school and job performance and social and psychological well-being during long-term follow-up visits.

B. Physical examination
Physical examination with serial neurologic examinations is the most useful tool for detecting toxicity.
1. Decreases in deep tendon reflexes, especially in the Achilles tendon, are among the earliest signs of chemotherapy-induced peripheral neuropathy.
2. Loss of proprioception and vibratory sensation also indicate peripheral neuropathy.
3. Changes in gait may indicate neurotoxicity. Observe toe walk, heel walk, and tandem walk. Changes in the ability to perform these tasks may indicate peripheral neuropathy or acute cerebellar syndrome.

C. Audiometry
Obtain audiometric evaluation before beginning cisplatin and before every other course of therapy.

D. Monitor cumulative dose calculation for cisplatin and vincristine.

IV. MODIFICATION OF THERAPY

A. Treatment Modifications

The following treatment modifications are only suggestions. Modification of treatment should be based on the child's diagnosis, stage of therapy, available alternatives, and the judgment of the clinician.

B. Vincristine
1. Doses $\geq$10–15 mg/m^2 may lead to neuropathy.
2. Grades 1 and 2 toxicity require no modification.
3. For grades 3 and 4 toxicity, hold the drug until symptoms subside or stabilize. Subsequent doses should be either decreased or omitted.
4. Trigeminal nerve toxicity results in jaw pain.
   a. Treat with acetaminophen.
   b. This symptom does not usually recur.
   c. Do not modify the dose.
5. Anticipate autonomic neuropathy resulting in constipation.
   a. Treat with laxatives such as lactulose, Pericolace, or Senokot S.
   b. Prevent with Senokot S or increase dietary fiber.
6. Treat symptoms of syndrome of inappropriate antidiuretic hormone. It is usually not necessary to not modify the vincristine dose unless serum sodium <130 mEq/L.

C. Cisplatin
1. Do not modify treatment for grade 1 or 2 toxicity.
2. For grade 3 or 4 toxicity, hold the drug until the symptoms subside or stabilize. Either decrease or omit subsequent doses.
3. High-frequency hearing loss occurs at cumulative doses of 270–450 mg/m^2.
4. Peripheral neuropathy occurs at cumulative doses of 300–600 mg/m^2.
5. May cause Lhermitte sign (sensation of tingling or electric shock in arms and legs when neck is flexed). Do not modify therapy.

D. Methotrexate
1. No modifications are needed for grade 1 or 2 toxicity.
2. For grade 3 or 4 toxicity, hold the drug until symptoms resolve or stabilize. Reduce or omit further doses.
3. Patients receiving high-dose methotrexate may develop acute encephalopathy with the following symptoms.
   a. Seizures
   b. Confusion
   c. Hemiparesis
   d. Dysarthria
4. High-dose methotrexate may be associated with the development of leukoencephalopathy.
   a. Symptoms include:
      i. Personality changes
      ii. Progressive dementia
      iii. Focal seizures
      iv. Changes in level of consciousness
   b. Follow the patient with serial magnetic resonance imaging scans.
   c. Omit further methotrexate treatment.
5. Acute encephalopathy sometimes occurs after intrathecal therapy.
   a. Symptoms include:
      i. Fever
      ii. Nausea and vomiting
      iii. Headache
      iv. Lethargy
      v. Paresis
   b. The decision to stop or continue intrathecal therapy must be made on an individual basis.

E. Ifosfamide
1. Symptoms of toxicity include:
   a. Hallucinations
   b. Confusion
   c. Cranial nerve dysfunction
   d. Cerebellar syndrome
   e. Seizures
2. Neurotoxicity is more common when serum albumin is low or infusions are rapid.
3. No modifications are needed for grade 1 or 2 toxicity.
4. Reduce or omit further doses for grade 3 or 4 toxicity.

F. L-Asparaginase
L-Asparaginase may cause a mild transient encephalopathy.
Also consider intracranial bleeding or clot.

G. 5-Fluorouracil
1. 5-Fluorouracil may produce the cerebellar syndrome.
2. Reduce or omit further doses.

Bibliography

Barbour GL, Crumb CK, Boyd CM, Reeves RD, Rastogi SP, Patterson RM: Comparison of inulin, iothalamate, and 99mTc-DTPA for measurement of glomerular filtration rate. *J Nucl Med* 17:317–19, 1976.

Barnett MJ, Richards MA, Ganesan TS, et al.: Central nervous system toxicity of high-dose cytosine arabinoside. *Semin Oncol* 12:227–32, 1985.

Berns JS, Haghighat A, Staddon A, et al.: Severe, irreversible renal failure after ifosfamide treatment: A clinicopathologic report of two patients. *Cancer* 76:497–500, 1995.

Branch RA: Prevention of amphotericin B-induced renal impairment. *Arch Intern Med* 148:2389–94, 1988.

Cantwell BMJ, Idle M, Milward MJ, Hall G, Lind MJ: Encephalopathy with hyponatremia and inappropriate arginine vasopressin secretion following an intravenous ifosfamide infusion. *Ann Oncol* 1:232, 1990.

Cersosimo RJ: Cisplatin neurotoxicity. *Cancer Treat Rev* 1989; 16:195–211, 1989.

Duarte CG, Preuss HG: Assessment of renal function—glomerular and tubular. *Clin Lab Med* 13:33–52, 1993.

Hurley RM: Assessment of renal function in the young. *Clin Lab Med* 13:257–67, 1993.

Packer RJ, Grossman RI, Belasco JB: High-dose systemic methotrexate-associated acute neurologic dysfunction. *Med Pediatr Oncol* 11:159–61, 1983.

Perry M, ed.: *The Chemotherapy Source Book.* 2nd ed. Baltimore, Williams & Wilkins 1996. pp. 1–1518.

Schwartz GJ, Brion LP, Spitzer A: The use of plasma creatinine concentration for estimating glomerular filtration rates in infants, children, and adolescents. *Pediatr Clin North Am* 34:571–87, 1987.

Steinherz LJ, Graham T, Hurtwitz R, et al.: Guidelines for cardiac monitoring of children during and after anthracycline therapy: Report of the Cardiology Committee of the Children's Cancer Study Group. *Pediatrics* 89:942–49, 1992.

Tuxen MK, Hansen SW: Complications of treatment; neurotoxicity secondary to antineoplastic drugs. *Cancer Treat Rev* 20:191–214, 1994.

8

The Management of Drug Extravasation

John S. Murphy, B.Pharm., and
Michael L. N. Willoughby, M.D.

I. DEFINITIONS

   A. Extravasation
       The unintentional instillation or leakage of a vesicant or irritant agent into the perivascular and subcutaneous spaces during parenteral administration that may result when an intravenous cannula slips from a vein into adjacent tissue, or when fluid leaks from a vein via a puncture or around a cannula site

   B. Vesicant
       An agent that, when extravasated, can produce ulceration and (often severe) local necrosis

   C. Irritant
       An agent that, when extravasated, produces burning or inconsequential inflammation without necrosis

II. CLASSIFICATION

   Agents may be classified according to the local reaction they produce when extravasation occurs (Table 8.1)

III. PREVENTION

   Establish standard operating procedures designed to prevent drug extravasation from occurring in the first place at each location

TABLE 8.1.
A Classification According to Local Reaction of Extravasated Drugs

Nonirritant
  L-Asparaginase (*Escherichia coli, Erwinia,* polyethylene glycol-asparaginase)
  Bleomycin
  Cytosine arabinoside
  Methotrexate
Irritant
  Carmustine
  Dacarbazine
  Epipodophylotoxins [e.g., etoposide (VP-16), teniposide (VM-26)]
  Melphalan (L-phenylalanine mustard)
  Oxazaphosphorines (e.g., cyclophosphamide, ifosfamide)
  Streptozotocin*
  Thiotepa
Vesicant†
  Actinomycin-D (dactinomycin)
  Amsacrine
  Anthracyclines (e.g., daunorubicin, doxorubicin, epirubicin, idarubicin)
  Mithramycin (plicamycin)*
  Mitozantrone (mitoxantrone)
  Mitomycin C*
  Nitrogen mustard (mustine, mechlorethamine)
  Taxol (paclitaxel)‡
  Vinca alkaloids (vinblastine, vincristine, vindesine, vinorelbine‡, vinzolidine‡)

---

* Agent rarely used in pediatrics.
† Specific antidotes are recommended for certain vesicants only.
‡ New agent. Not yet subject to "official" classification (probably vesicants).

---

where chemotherapy is administered. They should include the following recommendations:

A. Employ knowledgeable and highly skilled personnel.

B. Preferably inject hazardous agents into central lines or recently sited peripheral lines only. (The use of "butterfly" needles, which disclose infiltrations earlier, versus catheters, which are less easily dislodged, should be considered.)

C. Avoid "risky" cannulation sites (e.g., the lower extremities, veins over joints, wrists, the antecubital area, or superficial tendons and ligaments) and the selection of the vein itself. Candidate veins should be prominent, easily accessible, and visible at all times, with any evidence of compromised circulation taken into account.

D. Routinely use vasodilatory procedures (e.g., hot packs or glyceryl trinitrate patches).

E. Minimize venous exposure to "high risk" drugs by adequate dilution or injection into the side-arm of a fast-running drip.

F. Maximize patient cooperation.
   1. Encourage a confident yet relaxed approach to the patient by highly competent personnel.
   2. Perform cannulation procedures in a well-lit environment with all proper equipment at hand.
   3. Display awareness of high levels of anxiety, and have appropriate measures in place to deal with it.
   4. Instruct patients of the need to report, immediately, any untoward sensations associated with the injection/infusion.

G. Confirm and maintain venous patency during any injection. Stop immediately if there is any question of infiltration. Flush routinely before giving any high-risk agent and again after its completion, to ensure that no active drug is left to leak out when the needle is removed.

H. When two agents are to be administered at the same time but by different routes (e.g., vincristine intravenously and asparaginase intramuscularly, or methotrexate intrathecally and vincristine intravenously), it is important that they not be confused. The agents should be clearly separated and have contrasting labeling.

IV. MANAGEMENT

A. Rationale
   Should an extravasation occur, the aim of all management plans is to minimize long-term damage. All efforts, therefore, are directed toward minimizing tissue contact time. A truly standardized and universally accepted management plan does not exist, however, and disagreement as to the most appropriate course of action continues. Management is usually based on a limited number of animal experiments and anecdotal reports appearing in the literature as well as on personal experience. This means that for almost every recommendation there is an expression of concern. Only those steps that appear to have attained near "universal" acceptance are listed below.

B. Symptoms and signs of extravasation

Suspect extravasation if the patient reports pain, burning, or stinging at or around the site of the injection or along the tract of the vein. Additionally, the absence of blood return, interruption to the flow rate, erythema, and swelling or "bleb" formation at the intravenous site may be noted.

C. Steps

1. Stop the administration of the agent immediately but *do not remove the needle/cannula.*
2. If possible, attempt to draw back 3–5 mL of blood/drug solution into the tubing/needle, with the aim of removing as much of the infiltrated drug as possible.
3. Use a 25/26 gauge needle attached to a 1 mL TB syringe to aspirate (from several sites) any subcutaneous bleb of drug solution remaining after the completion of step 2.
4. With the needle/cannula still in place, decide whether it is appropriate to instill a specified antidote. Recommended antidotes are listed in Table 8.2.
   a. This is a highly contentious topic, with some widely accepted recommendations of earlier days now being disputed. Among these is the use of sodium bicarbonate solution and/or corticosteroids for anthracycline extravasations.
   b. There is, however, general agreement that hyaluronidase (1 mL) injected locally is effective for dispersing vinca alkaloids and minimizing the resultant tissue damage, and that sodium thiosulfate injection is an effective antidote to nitrogen mustard extravasation.

TABLE 8.2.
Vesicant Chemotherapeutic Agents and Antidotes That Have Been Recommended

Drug	Antidote	Dose (mL)
Actinomycin-D	Sodium thiosulfate 10%	0.1–4
Anthracyclines	Topical dimethylsulfoxide	
Mustine	Sodium thiosulfate 10%	3
Vinca alkaloids	Hyaluronidase	
	Injection	1
	Topical application	

Decisions regarding the injection of other "antidotes" should be made by institutional choice.

5. Remove the needle/cannula.
6. Apply pressure (or a firm bandage) to the area to stop bleeding and prevent the formation of a hematoma.
7. Apply cold packs or hot packs. There is general agreement that the use of ice packs is appropriate. The limb should be elevated during this procedure. For the vinca alkaloids, however, the use of warmth or hot packs carries general support. In addition to the well-documented risks of extravasation of intravenous vincristine, there exists a significant risk of accidental intramuscular administration, where it is confused with intramuscular L-asparaginase, especially during the induction phase of acute lymphomatic leukemia. The use of 8.4% sodium bicarbonate injected directly into the site followed by alternating hot and cold compresses has been considered to minimize possible damage.
8. Apply "topical" agent if appropriate. There is growing evidence that the topical application of dimethylsulfoxide to the site of an anthracycline extravasation is beneficial in reducing the likelihood of long-term tissue damage and subsequent need for extensive plastic surgery. Other topical applications have been recommended from time to time, including 1% hydrocortisone cream (to alleviate the local inflammatory effect of an extravasation) and hyaluronidase cream (for vinca alkaloids). Such creams or ointments would be best covered by a dressing (see Step 11). Decisions concerning the inclusion of topical applications should be made at the individual institutional level.
9. Document the incident at this point. This may include marking and/or photographing the site as well as completing the appropriate incident report. Document the ongoing resolution of the extravasation in the progress notes.
10. Order medication to relieve symptoms. Oral medications (including analgesics, sedatives, anxiolytics, and antihistamines) may be of value in individual cases.
11. Apply an appropriate dressing to protect the area from infection.
12. Reevaluate the site no later than 24 hours after the

extravasation. If the signs and symptoms are progressing despite conservative treatment, initiate surgical referral as soon as possible. The role of surgery soon after the occurrence of a large infiltration to remove the drug-laden tissue has its proponents, and the rationale (reduction of later necrosis) does have merit. There is solid consensus, however, on the importance of traditional debridement and plastic surgery in the management of serious extravasation.

13. Ensure that adequate follow-up for the next 1–2 weeks is instituted.

Bibliography

Bertelli G, Dini D, Forno GB, et al.: Hyaluronidase as an antidote to extravasation of vinca alkaloids: Clinical Results. *J Cancer Res Clin Oncol* 120:505–6, 1994.

Bertelli G, Gozza A, Forno GB, et al.: Topical dimethylsulfoxide for the prevention of soft tissue injury after extravasation of vesicant cytotoxic drugs: A prospective clinical study. *J Clin Oncol* 13:2851–55, 1995.

Boyle DM, Engelking C: Vesicant extravasation: Myths and realities. *Oncol Nurs Forum* 22:57–67, 1995.

Clark BS, Gallegos E, Bleyer WA: Accidental intramuscular vinicristine: lack of untoward effects and recommendations for management. *Med Pediat Oncol* 28:314–15, 1997.

Cox K, Stuart-Harris R, Abdini G, et al.: The management of cytotoxic-drug extravasation: Guidelines drawn up by a working party for the Clinical Oncologic Society of Australia. *Med J Aust* 148:185–89, 1988.

Reynolds JEF, ed.: *Martindale: The Extra Pharmacopoeia.* 30th ed. London: The Pharmaceutical Press; 1993.

9

Side Effects of Radiation Therapy in Children and Their Prevention and Management

Richard S. Pieters, M.D.

Radiation therapy has inherent side effects, early (during or immediately after treatment, termed acute), intermediate (weeks to months after treatment, termed *subacute*), and late. Early and intermediate effects are temporary, while late effects tend to be permanent. They can be minimized by careful fractionation and definition of the treatment volume. In general, tissues are most vulnerable to late effects during periods of rapid proliferation of that tissue, due to growth or maturation. Medical measures can also be taken to minimize or prevent the occurrence of either early or late effects and to manage those that do occur.

Since almost all children who receive radiation therapy are also treated with chemotherapy, sequentially and/or concomitantly, it is important to remember that each of the side effects of radiation therapy may be enhanced by chemotherapy (and vice versa), and thus occurs with greater severity or at a lower total dose. The sequelae of surgery and of radiation therapy also interact and may enhance each other.

General Principles: Management of the Side Effects of Radiation Therapy

I. EARLY EFFECTS

A. Nutritional support
Nutritional support during radiation therapy is vital for the prevention of cachexia, immune compromise, and inability to repair normal tissue damage. See Chapter 13.
1. Nutritional status needs to be assessed initially.
a. Weight loss probably indicates negative nitrogen balance, which must be corrected.
b. Counsel the patient and family regarding unusual or idiosyncratic dietary habits, to assure a nutritionally complete diet.
2. Caloric need during radiation therapy is approximately 110% of baseline.
3. An enteral diet is preferable to a parenteral diet.
a. Oral diet modifications may be necessary.
i. Taste may change secondary to the tumor or to treatment, which may alter diet.
ii. If the mucosa of the upper gastrointestinal tract is being irradiated, a soft, bland diet may be required (no spicy, acidic, or hot or cold food or drink).
iii. Standard oral supplements must be used if caloric requirements cannot be met otherwise (e.g., Sustacal, Ensure, or Carnation Instant Breakfast).
b. Nasogastric tube feeding is probably required if 10% weight loss occurs during treatment.
4. Intravenous hyperalimentation is indicated if the patient is unable to tolerate oral or nasogastric feeding.

B. Management of hematologic and immunologic toxicity
Radiation therapy of any part of the body can suppress blood counts, particularly white blood cells and platelets. Patients who have received chemotherapy, previously or concurrently, or whose treatment volume encompasses a significant percentage of marrow are at particular risk.
1. See Chapter 1.

2. Follow protocol guidelines for interruption of therapy due to hematologic toxicity.
3. In the absence of protocol guidelines, consider the rate of decrease in counts and clinical situation; consider holding treatment for absolute neutrophil count <1000 cells/μL or platelets <75,000.
4. The role of colony-stimulating factors during radiation therapy is not yet established.

C. Management of radiation-induced nausea and vomiting
Radiation-induced nausea and vomiting can be difficult to prevent. Nausea can be seen with radiation of the head or stomach; occasionally it is also seen when other parts of the body are irradiated. The mechanisms are different, so the treatments are different.
1. Management of nausea and vomiting due to cranial irradiation (see below, "Side Effects of Cranial Irradiation.")
2. Management of nausea and vomiting due to direct effect on the stomach
   a. Etiology: not well understood
   b. Treatment
      i. Sipping of decarbonated cola drinks may relieve symptoms
      ii. Antiemetic medications
          (1) Prochlorperazine (Compazine)
              (a) Dose:
                  Children (>10 kg or >2 years): 0.4 mg/kg/day, by mouth (PO) or per rectum, divided t.i.d.q.i.d.
                  Teenagers: 5–10 mg per dose t.i.d. to q.i.d.
              (b) Available:
                  Tablet: 5, 10, or 5 mg
                  Syrup: 5 mg/mL
                  Suppository: 2.5, 5, or 25 mg
          (2) Metoclopromide (Reglan)
              (a) Dose: 0.1 mg/kg PO q.i.d.
              (b) Available:
                  tablet: 5 or 10 mg
                  Syrup: 5 mg/mL
          (3) Cisapride (Propulsid)
              (a) Dose: children: 0.2–0.3 mg/kg per dose PO t.i.d. to q.i.d.
              (b) Available:

Tablet: 10 or 20 mg
Suspension: 1 mg/mL
(4) Ondansetron (Zofran)
(a) Dose: 0.15 mg/kg per dose; usually administered PO p4–6h, starting 1 hour before radiation daily.
(b) Available: tablet: 4 or 8 mg
3. Management of nausea and vomiting due to radiation of other parts of body
a. Etiology
This is believed to be due to delayed gastric emptying.
b. Treatment
Cisapride (Propulsid) and metoclopramide (Reglan) may have physiologic advantages by promoting gastric emptying.

II. LATE EFFECTS

A. Growth problems
1. Neuroendocrine effect of irradiation of hypothalamic pituitary axis
See below, Section IIIB under "Side Effects of Cranial Irradiation."
2. Direct effect on irradiated bone and soft tissue
a. Effect is age and dose dependent.
i. Irradiated bones may be smaller or shorter than nonirradiated bones.
ii. Spinal irradiation may affect height and may exacerbate kyphosis or scoliosis.
b. Irradiated muscle may atrophy.
3. Management of growth problems
a. Consider growth hormone replacement.
b. Monitor for scoliosis and kyphosis.
c. Consider early plastic surgical intervention to correct facial deformities. sufficient to cause psychosocial distress.
d. Offer psychosocial support
B. Soft tissue fibrosis over a joint
1. Etiology
This is caused by scarring after high-dose radiotherapy. The risk is increased if the field also includes a radical surgical site.

2. Prevention
If possible, plan surgical incisions to allow the radiation oncologist to avoid treating a full joint.
3. Treatment
Daily range-of-motion exercises for the rest of the patient's life will be necessary.

C. Peripheral edema
1. Etiology
a. Lymphatic obstruction
b. Venous insufficiency
2. Prevention
Place incisions vertically, not transversely, in extremities, to allow the radiation oncologist to treat the entire scar without treating the entire circumference of the extremity.

D. Carcinogenesis
1. Risk factors for second malignant neoplasm due to radiation therapy
a. The relative risk of a second malignant neoplasm due to radiation therapy is not yet well defined, as it varies from report to report and by original disease, age at treatment, and site treated.
b. Children treated for one malignancy have an increased risk of developing a second malignant neoplasm, even in the absence of radiation therapy.
c. Genetics (heredity) plays a role.
    i. Patients with basal cell nevus syndrome often develop basal cell cancers in the irradiated field 6 months to 3 years after treatment.
    ii. Patients with familial retinoblastoma are at increased risk of a second malignant neoplasm, even without irradiation.
d. About two-thirds of second malignant neoplasms are found in the field of radiation therapy. Bone and soft tissue sarcomas are considered radiation induced only if they occur in the radiated treatment volume.
e. Tissue sensitivity to carcinogenesis from radiation varies.
    i. Thyroid gland and breast are at risk after low doses.
    ii. Lung, liver, and lymphoid tissue are at risk after moderate doses.
    iii. Bone and muscle are at risk after higher doses.

f. Tissue stage of development alters risk; proliferating cells are most at risk. Girls whose breast tissue is irradiated between ages 10 and 16 (during pubertal development) have the greatest increase in risk of developing breast cancer; risk declines as the age at treatment increases.

g. Sex is a factor. The risk of a second malignant neoplasm is higher for females than males, even excluding breast cancer.

2. Management

a. Discourage smoking in survivors, especially if the respiratory tract has been irradiated.

b. Examine tissues at risk, i.e., those in radiation treatment volume (Table 9.1).

c. Perform scrupulous breast follow-up for women who received radiation to the breast during adolescence.

   i. Monthly breast self-examination

   ii. Regular clinical breast examinations; early annual mammography (exact age to start is controversial)

Side Effects of Skin Irradiation

I. EARLY EFFECTS

All radiation treatments treat skin. Severe skin reactions, sufficient to interrupt treatment, may occur at any site; intertriginous areas are most at risk.

A. Prevention

1. Avoid heat or cold, exposure to sun, sun block, and perfumes or perfumed ointments during treatment.

2. At most, use gentle soap on radiated surface. Preferably, rinse with lukewarm water and gently pat dry with soft towel, avoiding soap altogether.

3. Do not place adhesive or medical tape on irradiated fields.

a. If tape is absolutely required, use paper tape.

b. If tape is present on irradiated skin, soak it off.

4. Avoid scratching.

a. Corn starch applied generously as desired will provide some relief; wash it off frequently with lukewarm water.

b. Diphenhydramine (Benadryl) (1 mg/kg per dose PO; maximum 5 doses per day) may decrease itching.

TABLE 9.1.
Tissues at Risk for Secondary Neoplasm

Tissue Radiated	Second (Malignant) Neoplasm	Signs and Symptoms	Usual Time to Occurrence (years)
Bone marrow	Leukemia (acute myelogenous)	Fatigue, petechiae	7–10; rare past 15
Bone and soft tissues	Sarcoma	Pain, mass	≥8
Neck, mediastinum	Thyroid adenoma	Nodule	<10
	Thyroid carcinoma	Nodule, mass	≥10
Chest	Breast carcinoma	Mass, characteristic mammographic lesions	
	Lung cancer	Cough, mass on chest x-ray	≥8
Skin	Melanoma	Characteristic lesion	≥8
	Atypical basal cell carcinoma	Characteristic lesion	3–20
Brain	Brain tumor	Headache, vomiting, ataxia	≥8
Upper airways	Atypical squamous cell carcinoma	Pain, bleeding, mass, ulceration	≥8

    c. Care provider should observe closely.

    d. Keep fingernails clipped short.

    e. The patient may need to sleep with stockings over hands to prevent scratching while asleep.

    f. Do not scrub off radiation field marks; when treatment is complete, allow them to wear off.

B. Treatment

  1. For dry desquamation

    a. Start Sweem Cream, Aquaphor, or aloe vera lotion 4–6 times per day to the affected area.

    b. Rub in gently until gone.

    c. Treatment can be started as early as the start of radiation.

  2. For moist desquamation

    a. Clean gently; air dry; then use:

      i. Gentian violet solution USP; apply sparingly 2–3 times per day.

        or

      ii. Biolex spray and gel; apply to affected area 4 times per day.

    b. For large areas or failure to respond to above, use silver sulfadiazine (Silvadene) topical antibiotic cream, 1% 2 times per day.

II. LATE EFFECTS

A. Permanent increased sensitivity to sun

  1. Sensitivity is dose dependent.

  2. Sensitivity is greatest in the 1st year after radiation.

B. Treatment

  1. Avoid prolonged exposure to sun.

  2. Use sun block scrupulously.

  3. Remind the patient and family that a layer of cloth provides a sun protection factor of only about 7.

Side Effects of Cranial Irradiation

I. EARLY EFFECTS

    Nausea

A. Etiology
Nausea secondary to brain irradiation is due to brain edema with increased intracranial pressure.

B. Prevention
If peritumoral edema is present, start steroid treatment at least 4 hours before starting radiation; otherwise, starting just before radiation is acceptable.

C. Treatment: Dexamethasone (Decadron)
  1. Dose
     a. Not established
     b. Adults and teenagers: loading dose of 1 mg/kg intravenous (IV), then 4–6 mg IV or PO q.i.d., and then taper after the completion of radiation
     c. Younger children: can be individualized; 0.1 mg/kg per dose q6h (maximum 48 hours) reasonable initial dose, and then taper.
  2. Available
     a. Tablet: 0.25, 0.5, 1, 1.5, 2, 4, or 6 mg
     b. Injection: 4, 10, 20, or 24 mg/mL
     c. Elixir: 0.5 mg/5 mL
     d. Oral solution: 0.1 or 1 mg/mL

II. INTERMEDIATE EFFECTS

A. Delayed somnolence syndrome
  1. Presentation
     Patients exhibit extreme sleepiness, occurring several weeks to approximately 6 months after cranial irradiation.
  2. Etiology
     This is believed to be due to transient demyelinization. Syndrome occurs in up to 60% of patients treated for prophylaxis of acute lymphoblastic leukemia (ALL). Patients may be of any age.
  3. Treatment
     a. Syndrome is self-limiting, very gradually improving over several weeks to months
     b. Wake patient to eat, to maintain adequate nutrition.
     c. Corticosteroids may shorten duration. Use dexamethasone, dose as above, and taper gradually.

B. Headache/nausea
  1. Presentation

    a. Rare, occurring several weeks to approximately 6 months after cranial irradiation

    b. Severe headache, with associated nausea

2. Etiology: unknown
3. Treatment

    a. Self-limiting, with gradual improvement

    b. Use of corticosteroids to diminish severity of symptoms and possibly shorten duration (dexamethasone as above)

III. LATE EFFECTS

A. Cognitive impairment

1. Age at treatment, dose, and volume dependent
2. Variability between individual patients great
3. Quantitative processes more often affected than verbal
4. Management

    a. Perform early and regular neuropsychological testing.

    b. Inform parents of their child's legal rights to special educational help when indicated.

B. Neuroendocrine effects

1. Etiology

    a. Damage depends on the dose to the pituitary and hypothalamus. Growth hormone deficiency may be identified but is rarely clinically significant after cranial irradiation for central nervous system prophylaxis of ALL.

    b. Etiology is unknown, may be vascular insufficiency or late mitotic death.

    c. Hormones vary in sensitivity to radiation.

       i. Growth hormone is the most sensitive and first to be affected.

       ii. Gonadotrophins and adrenocorticotropin are intermediate.

       iii. Thyroid-stimulating hormone (TSH) is the least sensitive and last to be affected.

       iv. Transient hyperprolactinemia is seen.

    d. Anterior pituitary hormones are at risk; no posterior pituitary damage has been observed.

    e. Hypothalamus appears to be the site of damage.

    f. Premature onset of puberty is age and sex dependent.

    i. Girls

       Youngest girls at age of irradiation have earliest onset of puberty.

    ii. Boys

       Pubertal onset is earliest in those irradiated between 3 and 6 years of age.

2. Management

  a. Early referral and annual endocrine evaluation in follow-up are indicated to minimize effect on eventual height.

  b. Consider growth hormone replacement for those who have received >2700 cGy to pituitary hypothalamic axis.

  c. For patients with brain tumor, wait 2 years after therapy.

  d. Early puberty shortens the time available for growth hormone treatment, and the early pubertal growth spurt may mask the fact of ultimate short stature.

Side Effects of Head and Neck Irradiation

I. ACUTE EFFECTS

  A. Radiation mucositis

    1. Prevention

      a. Remove orthodontic braces before treatment.

      b. If a metal dental prosthesis or filling is in place, cover it with a substance such as chewing gum, dental rolls, dental wax, or fluoride carriers to avoid local scatter of electrons.

      c. Observe scrupulous oral hygiene; brush after each meal; rinse frequently as below.

    2. Treatment

      a. Rinse mouth with a lukewarm solution of 1 tablespoon of salt and 1 tablespoon of baking soda in a quart of water *and/or* diluted hydrogen peroxide solution for several minutes, 5 or 6 times a day.

      b. Consider Ulcerease.

        i. Swish or gargle 5–10 mL for 15 seconds, then spit out.

        ii. Use every 2 hours while awake.

    iii. Use with caution for child under 6 or those unable to avoid swallowing medication.

  c. Advise the patient to avoid spicy, very warm, very cold, or acidic food or drink and exposure to tobacco smoke.

  d. See Chapter 14.

  e. Vigorously address patient's nutritional status.

    i. Mucositis will discourage adequate nutrition.

    ii. Mucositis will resolve only when the patient is in positive nitrogen balance.

    iii. See Section IA under "General Principles: Management of the Side Effects of Radiation Therapy" above and Chapter 13.

  f. Use a prophylactic anti-inflammatory/antibiotic solution.

  Recipes vary; this one is representative. Use tetracycline syrup 2 g, *or* erythromycin syrup 2 g, Nystatin oral suspension, 2 million U, and hydrocortisone 50 mg. Mix in distilled water with flavoring to make 120 mL. Take 5 mL, swish and swallow q.i.d.

  g. Allow the patient to take a 3- or 4-day weekend off treatment. If mucositis is severe, a longer break until healing is well under way may be necessary.

  h. Manage pain.

    i. Give acetaminophen 10 mg/kg and/or codeine 1 mg/kg PO q4h.

    ii. A solution of diphenhydramine (Benadryl) and Maalox in equal parts has been effective as a soothing mouthwash; small amounts can be swallowed without ill effect. Do not exceed the maximum diphenhydramine dose of 5 mg/kg/day.

    iii. In an older child, who can expel the material, 2% viscous lidocaine (Xylocaine) may be used as a swish and gargle before and during meals as needed. Be aware of the increased risk of cardiac arrhythmia from lidocaine in the pediatric patient. Adding 2% lidocaine to above diphenhydramine/Maalox solution (1:1:1) is also useful.

    iv. Severe mucositis may require systemic opiates (see Chapter 11).

B. Radiation candidiasis

  1. Prevention

Scrupulous oral hygiene is needed; unfortunately, this is of limited efficacy.

2. Diagnosis

Clinical evidence of candidal infection is sufficient to start treatment.

3. Treatment

a. Manage candidal infection immediately and vigorously.

b. Each of the following has been used with success.

   i. Fluconazole

     (1) Dose

      Children: loading: 10 mg/kg PO or IV, then 3–6 mg/kg PO q.i.d.

      Teenagers: loading: 200 mg PO or IV, then 100 mg PO q.i.d.

     (2) Available

      Tablet: 50, 100, or 200 mg

      Injection: 2 mg/mL

      Suspension: 10 or 40 mg/mL

   ii. Nystatin oral suspension

     (1) Dose

      Infants and young children: swab and swallow

      Older children: 1–2 mL q.i.d., swish and swallow

      Teenagers: 5 mL swish and swallow q.i.d.

     (2) Available: suspension: 100,000 U/mL

   iii. Clotrimazole troche

     Dose: 10 mg (1 tablet) sublingually, 5 times daily

   iv. For refractory cases: ketoconazole

     (1) Dose

      Children: 5 mg/kg/day PO, rounded up to the nearest 50 mg (maximum 10 m/kg/day, divided b.i.d.).

      Teenagers: 200–400 mg PO q.i.d.or divided b.i.d.

     (2) Available

      Tablet: 200 mg

      Suspension: 100 mg/mL

c. Once a candidal infection has occurred during radiation therapy, it is important to continue oral candidal treatment as prophylaxis against recurrence until the end of radiation therapy.

C. Sialadenitis

1. Painful inflammation of salivary glands in direct radiation beam occurs occasionally, at variable intervals after the

start of radiation.

2. This condition is usually self-limiting, as it disappears when the affected glands cease to function.
3. Treat symptomatically with anti-inflammatory agents.

D. Loss of taste
1. This is most noticeable in patients with tongue in treatment field.
2. Some patients complain of metallic taste, others of cardboard taste of all food.
3. Eventually, sense of taste disappears.
4. Reassure the patient/parents that this is temporary; taste returns at least partially to normal.

E. Ear
1. Otitis externa
   a. Etiology
      i. Skin reaction
      ii. Superimposed infection
   b. Management
      See above, Section IB under "Side Effects of Skin Irradiation."
      i.   Wicks
      ii. Otic antibiotics
      iii. Steroid creams
2. Decreased hearing/sensation of water in ear
   a. Etiology: eustachian tube swelling and obstruction
   b. Treatment
      i. Give diphenhydramine (Benadryl).
          (1) Dose
              Children: 1 mg/kg per dose PO (maximum 5 doses per day)
              Teenagers: 10–50 mg per dose PO q6–8h
          (2) Available
              Tablet: 25 or 50 mg
              Syrup: 12.5 mg/5 mL
      ii. Consider inserting tympanic tubes.

II. LATE EFFECTS

A. Dry mouth
1. Etiology
   a. Doses greater than approximately 2700–3000 cGy in conventional fractionation obliterate salivary function

in treated glands; with chemotherapy this threshold may be lower.
   b. Severity of dry mouth depends on the volume of salivary glands irradiated.
2. Prevention
   Pilocarpine hydrochloride 5 mg PO q.i.d. daily during and 1 month after radiation therapy to the salivary glands has been shown to decrease the severity of dry mouth in adults. This use in pediatric patients has not been established.
3. Treatment (since prevention is not often possible)
   a. Perform life-long scrupulous oral hygiene.
   b. Carry water at all times for sipping.
   c. Consider pilocarpine hydrochloride, as above.
      i. Available: 5 mg tablet
      ii. Consistently use twice a day for at least 1 month before assessing response
      iii. Safety and efficacy of this drug in children not established
   d. Sugarless chewing gum helps many patients.
   e. Fat may help.
      A teaspoon of corn or olive oil as needed, especially at bedtime, has been reported to help.
   f. Room humidifier should be used at night in winter.

B. Radiation caries
1. Etiology
   Dry mouth, leading to altered oral flora, not a direct effect of radiation on the teeth
2. Prevention
   Life-long scrupulous oral hygiene (see Chapter 14)

C. Osteoradionecrosis
   This complication is seen less commonly in pediatric patients than would be expected from experience in adults; it is so devastating when it occurs that prevention is vital.
1. All patients requiring radiation to the mouth or parotid glands should be seen by a dentist as soon after diagnosis as possible to start a rigorous program of dental prophylaxis.
2. Healthy teeth should not be removed.
3. Permanent teeth in poor condition, requiring removal in

the foreseeable future, should be removed before treatment.
4. After dental extractions, delay radiotherapy approximately 2 weeks for healing.
5. For dental prophylaxis see Chapter 14.
6. Prophylactic antibiotics should be administered for all dental work performed after head and neck radiation therapy.

D. Ocular
  1. Cataracts
    a. Etiology
      i. This is a direct effect of radiation to the lens.
      ii. Dose dependent: >200 cGy in single fraction or 500 cGy fractionated to the lens virtually assures the development of cataract.
      iii. Busulfan and steroids can exacerbate the development of cataract.
    b. Treatment
      Surgical removal of lens
  2. Dry eye
    a. Etiology
      i. This is caused by loss of lacrimal gland function.
      ii. Dose dependent: >~3000 cGy in conventional fractionation may lead to permanent loss of function of the lacrimal gland.
      iii. Severity of dry eye depends on the volume of gland treated; sparing minor glands can diminish the problem.
      iv. Dry eye can cause corneal ulceration and severe pain.
    b. Treatment
      i. Use over-the-counter (OTC) eyedrops during the day. Preservative-free eyedrops are preferred, such as carboxymethylcellulose 1.0% ophthalmic solution
      ii. Use OTC viscous lubricant or white petrolatum/mineral oil lubricant ophthalmic ointment at bedtime.
      iii. Early ophthalmologic evaluation is vital to prevent complications of dry eye.
      iv. Painful, sightless dry eye can lead to enucleation as

           last resort.
    3. Retinitis
        a. Etiology
            i. Apparently vasculitis-microangiopathy
            ii. Dose and fraction size dependent
            iii. Latency 6 months to 3 years
            iv. Can lead to neovascular glaucoma
        b. Treatment
            i. Methods are not well understood.
            ii. Appears similar to diabetic retinopathy, so similar management seems reasonable.
            iii. Laser treatment has been used.
            iv. Early referral to a retinal ophthalmologist is indicated if retina receives >5000 cGy in conventional fractionation

E. Auditory
    1. Etiology
        a. Radiation alone rarely damages hearing.
        b. Cisplatin concomitantly or after radiation to middle ear can increase hearing loss.
        c. Cisplatin before radiation is not as ototoxic.
        d. Hearing loss progresses gradually, up to 6 years after radiation.
    F. Neuroendocrine
    See above, Section IIIB under "Side Effects of Cranial Irradiation."

Late Effects of Thyroid Irradiation

I. HYPERTHYROIDISM

Subclinical hypothyroidism will appear in 30–40% of patients treated with moderate to high dose (>2500–3000 cGy) radiation to the thyroid gland.

    A. Not dose related

    B. Occurs up to 18 years after irradiation

    C. Can occur in patients on thyroid hormone replacement

II. GRAVES OPHTHALMOPATHY

A. Etiology: not known

B. Does not require patient to be biochemically hyperthyroid.

III. THYROTOXICOSIS

A. Etiology: not known.

B. Condition transient; progresses rapidly to overt hypothyroidism.

IV. HYPOTHYROIDISM

A. About 50% of patients treated with mantle radiation for Hodgkin disease become subclinically hypothyroid. Therefore, thyroid function studies should be obtained at least annually if the lower neck has been irradiated.

B. Elevated TSH levels are occasionally transient.

C. Consider treatment for subclinical hypothyroidism.

D. Incidence of progression from subclinical to overt hypothyroidism is unknown.

E. Thyroid hormone replacement therapy may be indicated.

F. Hypothyroidism may increase the risk of accelerated atherosclerosis.

V. THYROID NODULAR DISEASE

A. Detection
   1. Careful palpation of thyroid at all follow-up examinations
   2. Thyroid scans and biopsy of suspicious nodules

B. Malignancy
   Ten to 20% of nodules are malignant.

Side Effects of Thoracic Irradiation

I. EARLY EFFECT

Esophagitis

A. Prevention

1. Sucralfate (Carafate) slurry, starting on the 1st day of irradiation, has been suggested to decrease incidence and severity.
   a. Dose: 10–20 mg/kg per dose PO q.i.d.
   b. Available: suspension: 100 mg/mL
2. Ranitidine HCl (Zantac) has also been suggested to decrease severity.
   a. Dose: Infants and children: 4–5 mg/kg/day, divided, b.i.d. or t.i.d.
   b. Available
      Tablet: 75 (OTC), 150 or 300 mg
      Syrup: 15 mg/mL

B. Presentation
   1. Symptoms include substernal pain on swallowing, sensation of lump in throat, and sore throat.
   2. Symptoms begin about 2 weeks into the course of thoracic radiation therapy.
   3. Symptoms usually ease after radiation to esophagus stops or even decrease when oblique fields start.
      a. Treatment
         i. Treat the same as oral mucositis.
         ii. If dysphagia persists or there is evidence of oral candidiasis, start candidal treatment (See above, "Section IB under "Side Effects of Head and Neck Irradiation").
         iii. If the dysphagia is severe, the patient may need a break from radiation treatment.

II. INTERMEDIATE EFFECTS

Radiation pneumonitis

A. Presentation
   1. This presents either during radiation therapy or up to about 6 months after treatment is completed; it is very rare with doses <3000 cGy.
   2. Symptoms are shortness of breath, dyspnea on exertion, and cough
   3. Fever is rare.
   4. Radiographic changes seen in most patients are infiltrates within the irradiated volume of lung.
   5. Decreased vital capacity and diffusing capacity are present.

6. Actinomycin D and Adriamycin may reactivate.
7. Abrupt steroid withdrawal may reactivate.

B. Treatment
1. Bed rest
2. Prednisone
   a. Dose: 0.5–2 mg/kg/day (maximum 80 mg/day), divided t.i.d. to q.i.d.
   b. Available
      Tablet: 1, 2.5, 5, 10, 20, or 50 mg
      Syrup: 1 mg/mL (5% alcohol)

III. LATE EFFECTS

A. Cardiac complications
1. Late cardiac complications
   a. Acute myocardial infarction
   b. Acute pericarditis
   c. Constrictive pericarditis
   d. Valvular disease
2. Risk factors
   a. Complications are dose, volume, and exact target dependent.
      i. Proximal coronary arteries tend to be in high-dose mediastinal fields.
      ii. Pericardial problems require that most of the heart be in treatment volume; this is rare today.
   b. Age dependent: Risk decreases as child's age at treatment increases.
   c. Acute pericarditis may be precipitated by abrupt steroid withdrawal.
   d. Malignant hypertension can exacerbate arteriosclerosis in irradiated vessels, precipitating myocardial infarction in patients at risk.
   e. Previous treatment with doxorubicin enhances the risk.
3. Presentation
   a. Acute myocardial infarction
      Remember this risk in patients who present with chest pain or congestive failure after chest irradiation.
   b. Acute pericarditis
      Pain

    c. Constrictive pericarditis
      Chest pain, poor tolerance of exercise, and normal heart size

B. Pulmonary fibrosis
  Presentation
  1. Radiographs: scarring in field of radiation, sometimes with retraction
  2. Rarely symptomatic
  3. Reduced diffusing capacity

Side Effects of Abdominal Irradiation

I. EARLY EFFECT

Nausea
  See above, Section IC under "General Principles: Management of the Side Effects of Radiation Therapy."

II. LATE EFFECTS

A. Renal toxicity
  1. Hypertension
    a. Etiology
      i. Parenchymal damage
      ii. Extrarenal vascular damage
    b. Treatment
      i. Medical treatment
      ii. Partial or total nephrectomy
  2. Renal failure
    Risk depends on volume of renal parenchyma treated, dose, fractionation, and age.

B. Bowel toxicity
  See below, Section II under "Side Effects of Pelvic Irradiation."

Side Effects of Pelvic Irradiation

I. EARLY EFFECTS

A. Radiation enteritis

Radiation enteritis is seen as a result of radiation to the pelvis or lower abdomen.

1. Presentation

    Radiation enteritis usually presents as diarrhea with frequent, watery, soft stools, and sometimes with cramping pain.

2. Prevention

    If the patient has a full bladder for as many radiation treatments as possible, the incidence and severity of radiation enteritis will decrease.

3. Treatment

    a. Diet

        i.   Restrict the roughage, or residue, in the diet.
        ii. If this is unsuccessful, restrict fat.
        iii. If this is still unsuccessful, restrict lactose; milk products can still be used if lactase-treated milk is provided (Lactaid, sweet acidophilus milk).
        iv. An elemental diet, which is absorbed in the upper small bowel to put the bowel at rest, may help.
        v.   The patient's weight must be maintained, as adequate nutrition is required to recover from radiation enteritis.

    b. Drug: loperamide (Imodium)

        i.   Avoid in the presence of significant abdominal distention.
        ii. Dose
             2–6 years (13–20 kg): 1 mg PO t.i.d.
             6–8 years (20–30 kg): 2 mg PO b.i.d.
             8–12 years (>30 kg): 2 mg PO t.i.d.
             Teenagers: 2 mg after each loose stool (maximum 16 mg/day)
        iii. Available
             Capsule: 2 mg
             Tablet: 2 mg
             Syrup: 1 mg/5 mL

    c. Interrupt radiation

        Radiotherapy may have to be interrupted for severe enteritis until it subsides.

    d. Failure

        If the above measures fail, hospital management is necessary. Admit the patient to the hospital for appropriate diagnostic evaluation, parenteral fluids, and other indicated therapies.

B. Proctitis
1. Presentation
   a. Perianal inflammation
   b. Exacerbated by diarrhea or constipation
2. Treatment
   a. Treat diarrhea/constipation.
   b. Recommend sitz baths after each bowel movement.
   c. Lukewarm water sprayed into the anus may help.
   d. Consider cortisone enemas.
   e. Manage pain.

C. Acute radiation cystitis
1. Presentation
   Acute radiation cystitis manifests as urinary frequency and dysuria. Anthracyclines or actinomycin-D given with bladder radiation increase the risk of hemorrhagic cystitis.
2. Diagnosis
   a. Symptoms are identical to those of urinary tract infection.
   b. Urinalysis with clean-caught urine culture and sensitivity is mandatory to rule out infection.
3. Prevention
   If the patient has a full bladder for as many radiation treatments as possible, the incidence and severity of radiation cystitis will decrease.
4. Treatment
   If urinalysis and culture are negative:
   a. Phenazopyridine HCl (Pyridium) for topical analgesic effect
      i. Dose
         6–12 years: 12 mg/kg/day PO divided, t.i.d.
         Teenagers: 200 mg PO t.i.d.
      ii. Available: tablet: 95, 100, or 200 mg
   b. Flavoxate (Urispas) (100–200 mg PO t.i.d. or q.i.d. if the child is >12 years) to relieve urinary spasm
      If obstruction of the bladder outlet is a risk, avoid flavoxate because of its anticholinergic effect.
   c. Oxybutynin chloride (Ditropan)
      i. Dose
         ≤5 years old: 0.4–0.8 mg/kg/day PO b.i.d.–q.i.d.
         >5 years old: 5 mg PO b.i.d. or t.i.d

        ii. Available
           Tablet: 5 mg
           Syrup: 5 mg/5 mL
    d. Interrupt radiation therapy only for gross hematuria.

II. LATE EFFECTS

A. Fertility
    1. Female
        a. Preservation of ovarian function
           i. Dose dependent: About 500 cGy seems to be enough to sterilize adult women.
           ii. Age dependent: Younger girls have a better chance of preservation of function at a given dose.
        b. Prevention
        Ovarian transposition and marking with metallic clips to place ovaries outside of the radiation field will allow the radiation oncologist to verify their location.
        c. Treatment
        Cryopreservation of oocytes is under investigation.
    2. Male
        a. Preservation of testicular function is dose dependent.
        b. Hormone function is less sensitive than fertility. Total body irradiation (TBI) will not damage hormone function, but the addition of testicular irradiation to TBI probably will.
        c. Oligospermia or azoospermia may recover after 18–24 months.
        d. Consider sperm banking when radiation therapy is planned to or near testes.
    3. Treatment for endocrine dysfunction from gonadal radiation
        a. If gonadal damage is expected, screen gonadotropins and sex hormones regularly after the age of expected puberty is reached.
        b. Monitor growth velocity and total growth closely.
        c. Recommend early endocrine consult.
        d. Give hormonal replacement as indicated.
B. Radiation enteritis
    1. Etiology
        a. Dose and volume dependent
        b. Vascular damage

      c. Risk increased by diabetes and underlying bowel disease

      d. Risk increased by prior abdominal surgery

  2. Presentation

      a. Diarrhea, bloody stool

      b. Small bowel obstruction

      c. Fistulization

  3. Treatment

      a. For diarrhea

        Consume a low-fat, low-residue, gluten-, cow's milk protein-, and lactose-free diet.

      b. For bleeding

         i. Rest bowel.

        ii. Consider photocoagulation or laser coagulation of telangiectatic, bleeding vessels.

       iii. Consider temporary colostomy.

       iv. Removal of bleeding segment of bowel is last resort.

      c. For small bowel obstruction

         i. Rest bowel completely.

        ii. Consider surgical bypass.

      d. For fistulization

         i. Rule out recurrence of tumor.

        ii. Consider surgical repair.

C. Chronic radiation cystitis

  1. Prevention

    Give radiation treatments when the patient has a full bladder, if possible, to minimize the volume of bladder wall treated.

  2. Presentation

    Chronic radiation cystitis is an infrequent late complication secondary to telangiectasia of blood vessels and can cause hemorrhagic cystitis with dysuria and frequency; at cystoscopy, telangiectatic mucosa is found.

  3. Treatment

      a. Hydrate to ensure good urine flow and observe to be certain the outlet is not obstructed.

      b. As conservative management, acidify the urine with cranberry juice or vitamin C until the pH is ≤ 6.

      c. Consider hyperbaric oxygen therapy.

      d. Consider installation of formalin or acetylcysteine solutions.

      e. Cystectomy is the last resort.

Side Effects of Total Body Irradiation

Total body irradiation is used only as a component of transplant preparative regimens, before bone marrow transplantation or peripheral stem cell infusion. The early side effects are managed by the transplant team as part of the acute effects of the total regimen. For the management of specific side effects felt to be due to radiation therapy, see the relevant section of this chapter.

The late side effects are covered in Chapter 17.

Bibliography

Bhatia S, Robison LL, Oberlin O, et al.: Breast cancer and other second neoplasms after childhood Hodgkin's disease. *N Engl J Med* 334:745–94, 1996.

Budtz-Jorgensen E: Etiology, pathogenesis, therapy and prophylaxis of oral yeast infections. *Acta Odontol Scand* 48:61–69, 1990.

Green, DM: *Long-Term Complications of Therapy for Cancer in Childhood and Adolescence.* Baltimore: Johns Hopkins University Press; 1989.

Haie-Meder C, Mlike-Cabanne N, Michel G, et al.: Radiotherapy after ovarian transposition: ovarian function and fertility preservation. *Int J Radiat Oncol Biol Phys* 25:419–24, 1993.

Halpern, EC, Constine LS, Tarbell NJ, Kun LE: Late effects of cancer treatment. In *Pediatric Radiation Oncology.* 2nd ed. New York: Raven Press; 1994.

Horning SJ, Adhikari A, Rizk N, et al.: Effect of treatment for Hodgkin's disease on pulmonary function: Results of a prospective study. *J Clin Oncol* 12:297–305, 1994.

Littley MD, Shalet SM, Beardwell CG: Radiation and the hypothalamic pituitary axis. In Gutin PH, Leibel SA, Sheline GE, eds. *Radiation Injury to the Nervous System.* New York: Raven Press; 1991.

Mulhern RK, Ochs J, Jun LE: Changes in intellect associated with cranial radiation therapy. in Gutin PH, Leibel SA, Sheline GE, eds. *Radiation Injury to the Nervous System.* New York: Raven Press; 1991.

Parson JT, Bova FJ, Fitzgerald CR, et al.: Tolerance of the visual apparatus to conventional therapeutic irradiation. *Radiation Injury to the Nervous System.* In Gutin PH, Leibel SA, Sheline GE, eds. New York: Raven Press; 1991.

Sher ME, Bauer J: Radiation induced enteropathy. *Am J Gastroenterol* 85:121–28, 1990.

Simon AR, Roberts MW: Management of oral complications associated with cancer therapy in pediatric patients. *ASDC J Dent Child* 58:384–9, 1991.

10

Chemotherapy-Induced Nausea and Vomiting

Donna L. Betcher, R.N., M.S.N., P.N.P.,
Darryl C. Grendahl, B.Pharm.,
Gina Cavalieri, R.Pharm., and
Ruth Daller, R.N., M.S.

Nausea and vomiting associated with cancer treatment remain important concerns for patients and medical personnel. Although new drugs have been developed, which have improved the quality of life for many patients, we continue to fail dismally for some.

The management of nausea and vomiting is complicated by the complex sequence of visceral and somatic events coordinated by a vomiting center in the medulla. The vomiting center may be stimulated through drugs, pathologic conditions, or radiation. Cortical stimulation can be affected by psychic factors such as unpleasant scenes or odors (e.g., the oncology clinic). Motion, nausea, and gastrointestinal irritation can also contribute to this complex problem.

Poor control of nausea and vomiting can lead to dehydration, electrolyte abnormalities, and the need for hospital admission to correct these problems.

I. COMMON ANTIEMETIC AGENTS

A. Phenothiazines
   Phenothiazines are commonly used antiemetic drugs that depress the chemoreceptor trigger zone (CTZ) and vomiting

center by blocking dopamine. They may cause extrapyramidal reactions. Administer diphenhydramine concurrently and for 24 hours after they are stopped to prevent extrapyramidal reactions.

1. Promethazine (Phenergan)
   a. Dosage
      i. Children: 0.25–0.5 mg/kg per dose or 7.5–15.0 mg/m^2 q6–8h prn
      ii. Adults: 12.5–25.0 mg q4–6h prn
   b. Preparations
      i. Vial: 25 or 50 mg/mL
      ii. Tablet: 12.5, 25, or 50 mg
      iii. Syrup: 6.5 or 25 mg/5 mL
      iv. Suppository: 12.5, 25, or 50 mg
2. Prochlorperazine (Compazine)
   a. Dosage
      i. Children >9 kg: 0.13 mg/kg intramuscular (IM).
      ii. Children >2 years: 0.1 mg/kg per dose q8–12h (maximum 15 mg/day)
      iii. Adults: 5–10 mg by mouth (PO) t.i.d. or q.i.d; 25 mg b.i.d.; 5–10 mg IM q3–4h (maximum 40 mg/day)
   b. Preparations
      i. Vial: 5 mg/mL
      ii. Spansule: 10, 15, or 30 mg (timed-released and dosed q12h)
      iii. Tablet: 5, 10, or 25 mg
      iv. Syrup: 5 mg/mL
      v. Suppository: 2.5, 5, or 25 mg
3. Chlorpromazine (Thorazine)
   a. Dose
      i. Children >6 months: 0.5 mg/kg (IM) or intravenous (IV) q6–8h; IV infusion at a rate of 0.5 mg/min IM maximum dose
      ii. Children <5 years: 40 mg/day
      iii. Children 5–12 years: 75 mg/day
      iv. Adults: 50–100 mg q6–8h (maximum 300 mg/day)
   b. Preparations
      i. Vial: 25 mg/mL
      ii. Spansule: 30, 75, 150, 200, or 300 mg
      iii. Tablet: 10, 25, 50, 100, or 200 mg
      iv. Liquid concentrate: 30 or 100 mg/mL

      v. Syrup: 10 mg/5 mL
      vi. Suppository: 25 or 100 mg

B. Serotonin antagonists
Serotonin antagonists work peripherally on the vagal nerve terminals and centrally on the CTZ of the area postrema. Serotonin (HT3) antagonists do not cause sedation and only rarely cause an extrapyramidal reaction. Headache and diarrhea are the most frequent side effects. HT3 antagonists work best for acute emesis and are less effective for multiple-day therapy. HT3 antagonists are not as effective in the pediatric population as with adults; however, they have become an important part of antiemetic management for children with cancer.
1. Ondansetron (Zofran)
   a. Dosage: 0.15 mg/kg IV or PO 30 minutes before and 4 and 8 hours after chemotherapy or a one-time dose of 0.45 mg/kg IV 30 minutes before chemotherapy
   b. Preparation
     i. Vial: 2 mg/mL, 20 mL multiple-dose vial
     ii. Tablet: 4 or 8 mg
2. Granisetron (Kytril)
   a. Dose: 10 µg/kg IV 30 minutes before chemotherapy
   b. Preparation
     i. Vial: 1 mg single-use vial
     ii. Tablet: 1 mg

C. Metoclopramide (Reglan)
Metoclopramide has both central (blocks the CTZ by blocking dopamine) and peripheral (accelerates gastric emptying) actions. In high doses, metoclopramide blocks serotonin receptors similar to the HT3 antagonists. Metoclopramide causes extrapyramidal reactions; administer diphenhydramine concurrently and for 24 hours after metoclopramide is stopped to prevent extrapyramidal reactions.
1. Dose: children: 1–2 mg/kg IV or PO 15–30 minutes before and 2, 4, 7, 10, and 13 hours after chemotherapy
2. Preparation
   a. Vial: 5 mg/mL
   b. Tablet: 10 mg
   c. Syrup: 5 mg/mL

D. Corticosteroids
The mechanism of antiemetic action is unknown.

Dexamethasone (Decadron)
1. Dose: children: <3 years = 2 mg, 3–5 years = 4 mg, 5–10 years = 6 mg, >10 years = 8 mg IV, 30 minutes before chemotherapy
2. Preparation
   a. Vial: 4, 10, 20, or 24 mg/mL
   b. Tablet: 0.25, 0.5, 0.75, 1, 1.5, 2, 4, or 6 mg
   c. Syrup: 0.5 mg/mL

E. Benzodiazepines
Benzodiazepines have no antiemetic effect but cause antegrade amnesia. They should always be used with an antiemetic.
1. Lorazepan (Ativan)
   a. Dose
      i. Children: 0.04 mg/kg per dose PO or IV q6h (maximum dose 2 mg)
      ii. Adults: 2–3 mg divided in 2 or 3 doses (maximum 10 mg/day)
   b. Preparation
      i. Vial: 2 or 4 mg/mL
      ii. Tablet: 0.5, 1, or 2 mg
2. Diazepam (Valium)
   a. Dose
      i. Children: 0.2 mg/kg IM or IV q6h (maximum 0.6 mg/kg per day in 3 or 4 divided doses)
      ii. Adults: 2–10 mg per dose b.i.d. to q.i.d.
   b. Preparation
      i. Vial: 5 mg/mL
      ii. Tablet: 2, 5, or 10 mg
      iii. Liquid: 5 mg/mL

F. Butyrophenones
Butyrophenones depress the CTZ. They cause extrapyramidal reactions and hypotension. Administer diphenhydramine concurrently and for 24 hours after they are stopped to prevent extrapyramidal reactions.
Droperidol (Inapsine)
1. Dose
   a. Children: 0.05–0.06 mg/kg per dose IM or IV q6h prn
   b. Children >12 years: 2.5–5 mg per dose q3–4h
2. Preparation
   a. Ampule: 2.5 mg/mL

     b. Vial: 2.5 mg/mL

G. Antihistamines

Antihistamines may block labyrinthine impulses to the CTZ and, in the case of diphenhydramine, decrease the toxicity of phenothiazines, metoclopramide, and butyrophenones by preventing or treating extrapyramidal reactions. They should be used concurrently with phenothiazines, metoclopramide, and butyrophenones.

  1. Diphenhydramine (Benadryl)
    a. Dose
      i. Children: 5 mg/kg/day PO or IV q6h or 1 mg/kg per dose; not for newborns.
      ii. Adults: 25–50 mg per dose q4–6h
    b. Preparation
      i. Vial: 10 or 50 mg/mL
      ii. Capsule: 25 or 50 mg
      iii. Tablet: 25 or 50 mg
      iv. Elixir: 12.5 mg/5 mL
  2. Trimethobenzamide (Tigan)
    a. Dose
      i. Children: 15–20 mg/kg per day PO/per rectum (PR) in 3 or 4 divided doses or 400–500 mg/m^2 in 3 or 4 divided doses; not recommended IM
      ii. Adults: 200 mg IM t.i.d. or q.i.d. 200–250 mg PO/PR t.i.d. or q.i.d.
    b. Preparation
      i. Injection: 100 mg/mL
      ii. Capsule: 100 or 250 mg
      iii. Suppository: 100 or 200 mg

H. Cannabinoids

Δ-Tetrahydrocannabinol is thought to exert an antiemetic effect by causing cetntral nervous system depression. Side effects include drowsiness, dizziness, and euphoria.

Dronabinol (Marinol)

  1. Dose
    a. Children: no data available
    b. Adults: start at 5 mg/m^2 1–3 hours before chemotherapy, then 5 mg/m^2 q2–4h (can increase by increments of 2.5 mg/m^2 up to 15 mg/m^2)
  2. Preparation: capsule: 2.5, 5, or 10 mg

II. MANAGEMENT OF CHEMOTHERAPY-INDUCED NAUSEA AND VOMITING

It is very important to attempt an aggressive plan at the start of therapy to prevent or minimize the initial experience of nausea, since there is a greater chance of preventing the development of anticipatory nausea and vomiting. *Never* give suppositories to neutropenic patients (always use them with discretion). See Figure 10.1.

FIGURE 10.1.
An algorithm for antiemetic treatment.

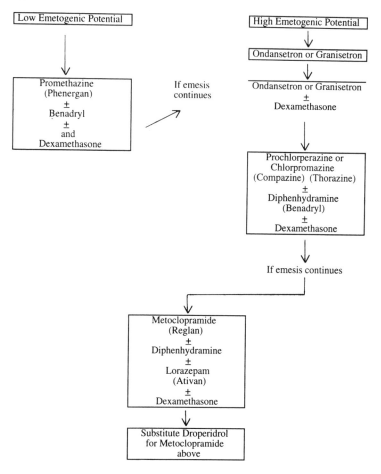

A. Drug combinations
Two or more classes of drug may be combined to optimize effectiveness (e.g., ondansetron and dexamethasone or metoclopramide, lorazepam, and diphenylhydramine).

B. Timing
Therapy must be started before chemotherapy and be continuous and individualized for each patient, depending on duration and intensity, chemotherapeutic agents, and the patient's age and psychological status.

C. Route of administration
The route of administration can be oral or intravenous. Serotonin antagonists are 65–70% absorbed when taken orally. Oral administration may be the preferred route. If the patient is unable to take oral medication, administer intravenously. Avoid rectal use whenever possible.

D. Duration
The duration of antiemetic treatment depends on the schedule of chemotherapy, expected delayed effect, and patient response. Continue diphenylhydramine at least 24 hours after phenothiazines, butyrophenones, and metoclopramide have been stopped.

E. Prevention and treatment of anticipatory or delayed vomiting
Behavioral techniques are required for anticipatory nausea and vomiting in addition to antiemetics. Some effective interventions have been: behavioral modification, guided imagery, hypnosis, and distraction. A careful history is important and an individualized self-care or assisted care plan can be especially effective for the preadolescent and adolescent populations.
  1. Benzodiazepines
     a. Diazepam (Valium)
     b. Lorazepam (Ativan)
  2. Behavior modification
     a. Hypnosis
     b. Relaxation
     c. Psychotherapy

III. THE RELATIVE EMETOGENIC POTENTIALS OF ANTINEOPLASTIC AGENTS

A. Classification according to frequency

Classification of emetogenic potential is based on the percentage of patients who experience nausea and vomiting after the chemotherapy without appropriate antiemetics and the number of times it occurs (Table 10.1).

1. *Low* emetogenic potential: <10% of the patients have any nausea and vomiting.
2. *Moderate* emetogenic potential: 50% of the patients will be nauseated and vomit several times.
3. *High* emetogenic potential: 100% of the patients will be nauseated and vomit more than 10 times.

B. Classification according to timing when it occurs
1. Anticipatory nausea and vomiting occur before the patient receives the chemotherapeutic agent.
   a. May be triggered by psychosocial/environmental factors
   b. Occurs more frequently if there was poor control of emesis after previous chemotherapy
2. Acute nausea and vomiting occurs 2–3 hours after chemotherapy is administered.
   a. Usually peaks 4–10 hours after the start of administration of chemotherapy and lasts 12–24 hours
   b. Usually associated with the more severe types of emesis
3. Delayed nausea and vomiting may occur from 1 to several days after chemotherapy is administered.
   a. Usually peaks 2–3 days after the administration of chemotherapy
   b. Often associated with less severe emesis

IV. NUTRITIONAL SUGGESTIONS TO MINIMIZE NAUSEA AND VOMITING

Regardless of what pharmacologic intervention is undertaken to prevent nausea and vomiting, reinforce common sense with caretakers regarding food intake.

A. Try foods such as:
1. Clear liquids/ice chips.
2. Toast, crackers, and pretzels.
3. Sherbet, yogurt.
4. Fruits and vegetables that are soft or bland.
5. Baked/broiled skinless chicken.
6. Angel food cake.

TABLE 10.1.
The Relative Emetogenic Potentials of Antineoplastic Drugs

Emetogenic Potential	Drug
High (90–100%)	Actinomycin D
	Cisplatin
	Cyclophosphamide (high dose)
	Cyclophosphamide/total body irradiation
	Cytarabine (high dose)
	Dacarbazine
	Melphalan/total body irradiation
	Methotrexate (high dose)
	Nitrogen mustard
	Nitrosoureas
	Pentostatin
	Streptozocin
Moderate (50%)	L-Asparaginase
	5-Azacytidine
	Busulfan/cyclophosphamide
	Carboplatin
	Cyclophosphamide (low dose)
	Cytarabine (low dose)
	Daunorubicin
	Doxorubicin
	Etoposide
	5-Fluorouracil
	Idarubicin
	Ifosfamide
	Methotrexate (low dose)
	Mitomycin C
	Polyethylene-glycolated asparaginase
	Procarbazine
	Tenoposide
	Thiotepa
	Vinorelbine
Low (<10%)	Bleomycin
	Chlorambucil
	Cladribine
	Fludarabine
	Melphalan PO
	Mercaptopurine IV and PO
	Taxol
	Thioguanine
	Vinblastine
	Vincristine

B. Avoid foods that are:
1. Fatty, greasy, or fried.
2. Spicy hot.
3. Characterized by strong odors

C. Try the following positive ideas.
1. Eat small amounts frequently, and avoid overeating.
2. Offer liquids throughout the day except at mealtime.
3. Serve beverages chilled.
4. Serve foods at room temperature or cooler; hot foods may add to nausea.
5. Avoid serving food 1–2 hours before chemotherapy or radiation treatments.

Bibliography

Berard CM, Mahoney C: Cost-reducing treatment algorithms for antineoplastic drug-induced nausea and vomiting. *Am J Health Syst Pharm* 52:1885–1997, 1995.

Sallan SE, Billet AL: Management of nausea and vomiting. In Pizzo PA, Poplack DG, eds.: *Principles and Practice of Pediatric Oncol.* Third Ed. Philadelphia: JB Lippincott; 1201-1208, 1997.

The Children's Hospital of Philadelphia. *Clinical Care Guidelines for Nutrition and Pediatric Oncology.* Philadelphia; July 1995.

Dilly S: Are granisetron and ondansetron equivalent in the clinic? *Eur J Cancer Clin Oncol* 28A (1 Suppl):S32–S35, 1992.

Gebbia V, Cannata G, Testa A, et al.: Ondansetron versus granisetron in the prevention of chemotherapy-induced nausea and vomiting. *Cancer* 74:1945–52, 1994.

Hesketh PJ, Harvey WH, Beck TM, et al.: A randomized, double-blind comparison of intravenous ondansetron alone and in combination with intravenous dexamethasone in the prevention of nausea and vomiting associated with high dose cisplatin (abstract). *Proc Am Soc Clin Oncol* 12:433, 1993.

Jurgens H, McQuade B: Ondansetron as prophylaxis for chemotherapy and radiotherapy-induced emesis in children. *Oncology* 49:279–85, 1992.

Navari RM, Madajewski S, Anderson N, et al.: Oral ondansetron for the control of cisplatin-induced delayed emesis: A large, multicenter, double-blind, randomized comparative trial of ondansetron versus placebo. *J Clin Oncol* 13:2408–16, 1995.

U.S. Department of Health and Human Services, Public Health Service, National Institutes of Health: *Eating Hints, Recipes, and Tips for Better Nutrition During Cancer Treatment.* Publication 92-2079, July 1992.

U.S. Department of Health and Human Services, Public Health Service, National Institutes of Health: *Managing Your Child's Eating Problems During Cancer Treatment.* Publication 92-2038; December 1991.

Van Hoff J, Hockenberry-Eaton MJ, Patterson K, et al.: A survey of antiemetic use in children with cancer. *Am J Dis Child* 145:773– 78, 1991.

11

The Management of Pain

Arnold J. Altman, M.D., Neil L. Schechter, M.D., and Steven J. Weisman, M.D.

Most children with cancer will be at risk for significant pain at some time during the course of their illness. Pain may be a product of the disease itself or the result of medical intervention in the form of diagnostic procedures, surgery, chemotherapy, or radiation therapy. An adequate standard of care requires that pain be systematically assessed and effectively managed on a routine basis for all children with cancer.

I. THE ETIOLOGY OF PAIN IN CHILDHOOD CANCER

Pain in childhood cancer has a number of possible etiologies. Because the epidemiology of childhood cancer is different from that of adult cancer, the pain experiences of children are different from those of adults. Pain in children with cancer can be from one or more of the following categories: 1) cancer related; 2) procedure related; 3) treatment related; and 4) another etiology, unrelated to the cancer or its treatment. In children, unlike adults, the majority of cancer pain is caused by procedures and treatments, with far less stemming from the disease itself. Many pediatric malignancies are both rapidly progressing and rapidly responding diseases. Thus, the patterns of pain seen in children are very different from those seen in adults, in whom chronic pain related to metastasis or neuroplexopathies predominates. Because most children have more than one type of pain, a pain problem list is often helpful.

A. Cancer-related pain
1. Bone pain is most common; it may be generalized, as in leukemia, or localized to specific sites, as in bony metastases.
2. Compression of central or peripheral nervous system structures is relatively common (e.g., headache from increased intracranial pressure or back pain associated with compression of the spinal cord).
3. Organ invasion or viscus obstruction causes disease-related pain.

B. Procedure-related pain
1. For many children, procedure-related pain is the most feared aspect of the disease
2. Pain ranges in severity from the significant pain associated with bone marrow aspirations and lumbar punctures to the milder pain associated with venipuncture, venous cannulation, and reservoir access.

C. Treatment-related pain
1. Chemotherapy-related pain
   a. Mucositis
   b. Peripheral neuropathy
   c. Aseptic necrosis of bone
   d. Steroid-induced myopathy
2. Radiation therapy-related pain
   a. Mucositis
   b. Radionecrosis
   c. Myelopathy
   d. Brachial/lumbar plexopathies
   e. Peripheral nerve tumors
3. Postsurgical pain
   a. Acute postoperative pain
   b. Postthoracotomy pain
   c. Postamputation pain

D. Pain unrelated to cancer
1. The diagnosis of cancer does not make a child immune to the other pain problems that children experience.
2. Pain associated with trauma, with traditional childhood illnesses such as otitis and pharyngitis, and with common recurrent pain syndromes such as migraine and recurrent abdominal pain syndrome are as likely to occur in children with cancer as in the general population.

II. MANAGEMENT OF PAIN ASSOCIATED WITH DIAGNOSTIC PROCEDURES

One of the goals of pain management during pediatric procedures is to make the child comfortable so that the child (and parents) will not dread the subsequent procedures. Thus, success is not a matter of merely restraining the child sufficiently to allow the procedure to be performed. Consider measures to control pain and anxiety an integral part of patient management. It is imperative that aggressive pain management be part of the initial diagnostic evaluation, since this may help prevent future difficulties with these and other procedures.

A. General principles
   1. In general, avoid unnecessary tests.
   2. Consolidate blood work so that all necessary studies are obtained at the same time; use central lines when possible.
   3. Persons performing a procedure should have a documented level of skill, and there must be appropriate supervision of less-experienced operators.

B. Environment
   1. Major procedures (e.g., bone marrow aspiration, lumbar puncture) should never be performed in the patient's bed.
   2. The environment of the treatment room should be relatively calm.
   3. Encourage a parent (or parent substitute) to attend the procedure and to participate actively in assisting the child. Do not demand that the parent restrain the child in any way. Instead, the parent should provide comfort or lead the child in any of a variety of distracting behavioral interventions.

C. Behavior management
   1. Use age-appropriate behavior management techniques. For infants, this may include stroking, swaddling, or use of a pacifier. Older children may be managed with distraction, story telling, bubble blowing, or hypnosis.
   2. A full review of these techniques is beyond the scope of this chapter but may be found in McGrath (1990).

D. Sedation
   Follow the standards for administering, monitoring, and documenting conscious sedation as developed by the American Academy of Pediatrics or the American Society of Anesthe-

siology (see Bibliography). Patients should have nothing by mouth (NPO) for clear liquids at least 2 hours before the procedure and NPO for solid foods at least 4–6 hours before the procedure. There must be a time-based record that documents vital signs and the level of sedation at appropriate intervals. Monitor all patients for pulse oximetry, blood pressure, heart rate, response to verbal command, and adequacy of pulmonary ventilation. Electrocardiogram (ECG) monitoring may be indicated for patients with significant cardiovascular disease.

E. Pharmacologic intervention
Warning: Before administering a sedative or opioid agent, ensure the immediate availability of oxygen, naloxone, flumazenil, and resuscitative equipment for the maintenance of a patent airway and support of ventilation. Pulse, respiration, blood pressure, and pulse oximeter measurements should be monitored by a person specifically assigned to this task.

1. Age 0–6 months
   a. Apply local anesthesia with EMLA cream by occlusive dressing at least 1 hour before performing the procedure. Infiltration of the deeper tissues with 1% lidocaine is helpful. Buffering of lidocaine with NaHCO3 (9 parts lidocaine:1 part $NaHCO_3$ USP) may alleviate some of the burning discomfort associated with the lidocaine injection. For procedures performed without EMLA cream, use buffered 1% lidocaine for the skin as well as deeper structures. The dose of lidocaine should not exceed 5 mg/kg (0.5 mL/kg).
   b. Consider using a 22-gauge lumbar puncture needle for both bone marrow aspiration and lumbar puncture.
   c. The use of opioids and sedatives for conscious sedation with this age group may be difficult. If analgesia is deemed necessary, consider small doses of a single medication. Consider completing the procedure under general anesthesia or deep sedation by an anesthesiologist.

2. Age >6 months
   a. Apply local anesthesia with EMLA patch by occlusive dressing at least 1 hour before the procedure. This may be supplemented by infiltrating 1% lidocaine intradermally and subcutaneously (to the level of the perios-

teum for bone marrow procedures); the dose of lidocaine should not exceed 5 mg/kg (0.5 mL/kg).

b. With patients who do not have an established intravenous (IV) route and for whom an IV line would not
otherwise be indicated, try the oral route first. With
patients who already have an IV line in place, use intravenous sedation.

c. Use a combination of a sedative (for anxiety) and an
opioid (for analgesia) Sedatives alone are inadequate.

i. Sedative
Give midazolam (Versed) IV solution: 0.2–0.4 mg/kg
PO 20–30 minutes before the procedure or 0.05
mg/kg IV 3–4 minutes before the procedure. When
deemed appropriate, midazolam can also be administered rectally at a dose of 0.2–0.5 mg/kg 5–10 minutes before the procedure. If intravenous access is
available, half the original dose may be repeated if
the child is not adequately sedated when the procedure begins. When using midazolam (or other benzodiazepines), flumazenil (Romazicon), a benzodi-
azepine reversing agent, should be available; the
dose of flumazenil is 0.01 mg/kg (maximum dose 0.2
mg) by slow IV push.
and

ii. Opioid
Give fentanyl 0.001 mg/kg (1 µg/kg) IV over 1–2 minutes, 3–5 minutes before the procedure. Half the
original dose can be repeated if the child is not adequately sedated when the procedure begins.
or
Give morphine sulfate 0.15–0.2 mg/kg PO 20–30 minutes before the procedure or 0.05 mg/kg IV over 1–2
minutes, 10 minutes before the procedure begins.

d. Consider transmucosal fentanyl citrate (Fentanyl
Oralet).
This transmucosal opioid delivery system has been
shown to be useful as a single agent for painful procedures in children with cancer. The dose is 5–15 µg/kg
with the unit dose chosen closest to that to be administered (100, 200, 300, and 400 µg sizes). The unit dose is
sucked (must not be chewed) in the buccal pouch 15-
20 minutes before the procedure is to be performed.

Do not administer with anxiolytics or other opioids. In general, this is not useful in toddlers, who may not be able to cooperate by sucking the lozenge.

e. If efforts to produce conscious sedation are inadequate or if multiple painful procedures (e.g., bilateral bone marrow aspirations and biopsies) are to be performed, consider general anesthesia. Some clinicians advocate agents such as ketamine, propofol, and nitrous oxide as appropriate for use for conscious sedation in children undergoing painful procedures. All of these agents may best be used by anesthesiologists with specialized training in their administration and in appropriate support of the airway.

   i. Ketamine is a dissociative general anesthetic agent that has many well-known side effects that are potentially difficult to manage. These include hypersalivation, increased cerebral blood flow, disturbing hallucinations, and prolonged recovery periods.

   ii. Propofol is an intravenous diisopropylphenol general anesthetic agent that can easily result in loss of all protective reflexes, markedly decreases systemic vascular resistance, and can cause severe myocardial depression.

   iii. Nitrous oxide is a clear, odorless inhaled anesthetic agent that is analgesic as well as amnestic. It can be administered in oxygen and has been used for painful procedures as well as in emergency rooms. It can induce general anesthesia with loss of protective reflexes. In addition, it must be used with a dedicated scavenging system to prevent environmental contamination.

III. MANAGEMENT OF PAIN ASSOCIATED WITH DISEASE

As with all forms of pain, the management of pain in the child with cancer requires a thorough investigation to establish a specific etiology. In the pediatric oncology setting, pain may be due to tumor infiltration or invasion of a number of structures, including bone, soft tissues, viscera, and nerves. Pain may also reflect treatment-related toxicity (e.g., vincristine neuropathy) or complications (e.g., infection). Once the mechanism for the pain is identified, more effective specific (e.g., local radiotherapy) and systemic therapy may be offered. The mainstay of the treatment of pain due to refractory tumor is administering analgesic medications. Incorporate behavioral interventions into the pain treatment plan of disease-related cancer pain.

A. General principles of the use of analgesics
  1. When feasible, try the oral route first.
  2. The goal should be to provide a level of comfort that the patient finds satisfactory; the patient should be the judge of adequate analgesia.
  3. Tailor the dosages of opioid analgesics to the clinical effect, rather than excessively adhering to "standard doses." The "right" dose is that sufficient to achieve relief of pain without undue toxicity.
  4. Effective use of opioids requires careful attention to, and management of, side effects (e.g., pruritus, constipation, or dysphoria).
  5. A stepwise approach using the "analgesic ladder" and tailored to the patient's needs and wishes is a useful technique (Figure 11.1 and Table 11.1).

B. Pharmacologic management
  1. Mild pain
     a. Initial management involves the use of nonopioids.
        i. Acetaminophen (Tylenol)
           Suggested dosage is: 10–20 mg/kg PO q4h.
        ii. Nonsteroidal anti-inflammatory drugs (NSAIDs) are useful for patients with bone pain (when the antiplatelet effect of NSAIDs is not contraindicated; e.g., the terminally ill patient). Frequently used agents include ibuprofen (Motrin) (5–10 mg/kg PO q6h), naproxen (Naprosyn) (5–7 mg/kg PO b.i.d. or t.i.d.), and tolmetin sodium (Tolectin) (5–7 mg/kg PO t.i.d. or q.i.d.). All can cause gastritis and are best administered with meals. Ketorolac (Toradol) is a commonly used NSAID currently approved for parenteral use. The dose for children is 0.5 mg/kg IV q6h. Choline magnesium salicylate (Trilisate) (10–15 mg/kg PO t.i.d. or q.i.d.) appears to have minimal effect on the bleeding time and causes relatively little gastritis.
     b. If pain is not relieved by the higher range of recommended doses, consider adding opioids or other modalities.

FIGURE 11.1.
An algorithm for the management of pediatric cancer pain

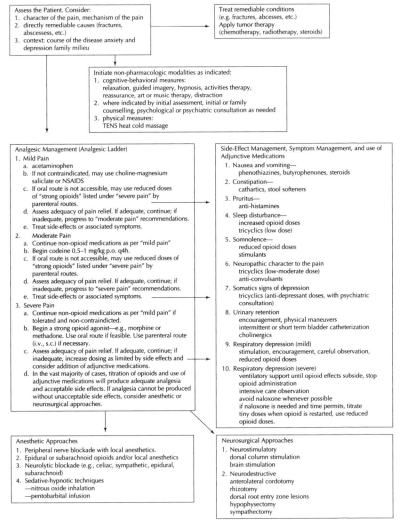

Source: Ideno, in Gottschlich, Matarese, and Shronts 1993, p. 83.

2. Moderate pain
   a. Continue acetaminophen (or NSAID).
   b. If pain is not controlled with the above, add a weak opioid (e.g., codeine). A standard starting dose of codeine is 0.5–1.0 mg/kg PO q4h; this may be increased to 1–2 mg/kg q4h.

TABLE 11.1.
Recommended Starting Doses for Analgesic Medications*

Medication	Dose (mg/kg)	Route	Schedule
Nonsteroidal anti-inflammatory drugs			
Acetaminophen	10–20	PO	q4h
(Tylenol)	15–20	PR	q4h
Choline-magnesium			
salicylate (Trilisate)	10–15	PO	q6–8h
Ibuprofen (Motrin)	5–10	PO	q6h
Ketorolac (Toradol)	0.5	IV	q6h
Opioids			
Codeine	0.5–1	PO	q4h
Fentanyl	0.001–0.002	IV	q1–2h
	(1–2 µg/kg)		
	0.002–0.004	IV	qh continuous infusion
	(2–4 µg/kg)		
Hydromorphone	0.02	IV	q3–4h
(Dilaudid)	0.1	PO	q4h
Methadone	0.1	IV	q6h × 2–3 doses; then q8–12h
	0.2	PO	q6–8h
Morphine	0.08–0.1	IV	q2–3h
	0.03–0.05	IV	qh continuous infusion
	0.2–0.4	PO	q4h
Morphine (MS Contin)	0.3–0.6	PO	q12h long acting; tablets should be taken whole and not broken, chewed or crushed
Oxycodone	0.15	PO	q4h
Adjuvants			
Amitriptyline (Elavil)	0.1–0.2	PO	qday at bedtime; advance to 0.5–2.0 mg/kg/day
Nortriptyline	0.1–0.2	PO	qday at bedtime; advance to 1.0–3.0 mg/kg/day
Methylphenidate (Ritalin)	0.1–0.2	PO	b.i.d.; slowly advance dose as tolerated
Dextroamphetamine (Dexadrine)	0.1–0.2	PO	qdose; slowly advance dose as tolerated

* For all medications, dosages should be modified based on individual circumstances. Many of these agents have not yet received specific approval for infants and younger children. Certain doses are based upon extrapolation from adult doses or from unpublished experience. For nonintubated infants aged 4 months or less, initial opioid doses should be reduced to $\frac{1}{3}$ to $\frac{1}{4}$ of the recommended doses. Opioids should be administered with the patient in a location that permits close observation and immediate intervention. For the management of severe ongoing acute or chronic pain, opioid doses should be increased until comfort is achieved or until side effects prohibit further dose escalation.

    c. If pain is not ameliorated, codeine may be replaced by a stronger agent, such as oxycodone (Roxicodone) 0.2 mg/kg q3–4h, oxycodone/acetaminophen (Percocet), or morphine (see below). A controlled-release preparation of oxycodone (Oxycontin) is also available, although its use in children is limited by their weight.

3. Severe pain

    a. Continue acetaminophen (or NSAID) in conjunction with a strong opioid.

    b. Morphine is the first-line opioid in most settings. The oral dose of 0.3 mg/kg q4h can be started.

      i. Time-released tablets (MS Contin) are convenient for patients who can swallow them. The recommended starting dose is 0.3–0.6 mg/kg PO q12h, but should be determined by the total amount of short-acting morphine required to achieve comfort. Methadone is also an effective long-acting agent that has the advantage of being prepared in liquid and tablet forms.

      ii. If the oral route is not feasible, continuous IV or subcutaneous (SC) infusions are effective.

      iii. Continuous morphine infusion (Table 11.2) is the preferred means of providing analgesia. Note that Table 11.2 describes a "bolus/raised rate" method for infants under 6 months (corrected age) and for all children over 6 months. This bolus/raised rate, increasing the rate by 10–15%, can be repeated every 1–2 hours until the pain is relieved. Each time the dose is increased, pain assessments and vital signs should be done every 30 minutes for 2 hours, followed by a return to assessments every 2 hours.

      iv. Patient-controlled analgesia (PCA) is also available for children of an appropriate age. Although its use has been described in children as young as 5 years of age, most children should be 7–8 years of age in order to be able to cognitively understand the mechanism of action of PCA. It can be used with a background continuous infusion. PCA is often started at a dose of 0.01–0.02 mg/kg q6–10 minutes with or without a basal infusion at 0.01–0.02 mg/kg/h. Consultation with an anesthesiologist or a pain service may be required.

TABLE 11.2.
The Management of Pediatric Pain with Morphine

Patient	Initial Bolus	Continuous Infusion	Repeat Bolus	How to Increase Patient Comfort			Other Issues
				Increase Continuous Infusion	Discontinue morphine Infusion*		
Infants <6 months old (corrected age)	0.03 mg/kg over 30 min	0.01–0.02 mg/kg/h min	0.02 mg/kg/h over 30	Increase rate by 10–15%	Decrease IV by 50%, add acetaminophen with codeine 0.2–0.4 mg/kg		1. Narcan at bedside with syringe and needle; respiratory depression/arrest dose 0.1 mg/kg
All children >6 months old corrected age	0.08–0.1 mg/kg over 30 min	0.04–0.05 mg/kg/h	0.05 mg/kg over 30 min	Increase rate by 10–15%	Decrease IV by 50%, add acetaminophen with codeine 0.5–1.0 mg/kg PO q4h or morphine 0.2 mg/kg PO q4h		2. Vital signs† q30 min for first 2 hours, then respiratory rate and sedation scale q12h
							3. If bolus given or rate increased, vital signs q30min × 4
							4. IV access at all times
							5. Pulse oximeter recommended, especially for children <6 months (corrected age)
							6. Bag, mask 0₂ setup, and tubing readily available on the floor.

*Usually 24 to 72 hours postoperatively, begin weaning IV medications and begin PO medications.
†Vital signs include heart rate, respiratory rate, and blood pressure.

v. To change between short half-life opioids, start the new opioid at 50% of equianalgesic dose. Titrate to the desired effect. To change from a short to a long half-life opioid (i.e., morphine to methadone), start at 25% of equianalgesic dose and titrate to the desired effect.

vi. It is necessary to taper opioids for any patient taking them for more than 1 week. Decrease the dose by 50% for 2 days; then taper by 25% q2 days. Opioid may be stopped when the dose is equianalgesic to an oral morphine dose of 0.3 mg/kg/day for patients <50 kg or 15 mg/day for patients >50 kg. Methadone is useful to wean patients off high-dose opioids.

c. Consider use of transdermal fentanyl.

i. The transdermal route allows for the continuous administration of fentanyl at one of four different dosing strengths (25, 50, 75, and 100 μg/h). Steady state is reached 8–12 hours after the patch is applied.

ii. Because this patch comes in only four sizes, it has limited applicability for children who are opiate naive, as they would receive excessive opiate, even with the smallest patch. Its use is not recommended for children under 12 years of age.

iii. Consider the transdermal patch for patients with relatively stable pain who are unable to take medications by the oral route and for whom intravenous access is limited.

4. Neuropathic pain (e.g., "phantom limb," vincristine neuropathy, herpes zoster, burning sensation)

a. Tricyclic antidepressants

i. Tricyclics have several uses in the management of children's cancer pain. Although classically regarded as best for pain of a burning character, many clinicians regard them as the agent of first choice for most forms of persistent or neuropathic pain.

ii. Tricylics are typically begun with a very small single daily dose an hour before bedtime. Amitriptyline (Elavil), imipramine (Tofranil), doxepin (Sinequan), and desipramine (Norpramin) have all been used. Starting dosages for amitriptyline and imipramine are 0.1–0.2 mg/kg at bedtime. The dose may be increased by 50% every 2–3 days up to 0.5–2.5 mg/kg at bedtime, although many patients will not tolerate the larger doses. Common side effects include dry mouth and somnolence; less common side effects, seen mostly with larger doses, are disorientation, urinary retention, constipation, and tachyarrhythmia. Hypertension may develop in patients with neuroblastoma. These side effects can frequently be managed by a temporary reduction and then a gradual increase in the dosage.

   iii. Use great caution in prescribing tricyclics for patients who have a history of palpitations or tachyarrhythmia or who have an increased risk of cardiac dysfunction (e.g., after the administration of anthracyclines). Carefully assess the effects of the medication on the ECG.

  b. Anticonvulsants

   i. Anticonvulsants are used for neuropathic pain, especially when it is of a shooting or stabbing character. Carbamazepine, phenytoin, and clonazepam have all been used. They are generally administered without initial loading, and dosages are advanced gradually until plasma levels lie in the therapeutic range used for seizure control or until limited by side effects (disorientation, somnolence, ataxia, gastrointestinal upset). Monitor patients regularly for hematologic, hepatic, or allergic reactions.

   ii. Gabapentin (Neurontin) is a new anticonvulsant agent that has been shown to have efficacy in treating neuropathic pain. Its safety and efficacy have not been established for children under 12 years old.

IV. MANAGEMENT OF POSTOPERATIVE PAIN

The goal of postoperative pain management is to keep the patient as comfortable as possible without compromising his or her safety. In addition to being more humane, adequate pain management will decrease hypoventilation and atelectasis secondary to splinting, allow increased patient mobility in the early postoperative period, and improve the patient's general well-being, which may have important immunologic and healing consequences.

A. General principles
   1. The medical, surgical, and nursing services should share the responsibility for patient comfort.
   2. Pain assessment is critical for good pain management; incorporate scheduled assessments, including bedside charting, into the pain plan.
   3. Pharmacologic management should use oral or intravenous routes; avoid intramuscular injections. Administer analgesics on a fixed schedule, not as needed.
   4. Behavioral approaches (distraction, hypnosis, and self-control techniques) have demonstrated efficacy; incorporate them into the care plan in conjunction with the child-life team and/or psychological providers.

B. Pharmacologic management
   The use of wound infiltration with local anesthetics by the surgeon, regional nerve blocks, or indwelling catheters for postoperative pain management is highly recommended. Epidural and regional plexus catheters can provide extremely effective and safe postoperative analgesia.
   1. Mild pain
      Examples might include the discomfort seen after the placement of a central line or after a simple biopsy of a superficial structure (lymph node).
      a. Oral analgesia
         Acetaminophen with codeine (1 mg/kg codeine) or NSAID (Table 11.1)
      b. Parenteral analgesia
         Morphine sulfate (0.08–0.1 mg/kg IV) q2–3h ± ketorolac (0.5 mg/kg) q6h
   2. Moderate and/or severe pain
      Examples might include appendectomy, incision and drainage of a deep abscess, complex orthopedic procedure, exploratory laparotomy, or thoracotomy.
      a. Regional analgesia
         Epidural or plexus catheters can be used to infuse local anesthetics with or without opioids. In some circumstances the anesthesiologist may use a single-shot technique, such as a single-shot caudal injection of bupivacaine and morphine. Alternatively, a single-shot axillary block may be placed. More commonly, an epidural catheter can be placed to permit bolus and

continuous-infusion delivery of low-dose solutions of opioids with or without local anesthetic.
  b. Parenteral analgesia
    i. Morphine infusions
        See Table 11.2 and Section IIIB3biii.
    ii. Patient-controlled analgesia
        See Section IIIB3biv.
    iii. Reassessment
        Carefully reassess all patients for pain on a regular basis to determine the need for continued infusion or PCA therapy. In general, with major surgical procedures, children will benefit from analgesia for 48–72 hours.
    iv. Discontinuing continuous morphine
        (1) Timing: Usual time to discontinue infusion is 48–72 hours after surgery if the patient is comfortable.
        (2) Transition to oral medications: Discontinue the infusion 30–60 minutes after an oral dose of acetaminophen with codeine or oral morphine.
        (3) If pain relief is inadequate on oral analgesics, resume intravenous therapy at previous doses.
        (4) Schedule oral analgesics around the clock or in a "reverse prn" fashion (the nurse checks and offers the analgesic for pain every 3–4 hours).
    v. Monitoring
        Record bedside charting of pain assessments along with respiratory rate and assess the level of sedation every 2 hours. Many clinicians will use continuous pulse oximetry for monitoring during continuous opioid therapy.
  3. Safety guidelines for the management of postoperative pain
    a. Naloxone (Narcan) should be readily available.
    b. Oxygen should be available at the bedside.
    c. For respiratory depression, see sections VB and VC.
    d. All continuous infusions should be delivered by infusion pump. Specific, easy-to-program pain-management pumps are available from several manufacturers.
    e. Infants under 6 months of age (corrected postgestational age) should be in a location that permits close observation and monitoring.

f. *Opioid doses in infants under 4 months of age must be reduced to $\frac{1}{3}$ to $\frac{1}{4}$ of the usual childhood doses.*

V. MANAGEMENT OF THE SIDE EFFECTS OF OPIOIDS

A. Somnolence
   1. Reduce opioid doses to the minimum required to produce adequate analgesia.
   2. Stimulants are useful in situations in which the administration of opioids is limited by somnolence.
      a. Both dextroamphetamine and methylphenidate have been shown to provide additive analgesia with a reduction in somnolence for patients with cancer. They are generally prescribed b.i.d., at morning and noon, in starting doses of 0.1–0.2 mg/kg. Evening dosing should be avoided because it may lead to sleep disturbances. After prolonged dosing, these medications should be tapered gradually to avoid withdrawal reactions.
      b. Dosing of stimulants in the fashion described above is preferred to premixed combinations (as in the Brompton cocktail), because of the importance of tailoring each component for the individual patient.
      c. Cocaine is not recommended, because of less evidence of analgesic effect and more evidence of dysphoric and toxic reactions.
      d. Caffeine has been advocated for use for analgesia in a similar fashion, and is a component of many proprietary headache remedies.
   3. If somnolence persists and is not desired by the patient, consider using regional analgesic techniques.

B. Respiratory depression
   Depression of respiration usually correlates reliably with the level of sedation, except in the very young infant.
   1. Constant monitoring of the patient is essential. When the patient is sleeping or left unattended, pulse oximetry can be used.
   2. For respiratory depression, full pharmacologic reversal is often not necessary. Administration of oxygen and reduction of the next dose of opioid may be all that is necessary. If the respiratory depression is more severe, support the airway, provide supplemental oxygen, and administer naloxone to the point of reversal of respiratory slowing

without compromising pain relief. It is important to recognize that rapid infusion of a large dose of naloxone can precipitate withdrawal, with the dramatic onset of severe pain and sympathetic instability in the child. Therefore, the naloxone dose should be 0.5–1 µg/kg q2min titrated to effect, provided that the patient is maintaining adequate oxygenation and ventilation.

C. Respiratory arrest
  1. Begin ventilatory assistance and call for help (code).
  2. Administer naloxone, 0.1 mg/kg IV, IM, or SC for infants and children under 5 years (or <20 kg). Older children (or those >20 kg) may be given 2 mg. Repeat in 1–5 minutes for 2 or 3 doses until effective. This can be repeated every hour as needed.
  3. Deliver 100% oxygen, support the airway, and closely monitor the patient. The effect of naloxone may not outlast the effect of the opioid and the patient may again become somnolent or apneic.

D. Nausea and vomiting
  Exclude primary conditions (e.g., bowel obstruction). Administer neuroleptics or, in certain cases, corticosteroids.
  1. Phenothiazines and butyrophenones are indicated in the treatment of nausea and vomiting. With the exception of methotrimeprazine (Levoprome), the neuroleptics provide little or no analgesia. They sedate and may mask the outward expression of pain more than they diminish the intensity of pain experienced. Commonly used agents include chlorpromazine (Thorazine) 0.15–0.5 mg/kg IV or PO q6h, perphenazine (Trilafon) 0.05–0.1 mg/kg IV or 0.1 mg/kg PO q6h, promethazine (Phenergan) 0.25 mg/kg q6h, and droperidol 0.01 mg/kg up to 0.625 mg q4–6h.
  2. The doses of these agents for the treatment of opioid-induced nausea appear to be much smaller (1/5 to 1/2 times) than those required to treat chemotherapy-induced nausea.
  3. Other antiemetics that are currently used for opioid-induced nausea and vomiting are metoclopramide (Reglan) 0.2 mg/kg PO or 0.1 mg/kg IV q6h, and ondansetron (Zofran) 0.1 mg/kg up to 4 mg q6h. Naloxone 0.001 mg/kg, if effective, can be administered by continuous infusion (see Section IIE).

E. Pruritus

Administer diphenhydramine (Benadryl) 0.5–1.0 mg/kg IV or PO q4–6h or naloxone 0.001 mg/kg q1–2 min for 2 or 3 doses until the effect is obtained. Naloxone can be successfully administered by continuous infusion after these doses. Infusions at 0.0005–0.001 mg/kg/h can successfully reverse the peripheral annoying side effects of the opioids without causing a reversal of the analgesic effects. In addition, trying another opioid, such as fentanyl, which does not release histamine, can be helpful with itching.

F. Urinary retention

Apply warm compresses over the bladder. The patient should ambulate, if possible. Patients who are adequately hydrated and have not voided in 8 hours and/or who begin to experience discomfort must be straight-catheterized. Some of these patients will require the placement of a urinary drainage catheter.

G. Constipation

Patients who receive opioids for more than 24 hours should be given a stool softener, such as Kondremul (1–2 teaspoons at night or b.i.d.), Senokot (1 pill or 1 teaspoon of granules) at bedtime, or Peri-Colace Syrup (1–3 teaspoons) at bedtime.

VI. NURSING RESPONSIBILITIES

A. General postoperative care

1. During the first 24–48 hours after surgery, it is very important to maintain a constant level of analgesia to provide pain relief for the patient. If a continuous infusion is not ordered, the nurse must make a special effort to offer and provide pain medications as needed. Assess the pain level at least every 4 hours and administer medications accordingly. Offering pain medications around the clock is often the best way to provide adequate pain relief.

2. Use nonpharmacologic interventions as appropriate. (If there is a concern whether an intervention is safe for a specific patient, check the patient's orders and, if there is still doubt, check with the physician.)

   a. Reposition the patient.

    b. Use basic comfort measures (e.g., blankets and closed curtains).

    c. Relieve thirst from dry mouth.

    d. Use distraction (e.g., television, movies, and music).

    e. Use parents and child life professionals to comfort the patient.

  3. If all of the above have been used and the patient is still in pain, then notify the appropriate physician.

B. Continuous infusion of opioids

  1. Assess and document the respiratory rate and level of sedation every $\frac{1}{2}$ hour when the infusion begins. If the assessments are stable after 2 hours, then assess the respiratory rate and the level of sedation every 2 hours. The acceptable respiratory rate for a given patient must be determined on an individual basis reflecting the patient's age and clinical status.

  2. If the rate of opioid is increased or a bolus is given, assess and document the respiratory rate and level of sedation (see below) every $\frac{1}{2}$ hour for 2 hours. If the assessments are stable after that time, then assess the respiratory rate and level of sedation every 2 hours.

  3. Sedation scale

    a. 0 = none: The patient is alert.

    b. 1 = mild: The patient is occasionally drowsy but easy to arouse.

    c. 2 = moderate: The patient is frequently drowsy and sleeping but still easy to arouse.

    d. 3 = severe: The patient is somnolent and difficult to arouse.

  4. If the patient's sedation level is 3, turn off the morphine drip (maintain IV access); stimulate and encourage the patient to breathe deeply; stay with the patient and have another nurse call the physician.

  5. If the rate of opioid is decreased, continue to assess and document the respiratory rate and level of sedation every 2 hours, but increase pain assessment to ensure that the patient is still receiving enough analgesic.

  6. If all of the above have been used and the patient is still in pain, notify the appropriate physician.

Bibliography

American Academy of Pediatrics, Committee on Drugs, Section on Anesthesiology: Guidelines for the elective use of conscious sedation, deep sedation, and general anesthesia in pediatric patients. *Pediatrics* 76:317–21, 1985.

American Academy of Pediatrics, Committee on Drugs: Emergency drug doses for doses for infants and children and naloxone use in newborns; clarification. *Pediatrics* 83:803, 1989.

American Academy of Pediatrics, Committee on Drugs: Guidelines for monitoring and management of pediatric patients during and after sedation for diagnostic and therapeutic procedures. *Pediatrics* 89:1110–15, 1992.

American Society of Anesthesiology, Task Force on Sedation and Analgesia by Non-Anesthesiologists: Practice guidelines for sedation and analgesia by non-anesthesiologists. *Anesthesiology* 84:459–71, 1996.

Berde C, et al.: Report of the Subcommittee on Disease-Related Pain in Childhood Cancer. *Pediatrics* 86, 1990 (suppl).

Cancer Pain Relief. Geneva, World Health Organization, 1996.

McGrath PA: *Pain in Children; Nature, Assessment and Treatment.* New York, Guilford Press; 1990.

Pediatric Cancer Pain Relief and Palliative Care. Geneva, World Health Organization; 1997 (in press).

Schecter, NL, Altman, AJ, Weisman SJ, eds. Report of the Consensus Conference on the Management of Pain in Childhood Cancer. *Pediatrics* 86, 1990 (suppl).

12

Oncologic Emergencies

Edythe A. Albano, M.D., and Arthur R. Ablin, M.D.

Pediatric oncologic emergencies arise as a result of space-occupying lesions, metabolic or hormonal derangements, and as a consequence of cytopenias. They can be the presenting feature of a new malignancy or can arise during treatment or recurrence. All these conditions are reversible if recognized and treated appropriately in a timely manner.

I. METABOLIC COMPLICATIONS

 A. Tumor lysis syndrome
  1. Overview
   a. Acute tumor lysis syndrome is a consequence of the rapid release of intracellular metabolites (uric acid, potassium, and phosphorus) in quantities that exceed the excretory capacity of the kidneys.
   b. Renal failure and hypocalcemia are common complications.
  2. Etiology
   a. Tumor lysis syndrome is seen in tumors that have a high growth fraction and that are exquisitely sensitive to chemotherapy.
   b. Burkitt lymphoma and T-cell leukemia-lymphoma syndrome and/or hyperleukocytosis are the most common causes. Evidence for the onset of tumor lysis can be found before beginning therapy, because of sponta-

neous tumor degradation, and also from 1 to 5 days after the initiation of treatment.

3. Evaluation
   a. Perform repeated physical examinations.
   b. Measure urine output, blood pressure, and weight 1–3 times daily.
   c. Monitor serum creatinine, uric acid, calcium, sodium, phosphate, and potassium every 8 hours until the risk period is over.
   d. If the patient remains oliguric, imaging studies of the kidney may be useful to rule out obstructive uropathy.

4. Prevention
   a. Urine output should be maintained at ≥5 mL/kg/h before initiating chemotherapy and at ≥3 mL/kg/h once chemotherapy is begun, and verified every 2 to 4 hours. If urine output falls, institute corrective measures promptly (more fluids and/or diuretics).
   b. Assure adequate hydration by replacing calculated deficits: intravenous (IV) fluids at 3000 $mL/m^2/day$; may need to increase fluids further to maintain urine output.
   c. Diuresis with furosemide (Lasix) (0.5–1 mg/kg) or mannitol (circulating fluid volume must be adequate: 5–15 g/m^2 as 25% solution over 5–10 minutes repeated every 6 hours as necessary to achieve desired urine volume).

5. Management
   a. Hyperuricemia (≥8 mg/dL)
      An elevated uric acid results from nucleic acid breakdown. Urates can precipitate in the acid environment of the kidney, causing renal failure.
      i. Allopurinol 300 $mg/m^2/day$ divided t.i.d.
      ii. Alkalinization of urine pH from ≥6.5 to ≤7.5 with $NaHCO_3$ 120 $mEq/m^2/day$ IV will increase the solubility of urates; pH >7.5 is associated with a precipitation of hypoxanthine as well as calcium phosphate crystals. Alkalinization should be discontinued once uric acid is controlled and/or if phosphorus is elevated.
   b. Hyperphosphatemia (≥6.5 mg/dL)
      Lymphoblasts have four times the content of phosphate of normal lymphocytes. When the calcium-phosphate product exceeds 60, calcium phosphate

precipitates in microvasculature and renal tubules, which can lead to renal failure.

   i. Low-phosphate diet

   ii. Aluminum hydroxide 150 mg/kg/day divided q4–6h

   iii. urine output ≥3 mL/kg/h

c. Hyperkalemia (≥6.0 mEq/L)

Potassium can be elevated because of tumor lysis or secondary to renal failure. Hyperkalemia leads to ventricular arrhythmias and death.

   i. Do not administer intravenous potassium until the tumor lysis is controlled.

   ii. Sodium polystyrene sulfonate (Kayexalate) removes 1 mEq potassium/L/g resin over 24 hours; give as 1 g/kg PO q6h with sorbitol 50–150 mL. This is not an emergency intervention. The duration of action depends on the rate of endogenous potassium release.

   iii. Administering calcium is the fastest means of reversing the cardiac effects of hyperkalemia. The onset of action is within minutes, but the duration of action is only about a ½ hour. Administer for life-threatening arrhythmias as calcium chloride 10 mg/kg IV. (Do not administer in the same line as sodium bicarbonate.)

   iv. Sodium bicarbonate at 1–2 mEq/kg IV will drive potassium into the cell. For every increase in 0.1 pH unit, potassium decreases about 1 mEq/L. The onset of action is in ½ hour; the duration of activity is several hours.

   v. Administering insulin and glucose will also move excess potassium into the cell. Glucose is administered continuously at 0.5 g/kg/h with insulin 0.1 U/kg/h. Monitor serum glucose closely and adjust infusion rates appropriately. In an emergency, glucose alone can facilitate potassium entry into the cell (1 mL/kg of 50% dextrose in a central line). Onset is in 20–30 minutes; the duration of activity is several hours.

d. Hypocalcemia (ionized calcium ≤1.5 mEq/L)

Hypocalcemia occurs secondary to hyperphosphatemia as a compensatory mechanism to maintain the calcium phosphate product at 60.

      i. For *symptomatic* hypocalcemia, administer 10 mg/kg of elemental CaCl in a drip over several minutes.

      ii. Discontinue administration when symptoms resolve.

   e. Dialysis

      Indications include fluid overload with congestive heart failure, anuria, symptomatic hypocalcemia with hyperphosphatemia, hyperkalemia with QRS interval widening which generally occurs with potassium >6, and elevated creatinine with poor urine output.

   f. Institute hyperleukocytosis interventions if appropriate.

B. Hypercalcemia

  1. Overview

    a. Hypercalcemia, a paraneoplastic syndrome, although rarer in children than in adults, has been reported in patients with leukemias, lymphomas, rhabdomyosarcoma, neuroblastoma, Ewing sarcoma, Wilms tumor, and rhabdoid tumors of the kidney.

    b. Mechanisms postulated to be the cause for the hypercalcemia are the following.

      i.   Production by the tumor of a parathyroid hormone-related protein

      ii. Production by the tumor of bone-resorbing substances (lymphotoxin and tumor necrosis factor)

      iii. Elevation of 1,25 dihydroxyvitamin D

      iv. Production of parathyroid hormone

    c. All the above cause excess release of calcium from bone into the blood. This results in polyuria, dehydration leading to diminished glomerular filtration with increased renal absorption of calcium, worsening the hypercalcemia.

  2. Evaluation

    a. The normal value of calcium corrected for albumin is 9–11 mg/dL (4.5–5.5 mEq/L). Mild hypercalcemia can be defined as 12–14 mg/dL (6–7 mEq/L) and severe hypercalcemia is >15 mg/dL (7.5 mEq/L). Add 0.8 mg/dL of calcium for every gram per liter reduction of serum albumen.

    b. Non-protein-bound ionized calcium (normal = 1.00–1.31 mmol/L) is of greater physiologic importance and does not need correction for serum protein.

c. Signs and symptoms of hypercalcemia are shown in Table 12.1.
3. Management
   a. Mild hypercalcemia
      i. Administer intravenous hydration with normal saline (3000 mL/m^2/day) and encourage oral intake. High fluid volume promotes the excretion of calcium, and saline interferes with the reabsorption of calcium in the proximal tubule of the kidney.
      ii. Furosemide 1–2 mg/kg IV t.i.d. or q.i.d. blocks the reabsorption of calcium in the ascending loop of Henle.
      iii. Monitor electrolytes frequently.
      iv. Maintain exercise and movement.
   b. Severe hypercalcemia
      i. Increase intravenous hydration to 6000 mL/m^2/day and continue furosemide as above.
      ii. Administer biphosphonates such as pamidronate 60 mg IV over 4 hours once for children over 50 kg. May repeat in 7 days as necessary. The dosage for smaller children has not been established. Action results in an inhibition of bone resorbtion.
      iii. For lymphoproliferative disorders, steroids (prednisone 2 mg/kg/day or its equivalent) may decrease serum calcium over several days of use.
      iv. Calcitonin, gallium nitrate, indomethacin, and mithramycin have all been used with some success but should be tried only if the above fails.
      v. Oral or intravenous phosphates seem to have more toxicity than benefit. They decrease bone resorption and can increase extraosseous bone formation,

TABLE 12.1.
Signs and Symptoms of Hypercalcemia

Neurologic	Gastrointestinal	Cardiac	Genitourinary
Headache	Nausea	Hypertension	Polyuria
Irritability	Vomiting	Bradycardia	Polydipsia
Seizures	Anorexia	Arrhythmia	Nocturia
Lethargy	Constipation		
Hypotonia	Ileus		
Coma	Abdominal pain		

possibly leading to increased renal toxicity. If they are used, monitor carefully.

vi. For patients refractory or resistant to other methods of treatment, dialysis, either peritoneal or hemodialysis, can be used.

C. Syndrome of inappropriate antidiuretic hormone
  1. Overview
     Antidiuretic hormone (ADH or arginine vasopressin) causes the resorption of free water at the renal collecting duct; thus, it is an important mechanism in regulating the volume and osmolality of extracellular fluid.

     a. ADH is released from the pituitary gland when osmoreceptors in the hypothalamus detect increased osmolality of the serum.

     b. Secretion of ADH also occurs when volume receptors in the left atrium, carotid sinus, and aortic arch detect decreased effective circulating volume.

     c. Volume depletion stimulates the secretion of ADH regardless of serum osmolality.

  2. Etiology
     The syndrome of inappropriate antidiuretic hormone (SIADH) exists when the release of ADH occurs in the absence of increased serum osmolality or volume depletion and is not suppressed by further volume depletion. It may occur with the following.

     a. Malignancies (e.g., leukemia, lymphoma, Ewing sarcoma, and brain tumor)

     b. Drugs (e.g., vincristine, vinblastine, barbiturates, and opiates)
        Cyclophosphamide produces a SIADH-like syndrome by acting directly at the kidney tubule to enhance the absorption of free water.

     c. Head trauma

     d. Infection of the central nervous system (CNS) or lungs

     e. Pain and/or stress

     f. Surgery

  3. Evaluation
     a. The urine is maximally dilute with a relatively high urinary sodium (>20 mEq/L) despite hyponatremia and low serum osmolality.

  b. Volume depletion, nephrotic syndrome, adrenal insufficiency, hypothyroidism, and congestive heart failure are absent.
4. Management
  a. Treatment of the underlying disorder
  b. Mild disease
    i. Fluid restriction, equaling urine output
    ii. Normal maintenance of Na^+ intake
  c. Severe hyponatremia (120–125 mEq/L) without life-threatening symptoms
    i. Furosemide 1 mg/k promotes a free water diuresis.
    ii. Replace urine loss milliliter for milliliter with normal saline.
    iii. Demeclocycline 6.6–13.2 mg/kg divided into 2–4 doses (maximum 600–1200/day) inhibits the action of ADH on renal tubules by interfering with the formation and action of cyclic adenosine monophosphate.
  d. Life–threatening neurologic symptoms (convulsions and stupor)
    i. Furosemide 1 mg/kg promotes a free water diuresis.
    ii. To correct sodium to 120 mEq/L, give 200 mL/m^2 of 1.5% NaCl in 6–8 hours, and then more slowly to normal over 24–72 hours.
    iii. It is important to avoid a rapid correction of serum sodium. Hypertonic sodium causes a sodium diuresis and may exacerbate the loss of sodium. Neurologic deterioration and death have occurred with too-rapid correction of serum Na^+.
D. Hypokalemia
  1. Overview
    a. Normal serum potassium is 3.5–5.5 mEq/L; electrocardiogram (ECG) changes are seen at ≤2.5 mEq/L.
    b. The principal effects are on cardiac rhythm, with symptoms occurring most commonly when the cause is acute.
    c. Patients may develop ileus or muscle weakness.
  2. Etiology
    a. Renal wasting secondary to drugs is the usual etiology in pediatric cancer patients.

    b. Commonly administered agents associated with tubular potassium loss include amphotericin B, antipseudomonal penicillins, aminoglycosides, ifosfamide, cisplatin, loop diuretics, and glucocorticoids.

3. Evaluation

    a. A semiquantitative assessment of potassium needs per day determines the potassium content of the patient's spot urine and the 24-hour urine output.

    b. Serum magnesium must be assessed, as potassium cannot be conserved without adequate magnesium.

4. Management

    a. Oral therapy is indicated for chronic hypokalemia.

    b. Intravenous replacement is indicated for an acute decrease (particularly <2.5 mEq/L) or if the patient cannot take an oral supplement.

    c. The potassium infusion rate should not exceed 0.5 mEq/kg/h.

    d. Potassium concentrations of 100 mEq/L are acceptable in a central line. Concentrations >40 mEq/L administered via peripheral vein are irritating or painful and can cause phlebitis.

    e. ECG monitoring throughout IV potassium replacement is essential.

    f. Potassium-sparing diuretics such as amiloride or aldactone may help conserve potassium.

II. HYPERLEUKOCYTOSIS

A. Overview

Hyperleukocytosis is defined as a total peripheral white blood cell (WBC) count >100,000/μl.

B. Etiology

Hyperleukocytosis occurs in 9–13% of children with acute lymphoblastic leukemia (ALL), 5–20% of children with acute nonlymphoblastic leukemia (ANLL), and most children with chronic myelogenous leukemia.

C. Pathogenesis

1. Blood viscosity

Hyperleukocytosis increases blood viscosity and is associated with aggregation of leukemic cells in the microcirculation.

2. Respiratory failure
   a. Stasis of leukemic blasts in the pulmonary vasculature can block oxygen diffusion.
   b. Release of intracellular contents of leukemic cells in the pulmonary vessels and interstitium can cause diffuse alveolar damage.
   c. This is seen almost exclusively in patients with ANLL.
3. Hemorrhage
   a. Central nervous system (CNS), gastrointestinal, pulmonary, and pericardial hemorrhages can occur, with devastating results.
   b. Hemorrage is significantly more common in ANLL than ALL. The mortality from CNS hemorrhage in ANLL patients with a WBC count >300,000/μl approaches 60%.
   c. Complicating coagulation defects are particularly common with M4 and M5 ANLL.
   d. Metabolic complications also occur, primarily related to tumor lysis, and are more common with ALL.

D. Evaluation
   1. Elicit signs and symptoms of hypoxia and acidosis, such as dyspnea, blurred vision, headache, somnolence, and confusion.
   2. Physical examination may show papilledema.

E. Management
   1. Avoid nonessential transfusions. Do not raise the hemoglobin >8–10 g/dL. Consider exchange transfusion to avoid further increase in blood viscosity.
   2. Leukapheresis has been proposed for symptomatic patients to rapidly lower WBC counts, particularly when WBC counts are >300,000/μl.
   3. Keep platelets >20,000/μl; transfusing platelets does not add appreciably to blood viscosity.
   4. Specific antileukemic therapy should be instituted as soon as life-threatening complications have been corrected.
   5. Consider whole-brain irradiation at 400 cGy in an attempt to prevent intracranial hemorrhage in patients with ANLL. This is a controversial therapy the value of which has not been proven, however.
   6. Aggressively manage metabolic abnormalities and any underlying coagulopathy associated with the leukemia.

7. Institute precautionary measures for tumor lysis syndrome: hydration, alkalinization, and allopurinol.

III. SUPERIOR MEDIASTINAL SYNDROME/SUPERIOR VENA CAVA SYNDROME

A. Overview
   1. Superior vena cava syndrome refers to the signs and symptoms resulting from compression of the superior vena cava.
   2. Superior mediastinal syndrome (SMS) occurs when tracheal compression also occurs.

B. Etiology
   1. Malignant tumors are the most common primary cause of SMS in children.
   2. Tumors arising from the anterior mediastinum and/or involving middle mediastinal lymph nodes, such as non-Hodgkin lymphoma, Hodgkin disease, leukemia, and germ cell tumors, compress the thin-walled, low-pressure vena cava and its tributaries, impairing venous return to the heart and increasing venous pressure distal to the obstruction, specifically in the head, neck, and upper thorax.
   3. Intravascular thrombosis occurs in 50% of cases.
   4. Obstruction of small and large airways occurs and edema further compromises air flow.

C. Evaluation
   1. Common symptoms include cough, dyspnea, chest pain, and orthopnea. Anxiety, confusion, somnolence, headache, visual disturbances, and syncope are less common but reflect a more profound impairment in physiology.
   2. A supine position often worsens the symptoms. Symptoms often progress rapidly over a few days.
   3. On physical examination, facial edema and possibly conjunctival edema are noted. Plethora or cyanosis of the face, neck, and upper extremities, distension of chest wall and other collateral veins, diaphoresis, wheezing, and stridor are all signs of SMS.
   4. A chest radiograph confirms the clinical picture. More detailed evaluation with chest computed tomography (CT) scan, echocardiography, and pulmonary function

studies may be needed to accurately define the degree of impairment and the anesthetic risk.

5. Carefully consider and evaluate before administering sedation or anesthesia, since severe morbidity and even mortality can be the end result.

   a. Establishing a tissue diagnosis is essential for planning definitive therapy; *however,* children with SMS often tolerate sedation and anesthesia poorly.

   b. With anesthesia, abdominal muscle tone increases, respiratory muscle tone decreases, bronchial smooth muscle relaxes, and lung volumes are greatly reduced. Even with intubation, these patients sometimes cannot be ventilated.

   c. Venous return is further reduced by the peripheral dilation caused by sedation, and sometimes cannot be restored.

   d. Attempt to make the diagnosis by the least invasive method. A complete blood count (CBC) or bone marrow aspirate may yield the diagnosis of lymphoma or leukemia. A pleurocentesis or pericardiocentesis, if an effusion is present, may yield diagnostic material. Serum α-fetoprotein or β-human chorionic gonadotropin can identify germ cell malignancies. In an older child a peripheral lymph node biopsy under local anesthesia can be attempted without sedation.

D. Management

When symptoms are life threatening, prebiopsy empiric therapy may be necessary.

1. Radiation is the most common emergency therapy using daily dosages of 200–400 cGy. A small radiation field concentrating on the trachea and vena cava is sufficient. Improvement can be seen within 18 hours. Histologic distortion and an inability to make a correct diagnosis is a potential complication. Anticipate radiation-induced edema. Both these problems can be minimized with small fields.

2. Intravenous steroids (methylprednisolone 50 mg/m^2/day divided 4 times daily) can reduce a lymphoid mass. Empiric chemotherapy may be necessary. Anticipate histologic distortion and tumor lysis.

3. Observe the patient in an intensive care unit. Elevate the patient's head and give supplemental oxygen.

4. Avoid overhydration. Maintain an adequate circulating blood volume. Avoid upper extremity venipunctures, which can bleed excessively due to high intravascular pressure.
5. Institute tumor lysis syndrome precautions.

IV. NEUROLOGIC EMERGENCIES

A variety of neurologic emergencies can arise in children with cancer. They can be seen at the time of presentation, while the child is undergoing therapy, or at relapse. The etiologies are numerous and include a direct effect of tumor or treatment sequelae. A detailed history with attention to the natural course of the malignancy and knowledge of the treatment is critical, as is a thorough neurologic examination.

A. Compression of the spinal cord
   1. Overview
      a. Although not life threatening, compression of the spinal cord causes severe neurologic morbidity. Prompt recognition of this process with appropriate intervention may prevent these complications.
      b. Back pain occurs in 80% of children with spinal cord compression. Consider any child with cancer plus back pain to have spinal cord compression until proven otherwise.
   2. Etiology
      a. Sarcomas, lymphomas, neuroblastoma, and leukemia at diagnosis or with relapse can cause spinal cord compression.
      b. Although the tumor may involve the vertebral body and secondarily compress the cord, it is more likely to cause spinal cord compression by infiltrating through intervertebral foramina from a paraspinous location.
   3. Evaluation
      a. Perform a detailed neurologic examination, with particular attention to extremity strength, reflexes, and tone. Percussion of the spine may elicit localized tenderness. Attempt to determine the sensory level.
      b. Close observation may be appropriate for the child with localized back pain and a normal neurologic examination. Evaluate persistent pain with a magnetic resonance imaging (MRI) scan.

c. For the child with an abnormal neurologic finding, an MRI scan of the entire spine is essential. There is probably no role for plain films, as fewer than half of existing abnormalities are found on plain films.

4. Management

a. Administer dexamethasone 1–2 mg/kg as a single loading dose (maximum dose 10 mg) followed by 1.5 mg/kg/day divided q6h (maximum dose 4 mg) to reduce edema. Neurologic function may improve with steroids but spinal cord decompression still needs to be carried out.

b. For spinal cord compression secondary to osteoporosis and vertebral collapse, laminectomy and fixation are necessary.

c. For spinal cord compression secondary to a radioresponsive tumor of a known etiology, administer radiation therapy in addition to steroids.

   i. The entire tumor volume should be included in the radiation field plus one vertebral body above and below the lesion.

   ii. Initiate radiation even for patients with a short life expectancy, as loss of function is devastating to the quality of life.

d. For chemosensitive tumors such as lymphoma, leukemia, and possibly neuroblastoma, administer appropriate chemotherapy in addition to steroids.

e. Decompressive laminectomy is indicated to establish a histologic diagnosis, for radioresistant-chemoresistant tumors, and for rapid neurologic deterioration during chemotherapy or radiation therapy.

B. Acute changes in mental status

1. Etiology

a. Metastatic disease, primary CNS infection (bacterial, fungal, or viral), sepsis/disseminated intravascular coagulation (DIC), and metabolic abnormalities are the most common causes of acute alterations in consciousness.

b. Although uncommon, acute changes in mental status can occur with chemotherapeutic drugs such as ifosphamide and high-dose cytosine arabinoside.

2. Evaluation

a. In an emergency, evaluate vital signs, breathing pat-

tern, pupil size with responsiveness to light, extra-ocular movements, spontaneous movements, and response to stimuli for evidence of herniation.
b. Elicit signs of increased intracranial pressure such as papilledema and focal neurologic deficits.
c. Obtain glucose, electrolytes, renal and hepatic function, and a DIC screen to rule out metabolic or hemorrhagic causes.
d. After the patient is stabilized, obtain an emergency CT scan if a mass lesion is suspected or the initial evaluation fails to identify the cause for the acute change in mental status.
e. Once a mass lesion has been ruled out and coagulopathy corrected, obtain lumbar puncture and appropriate studies for infection or tumor in cerebrospinal fluid.

3. Management
a. Correct life-threatening cardiorespiratory abnormalities.
b. Manage increased intracranial pressure with hyperventilation to partial pressure of carbon dioxide (pCO_2) of 20–25 mm Hg, IV dexamethasone (1–2 mg/kg) as a loading dose followed by 1.5 mg/kg/day divided every 6 hours (maximum dose 4 mg), and mannitol 25% at 0.5–1 g/kg.
c. Correct metabolic abnormalities and coagulation defects.
d. Treat potential infectious etiologies appropriately. If bacterial meningitis is a possibility, administer emergency antibiotic therapy at presentation.

C. Seizures
1. Etiology
a. Etiology is similar to that for acute change in mental status.
b. Metastatic disease late in the course of illness and complications of therapy are most common.
c. Antineoplastic drugs such as vincristine, intrathecal methotrexate, cisplatin, and L-asparaginase or the antibiotic imipenem can cause seizures.
d. Cranial radiation may increase the potential for seizures.
2. Evaluation

a. Evaluation is similar to that for acute change in mental status.
b. MRI may show abnormalities not seen on CT, particularly ones related to CNS damage from therapy.
c. An electroencephalogram (EEG) may localize the focus of seizure origin or show activity not suspected clinically.

3. Management
a. Prolonged seizure requires emergency management with cardiopulmonary support and anticonvulsant administration intravenously.
    i. Administer diazepam (Valium) 0.3 mg/kg (maximum dose 10 mg) at 1 mg/min. May repeat in 20 minutes (maximum 3 doses). Administer lorazepam (Ativan), which has a longer duration of activity, at 0.05 mg/kg IV over 2 minutes.
    ii. Administer phenytoin at 10–15 mg/kg IV at 1 mg/kg/min.
b. Antiepileptic medications will usually be required after a seizure. With correction of the underlying abnormality, they can often be discontinued relatively soon, particularly if the follow-up EEG is normal and there is no focal neurologic abnormality on imaging studies or persistent deficit on examination.

D. Cerebrovascular accident
1. Overview
Cerebrovascular accidents (CVAs) usually present as acute impairment in motor function, speech, and/or impaired mental status. Seizures are a common accompaniment.
2. Etiology
a. CVAs may be due to direct or metastatic spread of tumor, chemotherapeutic agents, CNS infection, hemorrhage, or thrombosis. Embolic causes are rare.
b. At the onset of illness CVAs are most commonly associated with disease-related coagulation abnormalities, while on therapy CVAs are usually drug related. For example, L-asparaginase during induction therapy for ALL is associated with coagulation abnormalities, and intracranial hemorrhage, thrombosis, or both may occur.

  c. At the end stages of disease, DIC, tumor, or infection can be associated with stroke.

  d. Radiation-induced vascular damage is associated with strokes months to years after treatment.

 3. Evaluation

  a. After the child has been stabilized, perform CT or MRI with and without contrast.

  b. If the initial scan is normal, a repeat study in 7–10 days may be needed.

  c. Evaluate coagulation status with CBC, DIC screen, and antithrombin III.

  d. Once a mass lesion has been ruled out and coagulation abnormalities have been corrected, proceed with lumbar puncture.

  e. MR angiography or arteriography can help diagnose partial sagittal sinus thrombosis or radiation vasculopathy.

 4. Management

  a. Supportive care is the mainstay of therapy; corticosteroids (dexamethasone) to reduce edema and mannitol to decrease intracranial pressure are warranted (see Section IIIB).

  b. Treatment of DIC includes platelet and fresh-frozen plasma infusions and possibly low-dose heparin; however, the use of anticoagulation for venous thrombosis is controversial (see Chapter 5).

  c. Some investigators recommend the twice-daily infusion of fresh-frozen plasma or antithrombin III concentrate for L-asparaginase-associated CVAs. This treatment has not been established as effective.

V. THE ACUTE ABDOMEN

 The classic physical examination findings of an acute abdomen in a neutropenic patient may be muted; however, pain is virtually always present. Steroids also mask the signs and symptoms of an acute abdomen. Physical examination at frequent intervals is essential for detecting subtle changes.

 A. Appendicitis

  Although rare, appendicitis is often associated with a delayed diagnosis and poor outcome, including death. It should always be considered in the differential diagnosis of typhlitis unresponsive to medical management and vincristine toxicity.

B. Typhlitis

1. Overview

   Typhlitis is a necrotizing colitis of the cecum with inflammation, often involving surrounding tissue, seen in neutropenic cancer patients, particularly those with leukemia.

2. Etiology

   The pathophysiology is related to the disruption of intestinal mucosa from chemotherapy and bacterial invasion of bowel wall in the setting of neutropenia.

3. Evaluation

   a. Perform a careful and thorough physical examination.

   b. Blood cultures are positive occasionally and usually show gram-negative enteric organisms.

   c. Obtain radiographic studies such as plain radiograph (four views of the abdomen), abdominal ultrasound, and/or CT scanning. Air in a thickened bowel wall, generally the cecum, and a soft tissue mass are findings of typhlitis.

4. Management

   a. Medical management is generally the mainstay of therapy and includes bowel rest, broad-spectrum antimicrobial coverage (consider double gram-negative coverage as well as anaerobic coverage), and supportive care.

   b. Vasopressors are occasionally needed, and hypotension at presentation is associated with a poor outcome.

   c. Indications for surgery include free air and persistent hypotension.

C. Hemorrhagic pancreatitis

1. Overview

   In the setting of abdominal pain, vomiting, and preceding treatment with L-asparaginase, consider pancreatitis.

2. Evaluation

   a. Serum amylase, lipase, and urinary amylase to creatinine ratio 1.5–2.0 times normal are consistent with pancreatitis.

   b. Obtain ultrasound and/or CT scanning of the abdomen.

    c. Serial studies may be necessary, particularly to monitor for abscess development, pancreatic dissolution, or the formation of a pseudocyst.

3. Management

    a. Bowel rest, nasogastric drainage, antibiotic coverage of bowel flora, fluid replacement, and hyperalimentation are necessary.

    b. Surgical drainage may be required if an abscess develops, pancreatic dissolution occurs, or a pseudocyst persists.

    c. Further asparaginase administration is contraindicated.

Bibliography

Angel CA, Rao BN, Wrenn E, et al.: Acute appendicitis in children with leukemia and other malignancies: Still a diagnostic dilemma. *J Pediatr Surg* 27:476–79, 1992.

Basade M, Dhar AK, Kulkarni SS, et al.: Rapid cytoreduction in childhood leukemic hyperleukocytosis by conservative therapy. *Pediatr Oncol* 25:204–7, 1995.

Bunin NJ, Pui C-H: Differing complications of hyperleukocytosis in children with acute lymphoblastic or acute nonlymphoblastic leukemia. *J Clin Oncol* 3:1590–95, 1985.

Byrne TN: Spinal cord compression from epidural metastases. *N Engl J Med* 327: 614–19, 1992.

Di Mario FJ, Packer RJ: Acute mental status changes in children with systemic cancer. *Pediatrics* 85:353–60, 1990.

Escalante CP: Causes and management of superior vena cava syndrome. *Oncology* 7:61–68, 1993.

Jones DP, Mahmoud H, Chesney RW: Tumor lysis syndrome: Pathogenesis and management. *Pediatr Nephrol* 9:206–12, 1995.

Lange B, O'Neill JA, Goldwein JW et al.: Oncologic emergencies. In Pizzo PA, and Poplack DG, eds. *Principles and Practice of Pediatric Oncology.* 2nd ed. Philadelphia: JB Lippincott; 1993. pp. 951–72.

Pollack ES: Emergency department presentation of childhood malignancies. *Emer Med Clin of North Am* 11:517–29, 1993.

Silliman CC, Haase GM, Strain JD, et al.: Indications for surgical intervention for gastrointestinal emergencies in children receiving chemotherapy. *Cancer* 74:203–16, 1994.

Sloas MM, Flynn PM, Kaste SC, et al.: Typhlitis in children with cancer: A 30-year experience. *Clin Infect Dis* 17:484–90, 1993.

13

Nutritional Support

Nancy Sacks, M.S., R.D., C.N.S.D.,
and Rita S. Meek, M.D.

The goals for nutrition intervention in the pediatric oncology patient are to prevent or reverse nutritional deficits, promote normal growth and development, minimize morbidity, and maximize the quality of life. Factors contributing to the origin and progression of cachexia in a young patient with cancer are shown in Figure 13.1.

I. CALORIE AND PROTEIN REQUIREMENTS

A. Recommended Daily Allowances (RDAs) (Table 13.1) can be used to determine estimated calorie and protein needs. Since the RDAs were developed as recommendations for healthy populations rather than sick individual patients, adjustments are usually necessary to maintain appropriate growth in sick patients. The allowances may need to be increased 15–50% to compensate for previous weight loss, malnutrition, or increased needs due to metabolic demands.

B. The estimation of basal metabolic rate developed by the World Health Organization may be more appropriate in acutely ill patients for determining energy requirements.

C. Premature infants may require 120 kcal/kg or more due to increased needs for growth.

II. INDICATIONS FOR SUPPLEMENTAL NUTRITION

A. To prevent malnutrition.

B. Specific childhood cancers associated with the poorest prog-

FIGURE 13.1.
Factors contributing to the origin and progression of cachexia in a child with cancer.

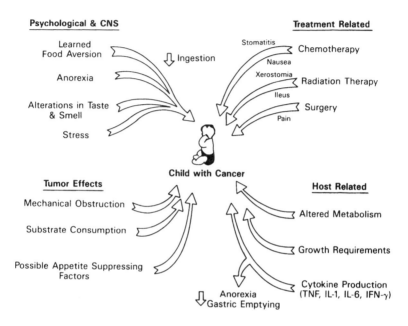

TABLE 13.1.
Recommended Daily Allowances for Calories and Protein

Category	Age (years)	Protein (g/kg/day)	Calories (kcal/kg/day)
Infants	0.0–0.5	2.2	108
	0.5–1.0	1.6	98
Children	1–3	1.2	102
	4–6	1.2	90
	7–10	1.0	70
Males	11–14	1.0	55
	15–18	0.9	45
Females	11–14	1.0	47
	15–18	0.8	49

noses tend to have the most intense oncologic treatment regimens and therefore are most likely to be associated with the development of protein energy malnutrition.

C. It can be anticipated that treatment (surgery, radiation, chemotherapy, and bone marrow transplantation) will cause changes that prevent adequate intake to maintain or restore nutritional status.

III. CRITERIA FOR NUTRITION INTERVENTION

Assess the patient's nutritional status at diagnosis and throughout therapy. Some quick and practical methods that may be used by physicians and nurses are the following.

A. Anthropometric
1. The current percentile for weight and/or height for age has fallen 2 percentile channels. Complete a growth chart for inpatients and outpatients at diagnosis and throughout therapy.
2. >5% weight loss from pre-illness weight or >5% weight loss over the last month.
   Percentage weight loss is derived from the highest previous weight. Weight is inaccurate when a child has edema, large tumor masses and organs extensively infiltrated with tumor effusions or organ congestion or when excess fluids have been administered (twice maintenance) for chemotherapy. These guidelines apply to initially obese as well as lean subjects.
3. <5th percentile weight for age
4. <5th percentile weight for height
5. <90% ideal body weight for height.
   This is calculated as the patient's actual weight divided by the ideal weight for height × 100. The latter figure is determined from the appropriate growth curve by first identifying the age for which the measured height is on the 50th percentile, then determining the corresponding 50th percentile weight for that height.
6. <5th percentile height for age
7. Degree of malnutrition
   The degree of malnutrition can be determined by assessing wasting—the patient's actual weight divided by the ideal body weight for height and assessing stunting—the

patient's actual height divided by the ideal height for age.
8. Other means
Other more sophisticated means of evaluating nutritional status can be performed by a registered dietitian, including assessment of muscle and subcutaneous fat stores.

B. Nutrient intake—when intake is <80% estimated needs

IV. ASSESSMENT OF BIOCHEMICAL DATA

A. laboratory tests that can be monitored before and during repletion include the following
   1. Obtain laboratory panel to screen for organ function to include: sodium, potassium, chloride, bicarbonate, glucose, creatinine, blood urea nitrogen (BUN), calcium, phosphorus, magnesium, total protein, albumin, triglycerides, cholesterol, alkaline phosphatase, alaline aminotransferase, γ-glutamyltransferase, and total bilirubin.
   2. Serum albumin <3.2 mg/dL may indicate decreased protein stores.
   3. Serum prealbumin level can be increased with impaired renal function (normal value varies with age). and decreased with altered hepatic function.

B. Providing nutrition to patients who are depleted can result in abnormalities such as:
   1. The refeeding syndrome
   This is seen in patients chronically deprived of adequate nutrition and is characterized by metabolic complications, severe fluid shifts, hypokalemia, and hypophosphatemia that occur in patients who are repleted enterally and parenterally. Monitor sodium, potassium, chloride, bicarbonate, BUN, creatinine, calcium, magnesium, and phosphorus.
   2. Tube feeding syndrome
   This is characterized by hypertonic dehydration, hypernatremia, and prerenal azotemia in patients receiving highly osmotic enteral feeds.

V. VARIOUS METHODS OF NUTRITIONAL SUPPORT

A. Before determining the most appropriate method of nutritional support, consider the following (see algorithm in Figure 13.2).

FIGURE 13.2.
An algorithm for nutritional support of children with cancer.

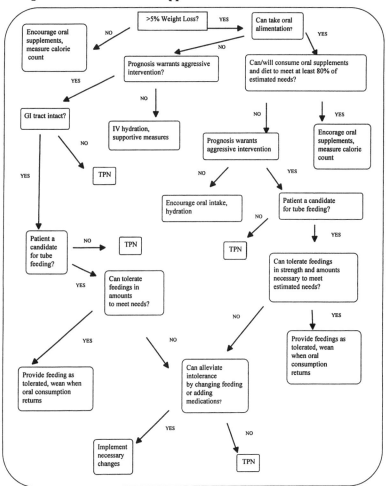

Source: Alexander and Norton, 1993, p. 1026

   1. Nutritional assessment/recommendations by registered dietitian
   2. Capabilities of family/patient for learning
   3. Insurance/home care coverage
   4. Ethical issues regarding disease (stage/prognosis)

B. Oral (volitional)
   1. Intervene early by involving a nutritionist at time of diag-

nosis or referral for nutritional assessment and counseling
2. Provide guidelines for managing complications of treatment (anorexia, alterations in taste, mouth dryness, dysphagia, early satiety, nausea, vomiting, stomatitis, mucositis, diarrhea, or constipation) and for increasing protein or calories. The National Cancer Institute (NCI) has publications available on nutrition for the child with cancer (1-800-4-CANCER).
3. Provide oral supplements for trial (e.g., shakes, bars). See classification of enteral feeding products (Table 13.2).
4. Provide specific macronutrients (modulars).
   i. Protein
   ii. Carbohydrate
   iii. Fat

C. Enteral tube feeding
   If oral feeding is not possible or is inadequate consider tube feedings. It is important to provide support from registered dietitians, physicians, nurses, and social workers to improve acceptance. (Patients and families need to know that their child can continue to eat with supplemental nutrition.)
   1. Initiate tube feedings:
      a. If the severity of mucositis and platelet count permits insertion of tube
      b. If a patient has a functional gastrointestinal tract along with the ability to tolerate feedings with manageable side effects of nausea, vomiting and diarrhea
      c. When a patient meets the criteria for nutrition intervention and oral intake is inadequate to meet estimated needs to provide for normal growth or to provide for repletion of nutritional status
   2. Determine the optimal access route for enteral nutrition based on anticipated duration of tube feeding, risk of pulmonary aspiration, and indications for specific access routes (Figure 13.3).
      a. Tube selection
         Use the smallest tube possible for greater comfort (6- or 8-French nasogastric tubes will work in most patients). A larger tube may be needed with fiber-containing formulas or highly viscous formulas. Silicone and polyurethane nasoenteric tubes decrease physical irritation and have less associated risk of pulmonary aspiration. Weighted tubes are designed to

TABLE 13.2.
Characteristics of Enteral Products

Product description	1–10 Years of Age — Tube Feeding and Oral	>10 Years of Age — Tube Feeding	>10 Years of Age — Oral
1. Standard or polymeric Intact macronutrients intended as meal replacements Requires normal digestive and absorptive capacity Usually lactose free unless otherwise indicated	Pediasure Kindercal Nutren Junior Resource just for kids	Isocal Osmolite Nutren (unflavored) Complete Modified Diet	Ensure Sustacal NuBasic Nutrashake* Carnation Instant Breakfast* Scandishake* Sustacal pudding*
2. High nitrogen Intact macronutrients with >15% total calories as protein Useful in patients with increased protein need (i.e., poor wound healing, radiation)		Isocal HN Osmolite HN Perative Replete	Ensure HN
3. Concentrated or high calorie Contain higher calorie per milliliter than standard and generally not well tolerated due to high osmolality May be used with fluid restriction		Nutren 1.5 (unflavored) Nutren 2.0 Two Cal HN Comply Magnacal	NuBasic Plus Sustacal Plus Ensure Plus Resource Plus

Table 13.2 continued

Product description	1–10 Years of Age	>10 Years of Age	
	Tube Feeding and Oral	Tube Feeding	Oral
4. Predigested/elemental Predigested or partially hydrolyzed peptide based diet that may be beneficial for child with impaired gastrointestinal function (diarrhea, mucositis, intestinal villous atrophy) Many contain medium-chain triglycerides to minimize fat intolerance Can have high osmolality	Peptamen Junior (vanilla or unflavored) Neocate One Plus (flavored or unflavored) Vivonex Pediatric	Peptamen Peptamen VHP Reabilian Tolerex Vivonex TEN Vivonex Plus	Vital HN
5. Fiber containing Contains fiber from natural sources or added soy polysaccharides to aid in bowel function	Kindercal Pediasure with fiber Nutren Junior with fiber	Jevity Ultracal Sustacal with fiber Nutren 1.0 with fiber	Jevity Ultracal Sustacal with Fiber Nutren 1.0 with Fiber
6. Disease specific Macro- and micronutrients modified for disease state	Liver: NutriHep Renal: Nepro, Suplena Pulmonary: Pulmocare, Nutrivent Altered fat absorption: Portagen, Lipisorb	1 year tube or oral	

Product description	Cow's Milk	Soy	Predigested
7. Infant formulas (variety of formulas available for premature infants and for infants with poor tolerance) Many infants are lactose intolerant after chemotherapy and benefit from lactose-free formulas Human breast milk should be used when possible (contains lactose and may not be tolerated well after chemotherapy)	Similac Enfamil Lactofree (lactose free) Gerber Carnation Good Start Similac PM 60/40	Isomil Prosobee	Pregestimil Alimentum Nutramigen
8. Modular components	Protein Casec Pro-mix ProMod NutriSource Protein Elementra	Carbohydrate Polycose Moducal Liquid Carbohydrate (LC) Sumacal NutriSource Carbohydrate NutriSource (long- or medium-chain triglycerides)	Fat Vegetable oil (long-chain triglycerides) Microlipid (long-chain triglycerides) Medium-chain triglycerides
9. Oral electrolyte solutions Provides electrolytes, calories and water during mild to moderate dehydration	Pedialyte Ricelyte Rehydralyte		

* Lactose containing.

FIGURE 13.3.
Determining the optimal feeding mode.

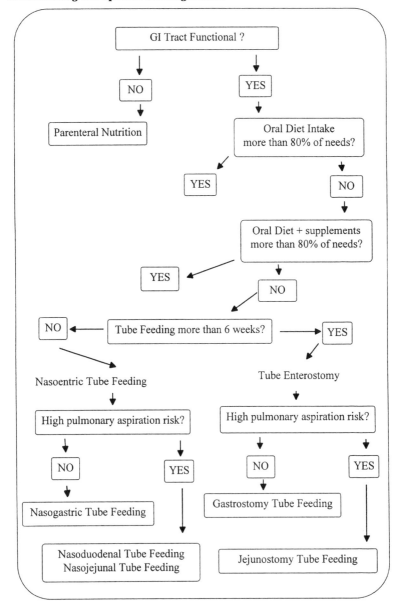

assist with postpyloric tube placement and maintenance of tube position. Placement is assessed by checking pH of aspirated contents or by x-ray.
  b. Nasoenteric—short-term use
    i. Silicone and polyurethane tubes
    ii. Tube lumen size range (6–10 french) based on age/size of child and viscosity of formula
    iii. Orogastric for infants <34 weeks gestational due to obligatory nose breathers
    iv. Nasogastric—easy intubation
    v. Nasoduodenal or nasojejunal, which require radiographic proof of placement and can be easily dislodged
  c. Enterostomy feeding tubes—long-term use
    i. Gastrostomy tubes are made of silicone, polyurethane, rubber, or latex. A Foley catheter may be used for Stamm, Witzel, or Janeway gastrostomies. Surgically or percutaneously placed gastrostomy tubes can be replaced with a button which is flush with the abdomen when a tract is formed.
    ii. Jejunostomy tubes are made of rubber, latex, silicone, polyvinyl, silicone rubber, or polyethylene and are surgically placed.
    iii. Complications with enterostomy tubes can include cellulitis and infections (particularly around the time of neutropenia).
3. Determine the method of administration.
  a. An enteral feeding pump provides reliable, constant infusion rate, decreases the risk of gastric retention, and may prevent gastrointestinal (GI) complications of nausea, vomiting, abdominal cramping/bloating, and diarrhea.
  b. With gravity flow feeding, the flow rate may be adjusted with a clamp that applies pressure on the tubing.
  c. Feeding schedules
    i. A continuous schedule is more likely to be tolerated than bolus feeds and requires a feeding pump.
    ii. A bolus (intermittent or gravity) schedule more closely mimics normal feeding.
    iii. A combination of continuous nocturnal feeds while the patient is sleeping and daytime boluses works well.

     iv. The feeding schedule will determine whether a portable or standard pump is required and which pump is reimbursable by insurance.

4. Determine formula based on composition, GI function, age, cost, and resources (e.g., insurance coverage). Use unflavored products for tube feeding. There are many products available for oral use and for tube feedings (see Table 13.2). Children do not generally accept oral products well. In addition, children generally are unable to gain weight with oral products and oral intake, and therefore usually require supplemental tube feedings.

5. Initiate tube feeding and monitor progression.
   a. If nothing by mouth (NPO) <3 days, begin full strength formula at 1–2 mL/kg/h. Increase by 1 to 2 mL/kg/h per day as tolerated until the goal is achieved.
   b. If NPO >3 days or if GI problems exist (e.g., mucositis, diarrhea, or gut atrophy), begin half-strength formula at 1–2 mL/hg/h. Advance concentration to full strength after 12–24 hours, then increase rate by 1–2 mL/kg/h per day to goal.
   c. One option is to provide ½ estimated needs continuously at night and the remaining ½ of calories in 2–3 boluses during the day. The daily volume can also be divided into q2–4h feedings if desired. Most patients will tolerate continuous feedings better than bolus feedings, particularly if they are nauseated.
   d. If fluid needs are not met with oral intake and tube feeding, provide extra free water as flushes or mixed with feeds.
   e. Flush tube frequently with water and before/after all medications.
   f. Supplementation with potassium, phosphorus, calcium, or magnesium should be divided throughout the day and mixed with feeds for better tolerance. To achieve maximal absorption, do not give calcium and phosphorus at the same time. Medications can be very hyperosmolar and can cause GI irritation. The intravenous form of some medications can be given in tube feedings with less irritation (e.g., magnesium).

6. Watch for mechanical complications of tube feedings.
   a. High gastric residual can be caused by delayed gastric emptying. Prokinetic medications (cisapride or

metoclopramide) may help as well as elevating the head of the bed at least 30° during and after feeding.

b. Nasopharyngeal and nasolabial irritation can be lessened with small bore tubes made of silicone or polyurethane and by taping the tube securely to avoid pressure on nares.

c. Skin irritation and excoriation at the ostomy site can be reduced with appropriate enterostomal therapy using topical or oral antibiotics during periods of severe neutropenia.

d. To avoid obstruction of feeding tube lumen, be sure to adequately flush the tube before and after medication and boluses, and every 4 hours during continuous infusion. Use liquid elixirs when possible. If the tube is clogged, mix 1 crushed Viokase enzyme tablet with 1 crushed tablet (324 mg) of sodium bicarbonate and 5 mL of tap water to prepare a pH 7.9 Viokase solution. Inject 5 mL of this enzyme solution through a Drum cartridge catheter inserted into the feeding tube. Allow to sit for 5 minutes and reirrigate feeding tube with 20–30 mL water.

e. Monitor during the administration of tube feeding.
   i. Check body weight, fluid intake/output, and GI function every day when initiating feedings, then two times per week when stable.
   ii. Assess biochemical indices (fluid balance, calcium, phosphorus, magnesium, and liver function tests). If refeeding syndrome or depleted stores are suspected, monitor laboratory values daily and increase calories slowly.
   iii. Enteral tubes can stay in place for 4–6 weeks before requiring replacement. Older adolescents may choose to place the tube daily for nocturnal feeds.

D. Total parenteral nutrition/hyperalimentation
Total parenteral nutrition (TPN) is indicated for patients when oral and/or tube feedings provide inadequate nutrients or when enteral feeds are contraindicated over a significant period of time. A nutritional assessment should be before starting TPN. A central venous catheter is essential if total nutritional requirements are to be met over several weeks or months.

The following guidelines are taken from the Parenteral Nutrition Ordering form developed by the Nutrition Support Service at the Children's Hospital of Philadelphia.

1. Guidelines for determining TPN requirements
   a. Determine fluid needs.
      1–10 kg: 100 mL/kg/day
      11–20 kg: 1000 mL + 50 mL each kg >10 kg
      20–30 kg: 1500 mL + 20 mL each kg >20 kg
      >30 kg: 35 mL/kg/day
   b. Determine parenteral calorie needs.
      i. For infants <1 year of age use the following guidelines.
         Preterm infant: 90–110 kcal/kg/day
         Full-term infant: 90–100 kcal/kg/day
         Older infant: 80–100 kcal/kg/day
      ii. For older children, see Table 13.1.
      iii. Basal metabolic rate can also be used with appropriate activity/stress factors to determine calorie needs.
   c. Determine protein needs (g/kg/day).
      i. Protein provides 4.0 kcal/g
      ii. Protein requirements are based on age and adjusted for needs.
         Preterm neonate: 2.5–3.5 g/kg/day
         Full-term neonate: 2.5–3.0 g/kg/day
         Infant: 1.5–2.5 g/kg/day
         1–10 years: 1.0–2.0 g/kg/day
         11–18 years: 0.8–2.0 g/kg/day
      iii. Use TrophAmine for children <6 months of age and Novamine for children >6 months of age.
   d. Determine fat/lipid needs (g/kg/day).
      i. 20% fat/lipid (Intralipid®) contains 2 kcal/mL and 10% contains 1.1 kcal/mL
      ii. Need to provide at least 0.5–1.0 g/kg/day to prevent essential fatty acid deficiency.
      iii. Fat/lipid intake should not exceed 4g/kg/day, or 60% of total calories. A reasonable goal is 30–40%.
   e. Determine carbohydrate/glucose needs.
      i. Dextrose provides 3.4 kcal/g
      ii. Usual rate of glucose administration is:
         Newborn: 5–12 mg/kg/min
         Children: 5–8 mg/kg/min

Adults: 2–5 mg/kg/min
   f. Determine electrolyte needs.
   The appropriate maintenance dose of specific electrolytes are indicated in Table 13.3. Needs may be altered for many causes and must be considered. (e.g., cisplatin causes increased losses of potassium, calcium, magnesium and phosphorus; amphotericin B causes increased losses of potassium and renal tubular acidosis requires acetate replacement in TPN).
2. Guidelines for advancing peripheral line TPN
   a. Day 1: Start with 10% dextrose, protein as required, and lipids at 1–2 g/kg/day.
   b. Day 2: Increase lipids by 1 g/kg/day to goal.
3. Guidelines for advancing central line TPN
   a. Day 1: Give 10% dextrose, protein as required, and lipids at 1–2 g/kg/day.
   b. Day 2: Increase dextrose solution and lipids to goal. If the patient is at risk for refeeding syndrome, increase calories more slowly (i.e., 10–15% per day).
4. Monitoring TPN
   a. Laboratory

TABLE 13.3.
Recommended Guidelines*

	Preterm	Term	Child (1–10 years)	Adolescent (>10 years)
Amino acids (g)	2.5–3.5	2.5–3.0	1.0–2.0	0.8–2.0
Intravenous fat emulsion (g)	1–3	1–3	1–4	1–4
Sodium (mE)	2–3	2–4	2–3	2–3
Potassium (mE)	2–3	2–3	2–3	2–3
Chloride (mE)	2–3	2–4	2–3	2–3
Acetate (mE)	<Use as necessary to balance in acidotic patient>			
Calcium (mE)	3–4.5	3–4	1–2	10/day
Phosphorus (mE)	2.7–4.0	1.5–3.0	0.7–1.4	0.7–1.4
<For potassium phosphate: mE K phosphate × 0.68 = mmol phosphorus>				
Magnesium (mE)	0.350.6	0.25–0.5	0.2–0.5	0.25–0.5
Iron (mg)				
patient >2 months	0.2	0.1	0.1	0.1
Heparin (U/mL)	0.5	0.5	1	1

*Estimated requirements may need to be adjusted, depending on medications. Values are kg/day, except as noted.

Obtain baseline screening panel (see Section IVA), then check weekly. Check more frequently with refeeding syndrome.
   b. Daily weight
   c. Intake and output daily
5. Cycling of TPN
   Many patients benefit from having TPN cycled over 10–12 hours to allow more time off for normal activity. A portable pump can be used to increase mobility while receiving TPN. The infusion rate of TPN solutions with >10% dextrose should be decreased by 50% during the last hour of the infusion to prevent rebound hypoglycemia.
6. Complications of TPN
   a. Hypoglycemia
      Avoid abrupt discontinuation of TPN (decrease rate before discontinuation).
   b. Hyperglycemia
      Decrease dextrose concentration or administer insulin with TPN as a separate infusion or provide subcutaneously.
   c. Fatty liver
      Avoid excessive carbohydrate infusion and provide a mix of dextrose, protein, and lipids.
   d. Cholestatic jaundice
      To avoid cholestatic jaundice, cycle TPN as soon as possible and provide enteral feeding.
7. Weaning
   Supplemental nutrition (TPN or tube feeding) can be slowly weaned as oral intake improves.

VI. ETHICAL ISSUES

Each patient/family situation needs to be reviewed concerning the goals, risks, and benefits of nutrition support. The choice to withdraw nutrition by families should be respected. Supplemental nutrition may not benefit patients in the terminal stage of their disease. When goals of the cancer therapy change, the level of nutrition intervention may also change.

Bibliography

Aker SN, Lenssen P: Nutritional Support of Patients with Hematologic Malignancies. In Hoffman R, Benz GJJ, Shattil SJ, Furie B, HJ Cohen, eds. *Hematology: Basic Principles and Practice.* New York: Churchill Livingstone; 1115–23, 1991.

Alexander HR, Norton JA: Nutritional supportive care. In Pizzo PA, Poplack DG, eds. *Principles and Practices of Pediatric Oncology.* 2nd ed. Philadelphia: JB Lippincott Company; 1993.

Grand RJ, Sutphen JL, Dietz WH, eds.: *Pediatric Nutrition: Theory and Practice.* Boston: Butterworth; 1987.

Ideno, KT. Enteral Nutrition. In Gottschlich MM, Matarese LM, Shronts EP, eds.: *Nutrition Support Dietetics Core Curriculum.* 2nd ed. Silver Spring, MD: American Society for Parenteral and Enteral Nutrition; 83, 1993.

Mathew P, Bowman L, Williams R, et al.: Complications and effectiveness of gastrostomy feedings in pediatric cancer patients. *J Pediatr Hematol Oncol* 18:81–85, 1996.

Mauer AM, Burgess JB, Donaldson SS, et al.: Special nutritional needs of children with malignancies: A review. *J Parenter Enteral Nutr* 14:315–24, 1990.

National Research Council: *Recommended Dietary Allowances.* 10th ed. Washington DC.: National Academy Press; 1989.

Nutrition Support Services Policies and Procedures. Philadelphia: The Children's Hospital of Philadelphia; June 1995.

Sacks N: Clinical care guidelines for the pediatric oncology patient. *Nutr Oncol* 2(8&9), 1996.

14

Mouth Care

Paula K. Groncy, M.D., Richard D. Udin, D.D.S.,
and Arthur R. Ablin, M.D.

The oral cavity is a frequent site of therapy-related complications, including mucositis, ulcerations, infections, bleeding, and xerostomia. Ulcerated mucosa may provide a pathway for intraoral bacteria to become blood borne. Good oral hygiene, including proper control of plaque to decrease the oral reservoir of microorganisms, plays a major part in the reduction of oral complications of therapy.

I. ORAL PROPHYLAXIS

A. Initial evaluation
1. Each child should have a thorough medical/dental history with an oral/dental and radiographic examination and a dental deplaquing/scaling before the initiation of therapy.
2. When this cannot be done, perform an initial screening dental evaluation to rule out any dental conditions that may cause complications during induction therapy or surgery.
3. Defer any treatment until white blood cell counts recover [absolute neutrophil count (ANC) >1000/μL] after initial chemotherapy.

B. Dental treatment (to eliminate/control the foci of infection)
1. Dental care is indicated in all patients before therapy whenever possible. The treatment of dental problems is mandatory for all patients before radiation therapy that will involve the head and neck

a. Definitive restoration of all carious teeth
b. Nonsurgical periodontal therapy
c. Removal of all nonrestorable or exfoliating teeth
   i. Primary closure of soft tissues should accompany extractions to promote healing.
   ii. In most cases 10–14 days for healing is sufficient before starting radiation therapy, although those who will receive 6500 cGy or more may need 14–21 days.
d. Endodontic therapy or pulpal treatment is contraindicated for primary teeth and may be contraindicated for permanent teeth.
e. Prosthetic/orthodontic devices should be removed.

2. During therapy
   Use conservative dental therapy as oral and medical conditions permit.
   a. Applications of fluoride gel via custom-fabricated flexible plastic trays are strongly suggested for all patients during radiation therapy to the head and neck (and for selected caries-prone patients during chemotherapy). Alternatively, nightly rinsing with an over-the-counter (0.05% neutral sodium fluoride) fluoride-containing rinse may be as effective (such as Act or Fluorigard). Commercial mouthwashes are not recommended, because they are not bacteriostatic, and many of them have a high alcohol content, causing burning, stinging, and desiccation of mucous membranes.
      i. Use neutral-pH preparations of either 1.1% neutral sodium fluoride (such as Previ Dent) or 0.4% stannous fluoride (such as Gel Kam).
      ii. Apply gel once daily after tooth brushing, preferably at bedtime. Spread a few drops on each tray and leave in the mouth for 5 minutes; the excess may be spat out, but do not rinse the mouth.
      iii. If the patient cannot use trays (because of sore mouth or gagging), he or she may apply fluoride gel with a toothbrush, disposable sponge (Toothette), or cotton-tipped applicator.
   b. When the ANC is expected to fall (e.g., with induction chemotherapy), all elective dental procedures are contraindicated.

   c. If emergency dental procedures are necessary in patients with an ANC <500–1000/µL or falling and expected to reach <500–1000/µL
      i. Consider prophylactic intravenous antibiotics.
      ii. Perform extractions 10 days before ANC is expected to fall to <1000. They should be performed as atraumatically as possible, using primary closure with multiple interrupted sutures. The placement of intra-alveolar packing agents in extraction sites is not recommended.

C. Daily regimen of oral hygiene
   1. Standard regimen (ANC >500/µL, platelets >100,000/µL)
      a. Brush teeth daily with a soft-bristle toothbrush (soak toothbrush in hot water to soften further).
      b. Floss with waxed or unwaxed dental floss, depending on the patient's and family's skills.
      c. "Pat and push" a thick paste of sodium bicarbonate and a few drops of warm water into the gingival sulcus and around the teeth using a soft toothbrush or use a fluoride-containing gel toothpaste.
      d. Use mouthwash of mild sodium bicarbonate (1/2 teaspoon baking soda per cup of water) or 0.12% chlorhexidine gluconate b.i.d.
      e. Use a new toothbrush after any infection.
   2. Conservative regimen (ANC <500/µL, platelets <50,000/µL, or if excessive bleeding occurs on the standard regimen)
      a. Cleanse oral hard and soft tissues with a mild solution of sodium bicarbonate (1/2 teaspoon per cup of water) using a 4 × 4 gauze pad or Toothette.
      b. Use mouthwash several times daily with the above solution. (See the note above regarding commercial mouthwash.)
      c. Use 0.12% chlorhexidine gluconate mouthwash
         i. Rinse the mouth 2–4 times daily.
         ii. Spit out the mouthwash after rinsing.
         iii. Do not eat anything for 30 minutes after rinsing.
         iv. For children <3 years old, use a gauze pad soaked in 0.12% chlorhexidine gluconate.

II. PREVENTION AND TREATMENTS OF MUCOSITIS

A. Prevention
   1. Good oral hygiene

The incidence and severity of mucositis have been related to the degree of preexisting mucosal disease, oral hygiene, and the nature of therapy.

2. Use 0.12% chlorhexidine gluconate rinse (see Section IC1c).

B. Treatment
1. Daily oral hygiene (conservative regimen)
2. Sucralfate slurry: swish and swallow
3. Topical agents
Topical agents may be tried and continued if they relieve symptoms. Their effectiveness is not proven, but for individual patients they may bring relief.
   a. Dyclonine HC 0.5% and diphenhydramine HC 0.5% in normal saline.
   Apply with a cotton-tipped applicator or swish and spit.
   b. Equal part 2% viscous lidocaine, diphenhydramine (12/5 mg/5 mL), and Maalox
   Swish and spit or apply with a cotton-tipped applicator.
   c. Cocaine applied topically
   d. Hurricaine
   e. Benzocaine in Orabase
   f. Diphenhydramine and Kaopectate
4. Dietary changes
   a. Dental/mechanical soft diet
   b. Avoidance of irritating foods (spicy, acidic, temperature extremes)
5. Systemic analgesics (see Chapter 11)

III. PREVENTION, DIAGNOSIS, AND TREATMENT OF ORAL INFECTIONS

Mucositis induced by chemotherapy or radiation therapy may be due to reactivation of latent herpes simplex virus (HSV), which occurs in 75% of seropositive patients. Secondary infection, usually with candida, can occur. Marginal gingivitis (recognized by an erythematous periapical line) is presumably caused by anaerobes.

A. Prevention
1. Good oral hygiene
2. Use of 0.12% chlorhexidine gluconate (see Section IC1c)
3. Prophylaxis against HSV (see Chapter 1)
4. Prophylaxis against fungal infection (see Chapter 1)

B. Diagnosis
   1. Direct microscopic examination (wet mount or gram stain)
   2. Cultures
       a. Aerobic and anaerobic bacteria
       b. Fungal
       c. Viral (HSV)

C. Treatment
Because candida and HSV may coexist, empiric treatment of both organisms is recommended until the results of direct microscopic examination and cultures are available.
   1. Candida
       a. Nystatin oral suspension 5 mL q.i.d. swish and swallow
       b. Ketoconazole 5–10 mg/kg/day in 2 divided doses (maximum 800 mg/day); 200 mg scored tablet
       c. Fluconazole 3 mg/kg/day (suspension: 10 or 40 mg/mL; tablet: 50, 100, 150, or 200 mg)
       d. Clotrimazole troche 10 mg 5 times daily
       e. Oral Amphotericin B solution (0.1 mg/ml) 15 mL q.i.d. swish and spit for patients refractory to the above .
   2. Herpes simplex virus
       a. Acyclovir
           i. Oral: 250–600 mg/m^2 4–5 times daily
           ii. Intravenous: 750 mg/m^2/day in 3 divided doses

IV. SALIVARY GLAND DYSFUNCTION

A. Definition
Salivary gland dysfunction includes decreased salivary gland flow, viscous ropy saliva, and decreased volume of saliva, resulting in a shift to highly cariogenic microorganisms, seen with some chemotherapeutic agents (e.g., doxorubicin) and x-ray therapy that incorporates the salivary glands in the radiation field.

B. Treatment
Custom vinyl trays for self-applied topical neutral sodium fluoride. If the patient cannot use trays (because of pain or gagging), he or she may apply fluoride with a toothbrush, Toothette, or cotton-tipped applicator. Alternatively, nightly rinsing with a 0.05% neutral sodium fluoride over-the-counter product may be used.

1. Good daily oral hygiene regimen
2. Helpful aids
   a. Saliva substitutes (Salivart, Xerolube)
   b. Mild sodium bicarbonate rinses (1/2 teaspoon baking soda per cup of water)
   c. Frequent sips of water (carry plastic squeeze bottle filled with water)
   d. Sugar-free chewing gum and/or sugar-free candy in moderation (effect of protracted use unknown)

V. ORAL AND/OR GINGIVAL BLEEDING

A. Oral hygiene
Discontinue mechanical hygiene and use good daily oral hygiene (conservative regimen). A major cause of gingival bleeding is gingivitis, and this must be considered and treated.

B. Abnormalities
Correct existing platelet/coagulation abnormalities if possible.

C. Topical agents:
1. Thrombin solution:
   Apply with 2×2 sterile gauze pad.
2. Avitene:
   Remove from jar using sterile dry hemostat; press onto bleeding site using 2×2 sterile gauze pad.
3. Instat:
   Cut sheet to size, then press onto gingival tissue using 2×2 sterile gauze pad.

D. Aminocaproic acid (Amicar)
1. Dosage: Initial 100 mg/kg per dose intravenous (IV), then 30 mg/kg/h IV until bleeding stops (maximum 18 g/m^2/24h); same dosage by mouth (PO)
2. Preparations
   a. 20 mL vial with 5 g of aminocaproic acid: 150 mg/mL
   b. 25% syrup: 1.4 g/5 mL
   c. Tablet: 500 mg

E. Tranexamic acid (Cyklokapron)
1. Dosage: 25 mg/kg PO t.i.d. or q.i.d. for 2–8 days or 10 mg/kg IV t.i.d. or q.i.d.

    2. Preparations
      a. Tablet: 500 mg
      b. Ampule: 100 mg/mL

Bibliography

Berg J, Bleyer A: Pediatric dentistry in care of the cancer patient. *Pediatr Dent* 17:257–58,1995.

Leggott PJ: Oral complications of cancer therapies: Chronic dental complications. *NCI Monogr* 9:173–78, 1990.

National Institutes of Health Consensus Development Conference Statement: *Oral Complications of Cancer Therapies: Diagnosis, Prevention and Treatment.* J of the Am Dental Assoc 119:179–83, 1989.

Simon AR, Roberts MW: Management of oral complications associated with cancer therapy in pediatric patients. *ASDC J Dent Child* 58:384–89, 1991.

15

Venous Access Devices in Children

Peter W. Dillon, M.D., and Eugene S. Wiener, M.D.

The establishment of long-term intravenous access is one of the challenges in treating children with cancer. It can be accomplished by using either external tunneled catheters or totally implanted subcutaneous ports. Collectively, these are referred to as implanted vascular access devices. With proper care and attention, these devices can function for a number of years if necessary. If central venous access is required for only a short period of time, then consider the use of temporary percutaneous intravenous central catheters.

Venous access devices are placed in most children entered in Children's Cancer Group protocols to ensure the delivery of medications, blood and blood products, and parenteral nutrition and to allow blood sampling in an atraumatic, reliable, and safe manner. Unfortunately, complications with these devices can occur. The most common complications are device-related infection and device thrombosis. The importance of such issues cannot be minimized in the care of the child with cancer, since device-related infection with associated septicemia can be a frequent life-threatening complication.

I. TYPES AND CHARACTERISTICS OF VENOUS ACCESS DEVICES

A. External catheters

External catheters are tunneled devices with cuffs that anchor the catheter in the subcutaneous tissues proximal

217

to the exit site. They are indicated for children requiring reliable and safe venous access. Access to the device is easier for parents to master, does not require the discomfort of a needle stick, and therefore presents advantages for young children. Children who are candidates for bone marrow transplantation require double- or triple-lumen catheters. Plasmapheresis catheters are usually large, double-lumen devices with a similar anchoring cuff. These devices require frequent changes of dressing and routine flushing with heparin. Activities such as showering or swimming should be avoided or require even more frequent dressing changes. With small children, consider the possibility of dislodgement from pulling or during play.

B. Subcutaneous totally implanted ports
Totally implanted ports have a lower incidence of device-related infections than external catheters and are cosmetically more acceptable. They are accessed by the insertion of a noncoring Huber needle through a self-sealing reservoir just beneath the skin. Extreme obesity or very young age may be a relative contraindication to their insertion, due to potential problems with insertion of the access needle. Because of the risk of bleeding or hematoma formation with each needle insertion for access, children with an uncorrectable coagulopathy or severe thrombocytopenia should not have a port inserted. Take great care to avoid extravasation from needle dislodgement or improper needle placement while administering agents with potentially toxic characteristics, such as parenteral nutrition solution and certain chemotherapeutic medications. When not in use, these devices require minimal care, with heparin flushes once every 2–4 weeks. Activities such as showering and swimming can be pursued.

C. Insertion
Insertion of these devices is accomplished surgically with either a percutaneous or a cutdown technique. The most common veins used for access are the subclavian, jugular (internal or external), facial, and saphenous veins. Rare sites of insertion include the lumbar, hepatic, and the azygous veins. The goal is to place the tip of the catheter in a central location at the junction of the right atrium with the superior or inferior vena cava. The procedure is usually accomplished

in the operating room guided by fluoroscopy or x-ray. At the time of insertion, the absolute neutrophil count should be >500µL and preferably >1000µL, and the platelet count should be >50,000µL. A broad-spectrum antibiotic is often administered at the time of insertion.

D. Removal
Removal of external devices can often be accomplished in the outpatient setting under local anesthesia, while removal of a port is usually done in the operating room.

II. DEFINITION OF COMPLICATIONS

A. Infection
1. Systemic device-related septicemia
Device-related septicemia is used to describe a bloodstream infection in a patient with a vascular access device associated with the clinical manifestations of sepsis and no other source of infection.
2. Local device-related infections
a. Exit site infection of external catheters
Purulent drainage at the exit site often associated with erythema and tenderness marks an exit site infection. Erythema alone does not indicate an infection, since this may result from mechanical irritation of the surrounding skin. Failure to respond to antimicrobial therapy and local wound care may indicate the involvement of the anchoring cuff in the infectious process.
b. Tunnel infection of external catheters and implanted ports
Erythema, tenderness, or swelling of the tunnel extending from the insertion site for external catheters and from the reservoir of implanted ports indicates a tunnel infection.
c. Reservoir infection of totally implanted ports
Reservoir infection is marked by erythema, tenderness, and swelling of the reservoir site. It seldom responds to antibiotic therapy and requires removal of the port to control the infection.

B. Device-related occlusion
1. Total occlusion: complete blockage of at least one lumen

of the device with combined inability to infuse fluid and withdraw blood

2. Partial occlusion: inability to withdraw blood through the device with continued ability to infuse fluids due to the catheter tip being lodged against the vein wall.

A rare case can develop with the ports where there is an ability to withdraw blood but great difficulty with the infusion of fluids due to a clot with a ball-valve mechanism in the reservoir of the device.

III. DETERMINATION OF COMPLICATIONS

A. Infection

1. Device-related septicemia is best determined by paired simultaneous blood cultures drawn through the device and from a peripheral site.
2. Quantitative blood cultures, if available, aid in the differentiation of device-related septicemia from bacteremia. Simultaneous quantitative blood cultures from the device and from a peripheral vein will show a differential colony count ≥10 times in the device blood culture or in the peripheral blood culture for device-related septicemia.
3. Exit site cultures may be helpful in establishing the kind of infection at the exit site or tunnel.

B. Thrombotic and mechanical complications

1. The inability to aspirate blood may not require treatment but may be an early indication of impending device thrombosis or occlusion with a fibrin sheath.
2. Dilated superficial collaterals, arm swelling, or axillary pain is suggestive of a major vein thrombus.
3. If catheter malfunction is suspected, obtain a posteroanterior and lateral chest x-rays to check for malposition, migration, or compression of the catheter. The classic "pinch-off" sign of the catheter portion of the device occurs between the clavicle and first rib.
4. To evaluate a device-related thrombotic event, echocardiography may be helpful in determining the presence of a thrombus at the end of the catheter. A contrast injection of the device will evaluate catheter patency and mechanical complications of the device, but a venogram through a distal peripheral vein of the arm is the best test for a thrombus in a major vein.

IV. THERAPEUTIC MEASURES

A. Device-related septicemia
1. Infection remains a significant cause of morbidity for patients with long-term venous access devices. The incidence of device-related infections reportedly ranges from 2% to >60%. Externally tunneled silastic catheters have a much higher rate of infection than totally implanted ports. The most common organism involved in a device-related bacteremia is *Staphylococcus epidermidis.* External catheters are also at higher risk for infections caused by gram-negative enteric organisms.
2. Device-related infections may be treated by administering an antibiotic through the infected device or removing the device and administering an antibiotic through a peripheral site. Consider removing the device if it is no longer required, if the patient is septic with signs of clinical instability, or if there is persistent device-related bacteremia unresponsive to appropriate antibiotic therapy in 24–48 hours.
   a. Neutropenic patient
      i. For suspected device-related septicemia, broad-spectrum gram-positive and gram-negative antibiotic coverage is indicated until the source of the infection is identified. The patient should be given vancomycin (40 mg/kg/day in patients with normal renal function), tobramycin (6–7.5 mg/kg/day in patients with normal renal function), and ceftazidime (100–150 mg/kg/day) (see Chapter 3).
      ii. It is essential to treat through the lumen(s) of the device rather than through a peripheral intravenous line.
      iii. Consider thrombolytic therapy with urokinase (5000 U/mL). The medication comes prepared in 1 mL vials. For most pediatric internal catheters, 1 mL will be an adequate amount. For most ports, 2 vials (2 mL) should be injected. The entire volume may be injected into the device at one time and allowed to dwell undisturbed for 30–60 minutes. It should then be aspirated rather than flushed through, to avoid an additional bacteremia. The device should then be properly flushed.
      iv. If cultures are positive, continue specific antibiotic

coverage for 7–14 days after cultures are negative. Obtain surveillance cultures at intervals during the course of therapy.

    v. If cultures remain positive after 48 hours of appropriate therapy or if clinical signs of deterioration develop and no other source of infection is clearly present, remove the device.

  b. Non-neutropenic patient

    i. For suspected device-related septicemia in the non-neutropenic patient, use vancomycin (40 mg/kg/day for patients with normal renal function) due to the high incidence of coagulase-negative staphylococcal infections. Monitor serum concentrations. In addition, an aminoglycoside (6–7.5 mg/kg/day for patients with normal renal function) or an advanced–generation cephalosporin such as ceftazidime (100–150 mg/kg/day) may be added until culture results are known. Some clinicians would use the cephalosporin alone until cultures indicate the need for vancomycin.

    ii. Consider administering urokinase (5000 U/mL) as described above.

    iii. If cultures are positive, continue specific antibiotic coverage for 7–14 days after cultures are negative. Obtain surveillance cultures at intervals during the course of therapy.

    iv. If cultures remain positive after 48 hours of appropriate therapy or if clinical signs of deterioration develop and no other source of infection is clearly present, remove the device.

3. Despite the high salvage rate (>75%) of infected devices and the importance of preserving access when limited sites are available, avoid prolonged efforts at salvaging the device in the ill, immune-compromised child.

4. A number of clinical studies have demonstrated a relationship between thrombus formation and device infection. Thrombolytic therapy, most often with urokinase, has been reported as a successful adjuvant in the therapy of infected catheters.

5. If fungal sepsis is present, a device can be infrequently salvaged (<10%). However, if access is limited, treatment may be initiated through an existing device. If subsequent

cultures remain positive or if the patient shows clinical signs of deterioration, remove the device.

6. If a device is removed because of sepsis, the insertion of a new device should await the completion of antibiotic therapy if possible. Additionally, in the neutropenic patient, neutrophil counts should be allowed to normalize as well. If peripheral access is impossible during this time period, a temporary central venous catheter or PICC line can be used. If necessary, a new device may be inserted during the course of antibiotic treatment if the patient has no signs of sepsis, surveillance blood cultures are negative, and the neutrophil count is acceptable.

B. Local device-related infections

1. Infection of the catheter exit-site and/or tunnel

   a. Exit site infections may be very difficult to control and often lead to the removal of the catheter if the catheter cuff is infected. However, local wound care of the exit site may prove beneficial in the treatment of an early site infection. Avoid transparent, occlusive plastic dressings, since these have been found to increase the risk of catheter colonization. Topical antibiotics (polymyxin, Neosporin, bacitracin, etc.) are also effective in minimizing catheter colonization, whereas povidone-iodine ointment is ineffective.

   b. Use systemic antibiotic therapy for the neutropenic patient and the patient who does not respond rapidly to local therapy. Obtain blood cultures and exit site cultures. Start therapy with dicloxacillin 25 mg/kg/day by mouth (PO) or nafcillin 150 mg/kg/day intravenous (IV). If there is progression in the exit site infection after 48 hours or if a tunnel infection develops, change to broad-spectrum antibiotics and remove the catheter.

   c. Tunnel infections of either an external catheter or an implanted port usually require the removal of the device, since systemic antibiotic therapy with broad-spectrum gram-positive coverage is seldom effective in controlling the infection.

2. Infection of the reservoir or pocket

   An infection of the reservoir or pocket of an implanted port is difficult to clear without removal of the entire device. When this is suspected, do not access the device. Initiate systemic antibiotic therapy with broad-spectrum gram-positive coverage through a peripheral site if salvage of the device is to be attempted.

C. Device-related occlusion
   1. Fibrinolytic therapy
      Most cases of total or partial occlusion of the device can be successfully treated with urokinase. In the case of a total occlusion, obtain a radiograph to rule out the possibility of mechanical complication such as catheter dislodgement or migration.
      a. Urokinase is available in premeasured 1 mL vials at a concentration of 5000 U/mL. Draw up enough urokinase into a syringe to fill the device. For most pediatric Broviac catheters, 1 mL will be an adequate amount, while most ports have a fill volume closer to 2 mL. For the larger devices, do not dilute the medication; more than one vial of the medication may be required.
      b. Inject the urokinase into the device and lock in place. If resistance during the injection becomes too high, initially inject one-third to one-half of the volume and lock in place. Inject the remaining volume 30 minutes later.
      c. Wait 60 minutes and then aspirate. If unable to withdraw, repeat with a second administration of urokinase.
      d. After successful treatment of the occlusion, immediately flush the device with saline and then heparinized saline as per institutional protocol to prevent rethrombosis.
      e. For persistent occlusive problems minimally responsive to bolus therapy, a continuous infusion of urokinase at 200 U/kg/h for 24 hours can be attempted. This approach does not require intensive monitoring of the patient or assessment of coagulation parameters.
   2. Precipitate occlusion
      The device that has been occluded by precipitation from total parenteral nutrition (TPN) or medication incompatibility may be treated by attempting to solubilize the precipitate by altering its pH through the administration of HCl or NaHCO3. Such a condition is to be suspected when precipitate is visible in the clear intravenous tubing line connected to the device.

   a. For TPN-associated occlusions, which usually involve
      $CaPO_4$ precipitation, do the following.
      i.   Mix 1 mL of sterile 0.1 N HCl with 9 mL standard
           heparin lock (Hep-Lock) saline (10 U/mL) for a final
           concentration of 0.01 N HCl.
      ii. Inject 0.5 mL of the solution into the device and lock
           in place.
      iii. Wait 30 minutes and then aspirate. If unable to with-
           draw, repeat the administration of 0.5 mL of the
           solution every 5 minutes until 30 minutes have
           elapsed or device patency is restored.
      iv. After successful treatment of the occlusion, immedi-
           ately flush the device with saline and then
           heparinized saline as per institutional protocol to
           prevent rethrombosis.
   b. For medication incompatibilities resulting in an occlud-
      ing precipitation, a similar protocol may be attempted
      using sodium bicarbonate at a concentration of
      1 mEq/mL.
D. Mechanical problems
   1. Reservoir extravasation from implanted ports
      Extravasation of injected fluids may occur as a result of
      inappropriate needle placement for port access before
      the infusion, needle dislodgement during the infusion, or
      malfunction of the device. Causes of device malfunction
      include the separation of the catheter from the reservoir,
      a fracture or break in the reservoir structure, and a frac-
      ture or break in the tunneled catheter portion of the port.
      a. When inappropriate needle placement or dislodge-
         ment is suspected do the following.
         i.   Attempt to reaccess the reservoir properly.
         ii. Flush the device with heparinized saline to prevent
              occlusion if the device is not to be used.
         iii. Use local therapy with warm compresses to help
              eliminate the surrounding swelling.
         iv. See Chapter 14 for treatment recommendations if a
              drug extravasation has occurred.
      b. If proper needle position has been confirmed and an
         extravasation due to a structural problem with the
         port is suspected, a contrast injection study of the
         device will help pinpoint the defect. Therapy usually
         requires complete removal of the port, although sal-

vage of the site can be attempted if there is no associated infection.

2. Extravasation within a tunnel of an external catheter
   a. A contrast injection study of the device will help pinpoint the defect.
   b. Therapy usually requires complete removal of the catheter, although salvage of the site can be attempted if there is no associated infection by insertion of a guidewire before its removal.
3. Dislodgement or malposition of the catheter
   Dislodgement or malposition of the intravascular catheter portion of the device generally requires replacement of the device. Occasionally, manipulating the guidewire under sterile conditions may be successful.
4. Fracture of the device
   a. External catheter
      i. Cracks or breaks of the external catheter can be repaired with kits available for the specific size and brand of the catheter. Carefully follow the instructions accompanying the kit.
      ii. Use sterile technique, including mask, gloves, and surgical preparation, to avoid contamination.
      iii. Temporary repair of an external catheter can be accomplished by the insertion of an appropriate-sized plastic IV catheter into the lumen of the catheter at the break point under sterile technique.
      iv. The catheter should then be flushed with heparinized saline solution to prevent occlusion. Permanent repair should be accomplished as soon as a kit is available.
   b. Internal catheter
      i. Fracture of the tunneled or intravascular portion of the catheter of either an external catheter or an implanted port may lead to intravascular embolization of that portion of the catheter.
      ii. The most common site of the catheter for this to occur is the point where the catheter passes between the clavicle and the first rib.
      iii. The embolized portion of the catheter usually travels to the right ventricle or to the pulmonary artery outflow tract.

iv. Retrieval of the embolized catheter can usually be accomplished in the cardiac catheterization laboratory.

Bibliography

Ascher DP, Shoupe BA, Maybee D, et al.: Persistent catheter-related bacteremia: Clearance with antibiotics and urokinase. *J Pediatr Surg* 28:627–29, 1993.

Bagnall HA, Gomperts E, Atkinson JB: Continuous infusion of low-dose urokinase in the treatment of central venous catheter thrombosis in infants and children. *Pediatrics* 83:963–66, 1989.

Dawson S, Pai MK, Smith S, et al.: Right atrial catheters in children with cancer: A decade of experience in the use of tunneled, exteriorized devices at a single institution. *Am J Pediatr Hematol Oncol* 13:126–29, 1991.

Fishbein JD, Friedman HS, Bennett BB, et al.: Catheter-related sepsis refractory to antibiotics treated successfully with adjunctive urokinase infusion. *Pediatr Infect Dis* 9:676–78, 1990.

Goodwin ML: Using sodium bicarbonate to clear a medication precipitate from a central venous catheter. *Journal of Vascular Access Networks* 1:23–26, 1991.

Groeger JS, Lucas AB, Thaler HT, et al.: Infectious morbidity associated with long-term use of venous access devices in patients with cancer. *Ann Intern Med* 119:1168–74, 1993.

Ingram J, Weitzman S, Greenberg ML, et al.: Complications of indwelling venous access lines in pediatric hematology patients: A prospective comparison of external venous catheters and subcutaneous ports. *Am J Pediatr Hematol Oncol* 13:130–36, 1991.

Lecciones JA, Lee JW, Navarro BE, et al.: Vascular catheter associated fungemia in patients with cancer: Analysis of 155 episodes. *Clin Infect Dis* 14:875–83, 1992.

Raucher HS, Hyatt AC, Barzilai A, et al.: Quantitative blood cultures in the evaluation of septicemia in children with Broviac catheters. *J Pediatr* 104:29–33, 1984.

Rubie H, Juricic M, Claeyssens S, et al.: Morbidity using subcutaneous ports and efficacy of vancomycin flushing in cancer. *Arch Dis Child* 72:325–29, 1995.

Schulman RJ, Reed T, Pitre D, et al.: Use of hydrochloric acid to clear obstructed central venous catheters. *J Parenter Ent Nutr* 12:509–12, 1988.

Weiner ES, McGuire P, Stolar CJ, et al.: The CCG prospective study of venous access devices: An analysis of insertions and causes for removal. *J Pediatr Surg* 27:155–64, 1992.

16

The Management of the Sexually Mature Young Adult Patient with Cancer

Arthur R. Ablin, M.D., and Paula K. Groncy, M.D.

The sexually mature teenager with newly diagnosed cancer presents a special challenge to the pediatric oncologist. This chapter touches briefly on ways the pediatric oncologist and coprofessionals may assist these young people to assume their new responsibilities of transition to adulthood while facing the additional burdens of cancer treatment.

I. AT DIAGNOSIS

A. A relationship based on respect, trust, and confidentiality between the patient and the physician and other health care providers must be established at the onset of treatment. The physician must set the model for open, honest, and trustworthy communication. It must be clear to the young patient that he or she has a personal physician who will represent the patient's interests and concerns.

B. These discussions with the teenage patient must take place privately, and may include the patient's parents when the patient gives permission.

C. In addition to explaining the disease, what may be known of its causes, treatment, prognosis, and impact on school, friends, and normal activities, address the issue of possible pregnancy with every sexually mature young adult, as well as the consequences, as we know them, of the cancer treatment for future fertility.

D. Before starting chemotherapy, strongly consider a pregnancy test for young women.

E. In addition to the usual content of the initial conference with the young man, before starting therapy, address the issue of possible oligo- or aspermia. Explore the possibility of banking frozen sperm, and reach a decision before starting chemotherapy. Discuss the difference between fertility and virility.

II. PREVENTION OF INFECTION

A. Abrasions
Vaginal abrasions and abnormalities of the vaginal mucosa have been reported with the use of tampons, especially super tampons. A potential for infection exists if a tampon is left in place longer than is recommended. Sanitary napkins or pads are recommended rather than tampons.

B. Intercourse
  1. For sexually active female patients with an absolute neutrophil count (ANC) <500 µL, sexual intercourse may constitute a risk for mucosal disruption and bacterial shower with subsequent infection. Abstention, especially during these times, is highly recommended.
  2. Both young men and young women should be made aware that infection may be spread with any episode of intercourse, no matter what the ANC.
  3. With sexually active teenagers, emphasize the use of both condoms and contraceptive jelly and verify a method for their procurement.
  4. When the vaginal mucosa is dry, water-based lubricants such as Astraglide may be used to decrease abrasions.
  5. Make known to the teenage patient the availability of confidential, nonjudgmental professional advice.

III. PREVENTION AND MANAGEMENT OF EXCESSIVE MENSTRUAL BLEEDING

A. Prevention
  1. While young women patients are on aggressive therapeutic

regimens, the suppression of menses by the use of oral contraceptive pills on a daily basis is strongly recommended.

2. Withdrawal bleeding may be allowed when chemotherapy is less aggressive, and it is anticipated that blood counts will be normal.

B. Management

With excessive bleeding, always rule out pregnancy, thrombocytopenia, and a coagulopathy. Also consider other causes, such as dysfunctional uterine bleeding.

1. With normal hemoglobin
   a. Observe, with frequent determinations of hemoglobin.
   b. If regular periods continue to be heavy or if hemoglobin drops to <12g/dL, then prescribe low-dose oral contraceptives (e.g., Ortho-Cept 21) daily.

2. With hemoglobin 8–12 g/dL
   a. Outpatient care is most likely possible.
   b. Start a moderate-dose oral contraceptive pill (Ortho-Novum 1/35 or Lo/Ovral) 1 tablet q.i.d. for 4 days, then 1 tablet t.i.d. for 3 days, then 1 tablet b.i.d. for 14 days, then 1 tablet daily.
   c. If no breakthrough bleeding occurs, the patient may switch to a low-dose pill, such as Ortho-Cept 21. If monthly menstrual bleeding is heavy, then daily continuous suppression of menses with a low- or moderate-dose pill is advised.

3. With hemoglobin <7 g/dL
   a. Hospitalization and consultation to control vaginal bleeding is indicated.
   b. Prescribe Premarin 25 mg IV every 4–6 hours until the bleeding stops (maximum 6 doses).
   c. After the bleeding stops, give Premarin 5 mg IV daily for 2–3 days.
   d. Start a high-dose contraceptive pill (Ovral) on the same schedule as Section 2b above immediately after Premarin on day 1. The patient may then switch to a moderate- or low-dose pill.
   e. If bleeding persists, give medroxyprogesterone (Provera) 10 mg/day by mouth (PO) until the bleeding stops.

IV. SEXUALITY AND CONTRACEPTION

A. Communication

Every young man and woman needs to make contact with someone with whom to discuss issues such as body image, sexual decision making, family conflicts, and handling peer pressure. This is especially appropriate for teenagers with cancer.

B. Contraception
1. Discuss the need for contraception with every teenage patient, both young men and young women.
2. Patients must understand that contraception does not protect against acquired immunodeficiency syndrome (AIDS) or other sexually transmitted diseases.
3. Even if the woman is on birth control pills, patients should use condoms. Counsel each young man and woman about the responsibilities of the other sex in addition to their own.
4. Apprise patients of the availability of emergency contraception, and encourage them to seek advice (Ovral 2 tablets to start and repeat in 12 hours or LoOvral 4 tablets to start and repeat in 12 hours).

Bibliography

Burt K: The effects of cancer on body image and sexuality. *Nurs Times* 91:36–7, 1995.

Polaneczky MM: Menstrual disorders in the adolescent: Dysmenorrhea and dysfunctional uterine bleeding. *Pediatr Rev* 13:83–7, 1992.

Sondheimer SJ: Update on oral contraceptive pills and postcoital contraception. *Curr Opin Obstet Gynecol* 4:502–5, 1992.

Tuttle JT: Menstrual disorders during adolescence. *J Pediatr Health Care* 5:197–203, 1991.

Van Winter JT, Simmons PS: Common menstrual problems in adolescents. *Postgrad Obstet Gynecol* 11:1–7, 1991.

17

The Care of the Pediatric Patient after Hematopoietic Stem Cell Transplantion

Kenneth De Santes, M.D., and John J. Quinn, M.D.

Bone marrow transplantation is a well-established treatment for acute and chronic leukemias, myelodysplasia, some solid tumors, aplastic anemia, hemoglobinopathies, and congenital immune deficiencies and cytopenias. More recently, transplants have been performed using peripheral blood or umbilical cord blood as the source of stem cells, so the term *hematopoietic stem cell transplant* (HSCT) will be used in this chapter. The complications that occur after a HSCT depend on multiple factors, including the pretransplant conditioning regimen, human leukocyte antigen (HLA) compatibility of the donor, stem cell source, graft manipulation (e.g., T-cell depletion, or tumor purging), as well as the child's age, underlying disease, and prior therapy (Table 17.1).

The conditioning regimen uses high-dose chemotherapy with or without regional or total body irradiation (TBI) and is usually completed in 4–8 days. After the stem cell infusion there is an obligatory period of pancytopenia, which has been shortened, to some extent, by the use of peripheral blood stem cells (PBSCs) and hematopoietic growth factors.

Discharge from the transplant center usually occurs when the patient achieves a stable absolute neutrophil count (ANC) 500–1000 neutrophils/μL, has resolved any acute infectious or transplant

TABLE 17.1.
Characteristics of Different Hematopoietic Stem Cell Grafts

Stem Cell Source	Risk of Graft-versus-Host Disease	Risk of Graft Failure	Timing of Engraftment	Risk of Prolonged Immune Deficiency
Bone marrow				
Autologous	None	Rare	Intermediate	Rare
Autologous, purged	None	Variable	Variable	Rare
Related, match	Moderate	Rare	Intermediate	Low
Related, match, T-cell depleted	Low	Low	Intermediate	Variable
Related, mismatch	High	High	Intermediate	Variable
Related, mismatch, T-cell depleted	Variable	High	Intermediate	High
Unrelated, match	High	Low	Intermediate	Variable
Unrelated, match, T-cell depleted	Variable	High	Intermediate	High
Unrelated, mismatch, T-cell depleted	High	High	Intermediate	High
Peripheral blood				
Autologous	None	Rare	Fast	Low
Allogeneic	Moderate	Low	Fast	Low
Cord blood				
Related, match	Low	Low	Slow	Low
Unrelated	Variable	Variable	Slow	Variable

related complications, and is obtaining adequate nutritional support. At the time of discharge all HSCT patients remain profoundly immunodeficient, especially those who develop graft-versus-host disease (GVHD), and many still require platelet and red cell transfusions. Economic pressures and the increased use of mobilized PBSC have resulted in earlier discharge from the transplant unit. Consequently, general pediatricians and pediatric oncologists who may have limited transplant experience are assuming greater responsibility for the care of these children. Management of the HSCT patient requires an understanding of the complications that can arise at different times after transplant, recognition of these problems, and the early implementation of appropriate therapy.

I. HEMATOLOGIC SUPPORT

A. Background

1. Patients may experience delayed hematologic recovery after HSCT for a variety of reasons, including infections, drugs, GVHD, autoimmune disease, late graft failure, and relapse of their underlying malignancy.
2. Manage cytopenias as follows.
   a. Identify and treat possible causes.
   b. Provide red blood cell and/or platelet transfusions.
   c. Use hematopoietic growth factors.
3. Blood products should *always* be irradiated before administration to eliminate the risk of GVHD.
4. If both patient and donor are cytomegalovirus (CMV) negative, then provide CMV-negative products whenever possible. If CMV-negative blood is unavailable, use a leukocyte filter to reduce the risk of transmitting CMV. Some centers also routinely use leukocyte filters to reduce the risk of alloimmunization.
5. If patient and/or donor are CMV positive, most blood banks will not release CMV- negative blood products; use leukocyte-filtered blood products.

B. Anemia

Most patients do not attain a normal hemoglobin level for several weeks to months after a HSCT. However, the persistence of severe anemia requiring transfusion support beyond 3 months or the development of anemia after achieving normal erythropoiesis requires investigation.

1. Possible causes, diagnostic procedures, and treatment options are listed in Table 17.2.
2. Consider transfusion with 10–15 mL/kg of irradiated, CMV-negative, and/or leukocyte-filtered packed red blood cells if:
   a. The hemoglobin falls below 7.0 g/dL.
   or
   b. Symptoms develop (e.g., fatigue, dizziness).

C. Thrombocytopenia

Most children become independent of platelet transfusions within 2 months of their transplant. The persistence of a transfusion requirement beyond 2–3 months, in the absence of an obvious cause (e.g., severe GVHD), requires investigation. Similarly, the development of thrombocytopenia after attaining a normal platelet count mandates further evaluation.

TABLE 17.2.
Hematologic Problems after Hematopoietic Stem Cell Transplant*

Disorder	Etiology	Diagnostic Studies	Treatment Options
Anemia	Autoimmune	Coombs' test, reticulocyte count	Steroids, IVGG, plasmapheresis, splenectomy
	HUS	RBC morphology, creatinine, platelet count	Consider stopping CSA
	Parvovirus infection	PCR for parvovirus	IVGG?
	Graft failure	Engraftment studies	Second transplant
	Unknown	EPO level, bone marrow aspirate	Consider EPO if level <500 U/L, RBC transfusion
Thrombocytopenia	Infection	Cultures	Antibiotics
	GVHD	Biopsy	Steroids, CSA, ATG
	Relapse	Bone marrow aspirate	Second transplant, immunotherapy
	ITP	Platelet-associated immunoglobulin	IVGG, steroids, splenectomy
	HUS	RBC morphology, creatinine	Consider stopping CSA
	Graft failure	Engraftment studies	Second transplant
	Unknown	Bone marrow aspirate	Platelet transfusion
	Drugs	Septra, ganciclovir, azathioprine	Consider alternative agent
Neutropenia	GVHD	Biopsy	Steroids, CSA, ATG
	CMV infection	CMV culture	Ganciclovir, IVGG, foscarnet
	Graft failure	Engraftment studies	Second transplant
	Unknown	Bone marrow aspirate	Consider G or GM-CSF if ANC < 500μL

*Abbreviations: ANC, absolute neutrophil count; ATG, antithymocyte globulin; CMV, cytomegalovirus; CSA, cyclosporine; EPO, erythropoietin; G-CSF, granulocyte-colony-stimulating factor; GM-CSF, granulocyte-macrophage-colony-stimulating factor; GVHD, graft-versus-host disease; HSCT, hematopoietic stem cell transplant; HUS, hemolytic uremic syndrome; ITP, immune thrombocytopenic purpura; IVGG, intravenous gammaglobulin; PCR, polymerase chain reaction; RBC, red blood cell.

1. Possible etiologies, suggested evaluations, and treatment options are listed in Table 17.2.
2. Consider transfusion with CMV-negative and/or leukocyte-filtered platelets if:
   a. The platelet count falls below 10,000–15,000/µL
   or
   b. Bleeding occurs.
3. If a patient experiences significant bleeding (e.g., gross hematuria), maintain the platelet count >50,000/µL.
4. If possible, use apheresis units to minimize donor exposures.

D. Neutropenia
Patients are generally not discharged from the transplant unit until they have recovered from the obligatory period of neutropenia soon after transplant.
1. The ANC may fluctuate for several months after transplantation but does not usually fall below 500/µL
2. Persistent severe neutropenia after discharge requires further evaluation and treatment (Table 17.2).
3. Some patients may benefit from intermittent doses of granulocyte-colony-stimulating factor (G-CSF) or granulocyte-macrophage colony-stimulating factor (GM-CSF) (3–7 days/week) to maintain an ANC >500/µL.

II. Nutritional Considerations

A. Background
Nearly all children require nutritional support at the time of HSCT and for several weeks to months thereafter. Close monitoring of nutrition is an important component of post-transplant care.
1. Reasons for poor dietary caloric intake soon after transplant may include:
   a. Anorexia, nausea, and mucositis consequent to the conditioning regimen
   b. Gastrointestinal GVHD.
   c. Infection or other complications that cause general malaise.
2. Resumption of normal dietary habits occurs slowly as the gastrointestinal tract recovers from the chemoradiotherapy and psychological food aversions begin to dissipate.

3. Progress is often hampered by damaged taste buds, xerostomia, and dietary restrictions placed on patients because of iatrogenic immunodeficiency.

B. Dietary restrictions and recommendations
There are few scientific data on which to base recommendations regarding dietary precautions after discharge from the transplant unit. Any restrictions imposed by the transplant center should be observed until immune function has significantly improved. The guidelines of one transplant center are presented below:
1. Avoid consuming unpasteurized dairy products and raw or undercooked meats, poultry, fish, or eggs.
2. Wash hands well before handling/preparing foods.
3. Wash hands well before eating.
4. Do not share eating or drinking utensils.
5. Once served, food should not stand at room temperature for more than 2 hours.
6. Take-out food is permitted but should be obtained from well-established chain restaurants.

C. Nutritional support and monitoring
Most children will require nutritional support after leaving the transplant unit.
1. This may be provided enterally or parenterally, depending on the child's clinical status and the preferences of the transplant team.
2. Support is usually weaned over 1–2 months as the patient's dietary caloric intake improves.
3. Obtain weight and dietary history every 1–2 weeks after discharge.
4. Parents should keep a log of their child's oral intake.
5. Pay special attention to new or worsening nausea, anorexia, vomiting, or diarrhea, since this may be indicative of:
   a. Infection.
   b. Gastrointestinal GVHD.
6. Once a child is taking ~75% of his or her caloric requirements by mouth, consider stopping supplemental enteral/parenteral support.
7. Consultation with a nutritionist may be quite helpful, especially for patients who require prolonged nutritional support.

III. PROPHYLAXIS AGAINST INFECTION

A. Background

The risk of infection after a HSCT is largely determined by the rapidity of myeloid and immune recovery. The rate of T- and B- cell immune reconstitution is variable and depends on the stem cell source, on HLA compatibility of the donor, on graft manipulation (e.g., T-cell depletion), and on whether GVHD develops as well as its treatment.

1. Between 30 and 100 days after transplant, most patients are still significantly immunocompromised and remain at increased risk of infection, especially those who develop acute GVHD.
2. Measures to reduce infection risk during this time may include:
   a. Using prophylactic antibiotics.
   b. Administering intravenous gammaglobulin (IVGG).
   c. Minimizing environmental exposures.
3. After day 100, severe infections are more commonly seen in patients with active GVHD or may be associated with a central venous catheter.
4. Complete immunologic reconstitution may not occur for 1 year or more after allogeneic transplantation, although significant recovery of immune function can usually be documented much earlier.
5. Each transplant center has its own policies to safeguard patients against infection. Some general guidelines will be discussed below.

B. Prophylactic antibiotics

1. Trimethoprim/sulfamethoxazole (TMP/SMX; 5 mg/kg divided b.i.d. 3 days/week) is usually administered for prophylaxis against *Pneumocystis carinii* for at least 6 months after transplant or until T cell function has significantly improved. Pentamidine (300 mg aerosolized or 4 mg/kg IV q28 days) may be used for patients who are allergic to TMP/SMX.
2. Fluconazole (3 mg/kg/day IV or PO) is frequently used for fungal prophylaxis before and soon after transplant, but often discontinued on discharge.
3. Acyclovir (250–500 mg/m^2 2 or 3 times a day) is often administered during the peritransplant period for prophy-

laxis against herpes viruses, but frequently discontinued on discharge.

4. Ganciclovir (5 mg/kg/day, 5–7 days/week) may be used for several months (often up to day 100 after transplant) for prophylaxis against CMV infection.
   a. This therapy is generally restricted to allogeneic transplant recipients who are at increased risk of developing CMV disease because they:
      i. Are CMV positive and have received an unrelated donor or T-cell-depleted graft.
      ii. Have received a transplant from a CMV-positive unrelated or mismatched related donor.
      iii. Have CMV isolated from the blood or other sites.
   b. Closely monitor patients receiving ganciclovir for renal and hematologic toxicity by performing at least weekly complete blood count (CBC) with differential and creatinine level.
   c. Consider discontinuing ganciclovir if the ANC falls below 750/µL. Administration of G-CSF or GM-CSF maybe helpful in maintaining the ANC >750/µL.
   d. Dose adjustment is required for renal insufficiency.
5. Children being treated for acute or chronic GVHD require more aggressive antibiotic prophylaxis (see Section IV).

C. Intravenous gammaglobulin
   The administration of IVGG after transplant appears to reduce the risk of infection, although the overall effect on survival remains uncertain.
   1. Many centers administer IVGG (400–500 mg/kg) monthly for varying periods of time or until there is evidence of adequate antibody production (as determined by serum levels of immunoglobin (Ig)A, IgM, and isohemagglutinin titers).
   2. Patients receiving a transplant for a congenital immune deficiency or those who develop chronic GVHD may especially benefit from monthly IVGG.
   3. Patients not receiving IVGG who are experiencing frequent infections should have serum levels of IgG and IgG subclasses measured. IVGG should be administered if hypogammaglobulinemia or a subclass deficiency is documented.

D. Environmental precautions

Few data are available regarding the efficacy of limiting environmental exposures to reduce infection risk after discharge from the transplant unit.

1. Most centers require patients to wear masks when traveling outside their home.
2. If possible, patients should avoid contact with:
   a. Crowds
   b. Ill friends or family members
   c. Construction sites (because of *Aspergillus* contamination)
3. Dietary modifications are discussed in Section II.
4. Environmental precautions are usually followed up to 1 year after transplant or until T cell function significantly improves. At that time most children can resume all prior activities, including return to school. Direct any questions regarding isolation procedures to the transplant center.

IV. GRAFT-VERSUS-HOST DISEASE

A. Background

GVHD may be present at the time of discharge from the transplant center or can develop subsequently. It can be divided into two phases.

1. Acute GVHD (aGVHD) develops during the first 100 days after transplant.
2. Chronic GVHD (cGVHD) either persists beyond or first manifests after 100 days after a HSCT. It may, in decreasing order of frequency:
   a. Evolve directly from acute GVHD (persistent cGVHD).
   b. Redevelop after the resolution of the acute phase (quiescent cGVHD).
   c. Be the first manifestation of GVHD (de novo cGVHD).

B. Acute GVHD

1. The primary target organs of aGVHD, in decreasing order of frequency, are skin, gastrointestinal (GI) tract, and liver (Table 17.3). Most patients have skin involvement, which often begins on the palms and soles, soon thereafter spreads to face, scalp, nape of neck, and ears, and then may involve the rest of the body.
2. Isolated GI or hepatic involvement is uncommon, although a subset of patients may be seen with only

TABLE 17.3.
Clinical Classification of Acute Graft-versus-Host Disease according to Organ Injury

	Skin	Liver (Bilirubin)	Gut
Stage			
1	Maculopapular rash on <25% of body surface	2–3 mg/dL*	300–600 mL/m^2 stool/day or nausea*†
2	Maculopapular rash on 25–50% of body surface	>3–6 mg/dL	>600–900 mL/m^2 stool/day
3	Maculopapular rash on >50% of body surface	>6–15 mg/dL	>900 mL/m^2 stool/day
4	Maculopapular rash on >50% of body surface with bullae and desquamation	>15 mg/dl	Severe abdominal pain with or without ileus
Clinical grade			
I (mild)	1 or 2	0	0
II (moderate)	3 or	1 or	1
III (severe)		2–3 or	2–4
IV (life threatening)	4 or	4	

Source: Modified from Pazepiorka D, Welsdorf D, Martin P, et al: 1994 Consensus Conference on acute GVHO grading. *Bone Marrow Transplantation* 15:825–28, 1995.
* Downgrade one stage if additional cause for elevated bilirubin or diarrhea is documented.
† Persistent nausea with histologic evidence of GVHD in the stomach or duodenum.

upper GI disease, manifesting as anorexia, nausea, and vomiting.

3. Diagnosis of aGVHD can usually be made by skin biopsy and involvement of the other organs inferred in the appropriate clinical context. For those uncommon patients whose skin is spared, rectal biopsy, endoscopic biopsy of an involved portion of the GI tract, or liver biopsy may be necessary to establish a diagnosis. A biopsy may also be required to exclude other causes of GI or hepatic dysfunction, such as CMV infection.

4. The prophylactic regimen used to prevent GVHD depends on the type of transplant (related versus unrelated) and individual preferences of the transplant center. Cyclosporine (CSA) is commonly used, often in combination with other agents such as methotrexate and/or methylprednisolone.

   a. CSA is usually given at a dose of 3.0 mg/kg/day intravenous (IV) divided q12h or 12 mg/kg/day by mouth

(PO) divided q12h. More frequent administration (e.g., every 6–8 hours or continuous infusion) may be required to achieve a therapeutic serum level, especially in very young children.

b. Pharmacologic monitoring should be used to ensure that a therapeutic serum level is attained (usually ~150–400 µg/L).

c. The CSA dose may need to be modified for renal insufficiency (Table 17.4).

d. If GVHD does not develop, then the CSA is usually tapered by 5% per week starting on day 50 after transplant.

e. A slower taper regimen is sometimes used for patients receiving unrelated donor grafts.

5. Treatment of newly diagnosed aGVHD or a flare-up of aGVHD will depend on which medications the patient received for GVHD prophylaxis or for prior therapy. Initiate or change therapy in consultation with the transplant center.

a. Steroids are the treatment of choice for aGVHD. If the patient has not been on steroids, then start prednisone or methylprednisolone, 2 mg/kg/day in divided doses.

b. Once there has been a satisfactory response, a slow taper of 0.5 mg/kg every 7–14 days can be instituted.

c. Patients who fail to respond to standard-dose steroids and CSA may be treated with high-dose "pulse" methylprednisolone (10–30 mg/kg/day) for several days or antithymocyte globulin (ATG, 20 mg/kg/day or qod × 7 doses). Other treatment modalities that have been used are listed in Table 17.5.

d. If there is GI involvement, especially significant diarrhea, the patient may need to be placed at gut rest and begin parenteral nutrition. If the diarrhea is secretory,

TABLE 17.4.
Cyclosporine Dosing for Renal Insufficiency*

Serum Creatinine	CSA Dose
<1.5 × baseline	Full dose
1.5-1.9 × baseline	50% dose
>2.0 × baseline	Hold dose

*General guidelines which may be modified based on patients clinical status.

TABLE 17.5.
Alternative Therapies for Acute Graft-versus-Host Disease

Agent	Example(s)
Newer immunosuppressive drugs	FK506, CellCept
Anti-T cell monoclonal antibodies	OKT3 (anti-CD3)
Anti-T cell immunotoxins	XomaZyme (anti-CD5)
Antibodies that block cytokines	Anti-tumor necrosis factor, anti-interleukin (IL)-2
Antibodies that block cytokine receptors	Anti-IL-1R, anti-IL-2R

octreotide therapy may also be beneficial (1 μg/kg q12h; may slowly increase dose up to 10 μg/kg as needed). As the disease comes under control, gradually reintroduce enteral feeding.

6. The immunosuppressive agents used for prophylaxis or to treat GVHD can cause numerous complications. The side effects of steroids are well known to most medical personnel and will not be reviewed here. CSA commonly causes neurologic symptoms and renal dysfunction (Table 17.6). Monitor trough serum CSA levels, creatinine, electrolytes, and magnesium on a regular basis. The most frequent toxicities requiring intervention are the following.
   a. Hypomagnesemia
      i. Potentiates the neurotoxicity of CSA
      ii. Often requires treatment with intravenous or oral magnesium
   b. Hypertension
      i. Especially common in patients on concomitant steroids
      ii. Often responds well to vasodilating calcium channel blockers (e.g., nifedipine)
      iii. May require additional antihypertensive agents (e.g., labetalol or clonidine)
   c. Renal insufficiency
      i. May be alleviated by improving hydration status
      ii. Dose adjustment of CSA may be required
7. Prevention and treatment of infections is crucial for successful management of aGVHD.
   a. Maintain prophylaxis against *P. carinii* (TMP/SMX), fungal infection (fluconazole or clotrimazole), and herpes viruses (acyclovir or ganciclovir if CMV prophylaxis is indicated).

TABLE 17.6.
Toxicity of Cyclosporin

Neurotoxicity
  Common
    Tremor
    Headache
    Dysesthesia
  Uncommon
    Seizures
    Ataxia
    Somnolence
    Leukoencephalopathy
Renal toxicity
  Common
    Elevated creatinine
    Hypomagnesemia
    Hypertension
  Uncommon
    Acute renal failure
    Hemolytic uremic syndrome with:
      Renal insufficiency
      Microangiopathic hemolytic anemia
      Thrombocytopenia
Hirsutism
Hepatic insufficiency

    b. Early recognition and prompt treatment of complicating bacterial, fungal, and viral infections is essential.

C. Chronic GVHD
  1. cGVHD can be classified as limited or extensive (Table 17.7). It may affect the same target organs as the acute form, but may also involve the mouth, eyes, and lungs as well as other organ systems (Table 17.8). The clinical manifestations often resemble those of a persistent autoimmune disease.
  2. Screening tests for cGVHD include biopsy of involved organs; assessment of pulmonary, hepatic, and immunologic function; CBC; and Schirmer test (Table 17.8).
  3. Immune deficiency persists with propensity to opportunistic infections and infections with encapsulated bacteria. This is the usual cause of death in these patients.
  4. If there is progressive bronchiolitis obliterans, death may be due to respiratory failure.
  5. Treatment of cGVHD is most efficacious when adminis-

TABLE 17.7.
Clinical Grading of Chronic Graft-versus-Host Disease

Limited (better prognosis)
   Localized skin involvement or hepatic dysfunction
Extensive (worse prognosis)
   Generalized skin involvement or localized skin involvement
     plus any of the following:
       Chronic hepatitis or cirrhosis
       Keratoconjunctivitis
       Oral mucosal involvement
       Involvement of any other organ (e.g., lung or GI tract)

TABLE 17.8.
Chronic Graft-versus-Host Disease: Clinical Features and Screening Studies

Organ/System	Clinical Features	Screening Studies
Skin	Lichenoid or sclerodermatous changes, dyspigmentation, erythema, scaling, alopecia, onychodystrophy	Punch biopsy of skin
Oral cavity	Lichen planus, xerostomia	Lower lip biopsy
Ocular	Sicca, keratitis	Schirmer test
Liver	Icterus	Bilirubin, alkaline phosphatase, γ-glutamyl transpeptidase
GI tract	Dysphagia, malabsorption, diarrhea, weight loss	Endoscopy with biopsies
Pulmonary	Bronchiolitis obliterans producing obstructive/restrictive lung disease	Pulmonary function tests, oxymetry
Immunologic	Opportunistic infections, encapsulated bacterial infections, frequent sinopulmonary infections	T-cell function and subsets, quantitative immunoglobulins, IgG subclasses
Hematologic	Eosinophilia, thrombocytopenia	CBC

tered early in its course. Screening tests help identify patients in need of therapy. For those patients whose cGVHD is not a direct progression from unresolved aGVHD, clinical manifestations of cGVHD may become apparent as post-transplant immunosuppressive therapy is tapered.

6. Patients who develop cGVHD during a CSA taper should be placed back on a full therapeutic dose (12 mg/kg/day

PO). If resolution does not occur, then the first-line therapy for cGVHD, as for aGVHD, is corticosteroid administration. To minimize the long-term side effects of therapy, place patients on alternate-day treatment as soon as possible.

  a. A commonly used regimen consists of prednisone 1 mg/kg/day PO and CSA 12 mg/kg/day PO in 2 divided doses. As the disease comes under control, switch the patient to an alternate-day regimen so that on any given day only one of the two drugs is administered.

  b. Patients who fail to respond to the above regimen may be tried on alternative therapies (Table 17.9).

  c. Patients with refractory oral disease may respond to steroid rinses or Psoralen and ultraviolet A therapy to the oral cavity.

7. Additional supportive care measures are critical.

  a. Continuation of prophylaxis against *P. carinii* and infection with encapsulated bacteria with daily TMP/SMX or TMP/SMX 3 days/week plus an oral penicillin or cephalosporin

  b. Oral antifungal prophylaxis

  c. Protection from sun exposure by covering commonly exposed areas and using sunscreen

  d. Artificial tears for patients with eye involvement

  e. Monthly IVGG at a dose of 400–500 mg/kg may be beneficial, especially for patients with hypogamma-globulinemia or IgG subclass deficiencies

  f. Hypervigilance for viral, fungal, and bacterial infections

V. ENDOCRINE CONSIDERATIONS

A. Background
Abnormalities of linear growth, sexual maturation, and endocrine function may be encountered after a HSCT and are related to the pretransplant conditioning regimen, age at transplant, development of cGVHD, the patient's underlying disease, and prior therapy.

B. Growth
The most important factor influencing growth in the HSCT patient is the pretransplant conditioning regimen.

1. TBI may directly damage growth plates and cause growth hormone deficiency (especially in patients treated with

TABLE 17.9.
Alternative Therapies for Chronic Graft-versus-Host Disease

Agent	Toxicity	Comments
Azathioprine	Bone marrow suppression	Monitor CBC regularly. Thrombocytopenia is a relative contraindication
Psoralen and ultraviolet A therapy	Erythroderma, xeroderma, hyperpigmentation pruritis, nausea	Used for cutaneous cGVHD. Psoralen may be given orally or in bath. Avoid concomitant photosensitizing drugs
Thalidomide	Somnolence, dizziness, rash, constipation, headache, xerostomia, xeroderma, peripheral neuropathy	Drowsiness abates after a few weeks. Discontinue drug if patient develops evidence of peripheral neuropathy. May be helpful to monitor plasma levels
Etretinate	Scaling of skin, chelitis, xerosis, eye irritation	Has been used for sclerodermatous cGVHD. May be teratogenic
Hydroxy-chloroquine	Retinopathy, keratopathy	Experience with this drug is very limited
Clofazimine	Nausea, diarrhea, constipation, hyper-pigmentation of skin/conjunctiva	Experience with this drug is very limited
Total lymphoid irradiation	Leukopenia	Experience with this modality is very limited

prior cranial irradiation) and probably other endocrine abnormalities resulting in impaired growth.

2. Busulfan, which is often used in lieu of TBI, may cause a similar degree of growth retardation.

3. Conditioning regimens that use cyclophosphamide alone do not appear to affect growth adversely.

4. Relatively few data are available regarding the growth of children with solid tumors who undergo conditioning with chemotherapy alone. However, patients with neuroblastoma appear to be at especially high risk of significant growth retardation.

5. After transplantation, measure height at least yearly until final adult stature is attained.

   a. Children experiencing subnormal growth velocity should be evaluated by a pediatric endocrinologist.

b. Preliminary experience with growth hormone administration to HSCT patients suggests that early implementation of replacement therapy may alleviate, to some extent, the detrimental effects of chemoradiotherapy.

C. Sexual development
1. The use of TBI has been associated with a high risk of gonadal failure, resulting in:
   a. Delayed pubertal development.
   b. Infertility.
2. Busulfan also appears to cause gonadal dysfunction with similar effects on sexual development and fertility. Many children treated with busulfan also have an underlying disease that may contribute to the gonadal failure (e.g., ß-thalassemia).
3. Most children treated with cyclophosphamide alone appear to regain normal gonadal function 6–12 months after transplant, and fertility is usually unimpaired.
4. Determine Tanner developmental scores yearly after transplant until adulthood. Some centers also perform yearly sex hormone determinations starting at the age of expected puberty.
5. Patients manifesting delayed pubertal development or showing other signs of gonadal dysfunction should be evaluated by a pediatric endocrinologist.

D. Thyroid function
1. Hypothyroidism develops in approximately 10–30% of patients exposed to fractionated TBI and can occur many years after the transplant.
2. In most cases, compensated hypothyroidism is diagnosed [elevated thyroid-stimulating hormone (TSH) with normal thyroxine (T_4) index], but occasionally overt hypothyroidism occurs (low T_4 index).
3. Rarely, hypothyroidism has been reported in patients conditioned with chemotherapy alone.
4. Obtain thyroid studies (TSH and T_4 index) yearly for patients exposed to TBI and palpate the neck to detect any nodules suggestive of a secondary malignancy.
5. The management of compensated hypothyroidism is controversial, but consider hormone replacement therapy for patients manifesting a significant and persistent elevation of TSH.

6. Overt hypothyroidism requires treatment with thyroid hormone, which should be administered after consultation with a pediatric endocrinologist.

VI. DELAYED ORGAN TOXICITY

A. Background

Delayed organ toxicity (Table 17.10) in the HSCT patient is often multifactorial.

1. Previous chemotherapy and radiotherapy may have already produced toxicity or increased the risk of toxicity from the conditioning regimen.
2. Doses of radiation and chemotherapy used for conditioning often approach the tolerance limits of nonhematopoietic tissues.
3. Toxicity may also result from or be exacerbated by drugs used for the prevention and treatment of infection or GVHD.

B. Renal and bladder toxicity

1. Renal toxicity can be a consequence of administering any of the following drugs singly or in combination.
   a. Aminoglycoside antibiotics
   b. Amphotericin B
   c. Ganciclovir and acyclovir
   d. Foscarnet
   e. Pentamidine
   f. CSA and FK506
2. Whenever possible, minimize the number of potentially nephrotoxic drugs.
3. Renal toxicity can also result from endothelial cell damage produced by the conditioning regimen (TBI) or cyclosporine/FK506 or both. Pediatric patients seem to be particularly prone to an hemolytic uremic-like syndrome, which develops after transplant and is characterized by renal insufficiency, microangiopathic hemolytic anemia, and thrombocytopenia.
   a. Patients at highest risk include:
      i. Recipients of TBI (especially when dose exceeds 1200 cGy).
      ii. Infants and young children.
      iii. Allogeneic HSCT recipients receiving CSA/ FK506.

TABLE 17.10.
Delayed Complications after Hematopoietic Stem Cell Transplant*

Organ	Process	Onset after Transplant	Diagnostic Tests	Risk Factors
Kidney	Hemolytic uremic syndrome	Months	CBC, creatinine	Young age, TBI, CSA
Bladder	Hemorrhagic cystitis	Weeks–months	Urinalysis, viral culture	Cyclophosphamide, busulfan
Eye	Sicca syndrome	Months–years	Schirmer test	cGVHD
	Cataracts	Months–years	Slit lamp exam	TBI, steroids
	Retinopathy	Months	Fundus exam	CSA
Heart	Myocardial failure	Years	Echocardiogram, RNA scan	Anthracyclines, chest radiotherapy
Liver	Cholestasis	Months–years	Liver function tests	cGVHD, prolonged use of parenteral nutrition
	Hepatitis	Months–years	Liver function tests, hepatitis C, PCR, HBSAg	Infection with hepatitis C or hepatitis B
Lung	Restrictive changes	Months–years	Pulmonary function tests	Bleomycin, BCNU, chest radiotherapy or thoracotomy, conditioning with BCNU or busulfan
	Obstructive changes	Months–years	Pulmonary function tests, chest CT, lung biopsy	cGVHD

*Abbreviations: BCNU, carmustine; cGVHD, chronic graft-versus-host disease; CSA, cyclosporine; CT, computed tomography; GVHD, chronic graft-versus-host disease; HBSAg, hepatitis B surface antigen; PCR, polymerase chain reaction; RNA, radionucleotide cardiac cineangiography; TBI, total body irradiation.

    b. Treatment is primarily supportive care.

       i. Transfuse with packed red blood cells if hemoglobin <7.0 g/dL.

      ii. Transfuse with platelets if significant bleeding occurs.

     iii. Discontinue CSA/FK506 if possible.

4. Bladder toxicity is most often due to severe hemorrhagic cystitis.

   a. Early-onset (days to weeks after transplant) hemorrhagic cystitis usually results from the administration of cyclophosphamide, but can occasionally occur after busulfan (i.e., even in patients who do not receive cyclophosphamide).

   b. Late-onset hemorrhagic cystitis (weeks to months) may be due to infection with adenovirus, papovavirus, or CMV.

   c. Management is largely symptomatic.
     i. Adequate hydration to maintain a good urine output
     ii. Bladder irrigation if blood clots develop
     iii. Smooth muscle relaxants to alleviate bladder spasm
     iv. Platelet transfusions for thrombocytopenic patients

   d. Other therapeutic options may include:
     i. Ribavirin therapy for patients with adenovirus.
     ii. Ganciclovir therapy for patients with CMV.
     iii. Aminocaproic acid. (Cystoscopy is required to remove all clots within the bladder before administration.)
     iv. Intravesicular instillation of various prostaglandins (PGE_1, PGE_2, or $PGF_{2\alpha}$)
     v. Intravesicular instillation of formalin. (Ureteral reflux is a contraindication.)

C. Ocular toxicity

  1. Anterior segment pathology

   a. Conjunctival involvement in acute and chronic GVHD. Patients with keratoconjunctivitis sicca have:
     i. Burning.
     ii. Irritation.
     iii. Photophobia.
     iv. Painful punctate erosions.

   b. Posterior subcapsular cataracts usually develop 2–6 years after transplant. Patients at risk are those who received TBI (especially with dose of 1200 cGy or more) and/or required prolonged systemic corticosteroid therapy.

  2. Posterior segment pathology

This consists primarily of an ischemic retinopathy characterized by cotton wool exudates and occasionally by disc edema.

    a. It occurs in patients treated with CSA.

    b. It develops within the first 6 months after transplant.

    c. If CSA can be discontinued, the retinopathy is usually reversible.

D. Cardiac complications

    1. Therapies received before HSCT are the most important determinants of late cardiac complications. As discussed in Chapter 7, cumulative anthracycline dose and mediastinal irradiation both individually and collectively determine the risk of cardiac complications. Follow HSCT patients who have these risk factors as recommended in Chapter 7.

    2. TBI can further increase the risk of late cardiac complications. Cardiac irradiation during TBI will add to the toxicity of prior anthracyclines or mediastinal irradiation or both.

E. Hepatic complications

    1. Allogeneic HSCT patients with cGVHD often have liver involvement.

        a. Patients are usually asymptomatic but may have biochemical abnormalities.

            i.   Hyperbilirubinemia

            ii. Elevated γ-glutamyl transpeptidase

            iii. Elevated serum alkaline phosphatase

            iv. Modest elevation of transaminases

        b. Most patients respond to immunosuppressive therapy (see Section IVC6).

        c. Occasionally patients develop progressive cholestasis and ultimately biliary cirrhosis.

            i.   Histologically this entity can be difficult to distinguish from chronic active hepatitis.

            ii. Ursodeoxycholic acid may lower bilirubin levels and alleviate pruritus.

    2. Autologous and allogeneic HSCT recipients may also develop chronic active hepatitis. They may have:

        a. Fluctuating transaminase levels.

        b. Evidence of hepatitis C virus infection (positive antibody titers in patients not receiving IVGG and/or detection of hepatitis C virus RNA by polymerase chain reaction in serum or liver).

c. Evidence of hepatitis B virus infection (hepatitis B surface antigen, IgM anti-hepatitis B core antigen).

3. In allogeneic HSCT patients, chronic active hepatitis may be difficult to distinguish clinically from chronic hepatic GVHD. A liver biopsy may sometimes be helpful in arriving at a definitive diagnosis. Patients with progressive hepatitis may be candidates for clinical trials of antiviral therapy.

F. Pulmonary complications
   1. Pulmonary complications may result from prior lung infections or therapies received before transplantation, such as:
      a. Chemotherapy with carmustine (BCNU), bleomycin, or busulfan.
      b. Radiotherapy to the mediastinum or lungs or both.
      c. Thoracotomies to remove pulmonary metastases.
   2. Mild restrictive abnormalities in pulmonary function that did not produce any clinical symptoms have been reported in the following patients.
      a. Recipients of autologous HSCTs conditioned with high-dose chemotherapy only.
         i. In most cases, therapies administered before HSCT were thought to be responsible for the abnormalities in pulmonary function.
         ii. In other cases, BCNU or busulfan administered as part of the conditioning regimen may have contributed to the abnormalities.
      b. Recipients of autologous or allogeneic HSCTs who received TBI.
   3. Obstructive abnormalities varying from mild to severe occur primarily in recipients of allogeneic HSCTs as a manifestation of cGVHD.
      a. Patients at greatest risk are those with cGVHD who:
         i. Received allografts from mismatched related or matched unrelated donors.
         ii. Have hepatic involvement.
      b. Chest X-ray often either is normal or demonstrates mild hyperinflation unless there is:
         i. Intercurrent infection.

      ii. Extensive interstitial involvement.

      iii. Pneumothorax/mediastinum.

   c. More severely affected patients have:

      i. Cough.

      ii. Dyspnea.

      iii. Wheezing.

      iv. Pneumothorax/mediastinum.

      v. Propensity to recurrent bronchopulmonary infections.

   d. Diagnosis

      i. Pulmonary function tests may demonstrate obstruction

      ii. Chest computerized tomography scan may demonstrate bronchiolitis obliterans.

      iii. Bronchioalveolar lavage and/or lung biopsy may be needed to exclude infection as the primary cause of the patient's pulmonary process.

   e. Therapy

      i. Immunosuppression is the primary mode of treatment (see Section IVC6).

      ii. Treatment of intercurrent sinopulmonary infections is essential.

      iii. Symptoms may be worsened by coexistent gastroesophageal reflux; if demonstrated by endoscopy or pH probe, the patient should commence treatment.

VII. IMMUNIZATIONS

  A. Background

    1. Immunization practices are covered more thoroughly in Chapter 2. The following recommendations relate to how these practices have to be specifically modified for the HSCT patient.

    2. Patients undergoing autologous or allogeneic HSCTs sometimes have immunologic reconstitution with cells that retain immunologic memory for antigens to which they had previously been exposed. However, this is far from certain. Furthermore, infants and young children who serve as their own stem cell donors or as stem cell donors for allogeneic HSCTs will have received few, if any, immunizations before the transplant.

    3. Recipients of cord blood transplants and T cell-depleted

transplants receive stem cell products largely devoid of memory cells.

4. Most HSCT patients will require a complete set of immunizations after the transplant.

5. Immunizations will not be effective until immune reconstitution has occurred. As a rule, recipients of allogeneic HSCTs have slower return of immunologic function than recipients of autografts. Immune function may be impaired for prolonged periods of time (24 months or more) after T cell-depleted or partially HLA-matched HSCTs, and may never return to normal in patients with cGVHD.

B. Guidelines for immunization

1. General recommendations for post-transplant immunizations are summarized in Table 17.11. Some centers also immunize with the acellular pertussis vaccine, although this is not recommended for children ≥7 years old.

2. Children receiving IVGG should not begin immunizations until 3 months after the last dose is given.

3. Do not administer live polio vaccine to the patient or to household contacts of the patient.

4. For patients who do not have cGVHD and who are not on immunosuppressive therapy, the following guidelines apply.

   a. Diphtheria-tetanus (DT) vaccine for children through 6 years, Td for children after their seventh birthday and inactivated polio vaccine (IPV) can commence 12 months after transplant.

   b. Pneumococcal, *Haemophilus influenzae* type b, and influenza vaccines can be given 12–24 months after transplant.

   c. Measles, mumps, rubella (MMR) can generally be administered 24 months after transplant. It may be prudent to document a response to DT or Td and polio vaccines before immunizing with live virus.

   d. Obtain post-immunization antibody titers to ensure that the patient is adequately protected.

5. For patients with cGVHD or patients on immunosuppressive therapy, the following guidelines apply.

   a. Do not administer any live virus vaccines such as MMR.

TABLE 17.11.
Recommended Immunizations after Hematopoietic Stem Cell Transplant*

GVHD or Immunosuppressive Therapy

Vaccine	No: Time after Transplant	Yes: Time after Transplant (mo)
DT	12, 14, 16, and 24 months	Same
IPV	12, 14, 16, and 24 months	Same
Pneumococcal	12 and 24 months	Same
HibCV	12 and 24 months	Same
Influenza	Yearly, beginning at 12 months	Same
MMR	24 months	Do not administer
OPV	Do not administer to patient or household members	Do not administer to patient or household members

*Abbreviations: DT, diphtheria tetanus; HibCV, *Haemophilus* type b conjugate vaccine; IPV, inactivated polio vaccine; MMR, measles mumps rubella; OPV, oral polio vaccine.

b. The above schedule for DT or Td vaccine, IPV, pneumococcal, *H. influenzae* type b, and influenza vaccines can be used, but efficacy is much less certain.
c. Alternatively, the patient can be maintained on monthly IVGG.

VIII. NEUROPSYCHOLOGICAL FUNCTIONING

Children undergoing a HSCT may be exposed to agents that can damage the central nervous system (CNS) (e.g., TBI, busulfan, CSA) and may also have been previously treated with cranial irradiation and/or intrathecal chemotherapy. In addition, most patients endure a prolonged hospitalization and social isolation after discharge because of their immunocompromised status. It is, therefore, not surprising that many children will show a modest decline in IQ and Adaptive Behavioral Scores after transplant.

A. Factors influencing cognitive functioning
   The degree of cognitive impairment, if any, depends on:
   1. Age at transplant.
   2. Age when previously exposed to neurotoxic agents.
   3. Extent of prior exposure to neurotoxic agents.
   4. Transplant conditioning regimen.
   5. Child's underlying disease.

B. Neuropsychologic testing
1. In the majority of patients, specialized testing is required to detect any deficits in neuropsychologic functioning. However, some children will experience significant cognitive problems, which usually manifest as poor academic performance.
2. Age-appropriate developmental testing should be conducted by a child psychologist yearly for at least 3 years after a HSCT to ascertain any learning disabilities that may impede scholastic performance and allow for the early implementation of school-based interventions.

C. Leukoencephalopathy
Severe leukoencephalopathy is occasionally seen in patients who have received extensive prior CNS therapy.
1. The risk may be increased by administering post-transplant intrathecal chemotherapy.
2. Symptoms (e.g., lethargy, confusion, dysarthria, ataxia, and seizures) usually develop within a few months after exposure to TBI.
3. Patients should be evaluated by magnetic resonance imaging that shows white matter destruction and ventricular dilatation.
4. A lumbar puncture may be helpful to confirm the diagnosis (elevated myelin basic protein) and rule out a CNS infection.

D. Other causes of neurologic dysfunction
1. Infection.
2. Drug toxicity.

E. CNS infections
CNS infections are relatively uncommon after transplant and are:
1. Usually caused by *Aspergillus* or *Candida* species.
2. Occasionally caused by other fungal species (e.g., cryptococcus) or bacterial or viral pathogens, most commonly in patients with cGVHD.

G. Drug toxicity
CSA may cause a variety of neurologic symptoms (Table 17.6). Monitor CSA levels to reduce the risk of severe neurotoxicity.

IX. SURVEILLANCE FOR RELAPSE

A. Leukemias
   The risk of relapse after transplant depends on the type of leukemia, disease status before transplant, the marrow donor (autologous versus allogeneic, related versus unrelated), and other factors.
   1. Perform a CBC and physical examination monthly for 1 year after transplant.
   2. Follow stable patients every 3 months during the 2nd year, every 4 months during the 3rd year, and every 6–12 months thereafter until 5 years after transplant (Table 17.12).
   3. Performing routine surveillance bone marrow examinations is of questionable benefit, unless required for research purposes. One exception may be chronic myelogenous leukemia patients, for whom the detection of persistent Ph^+ cells after transplant has prognostic significance and may alter patient care.

B. Solid tumors
   Children with high-risk or recurrent solid tumors may be candidates for a HSCT. The risk of relapse after transplant depends on the patient's disease, disease status at the time of transplant, conditioning regimen, and biologic characteristic of the tumor. The frequency of disease evaluations after transplant is usually determined by protocol; however, some reasonable guidelines are presented in Table 17.12.

TABLE 17.12.
Relapse Surveillance after Hematopoietic Stem Cell Transplant

Years after Transplant	Time Interval between Studies (months)	
	Leukemias*	Solid Tumors†
1	1	3
2	3	4
3	4	6
4	6–12	12
5	6–12	12

* CBC, physical examination.
† Radiologic studies, biochemical markers, physical examination.

X. SECONDARY MALIGNANCIES

A. Background
The lifetime risk of a secondary malignancy occurring in a HSCT patient appears to be 7–11 times greater than that observed in the general population. The malignancies can be classified as follows:
1. Non-Hodgkin lymphoma
2. Myelodysplasia/acute nonlymphoblastic leukemia
3. Solid tumors

B. Non-Hodgkin lymphoma
1. Non-Hodgkin lymphoma (NHL) is the most common secondary malignancy and occurs in patients who have had allogeneic HSCTs.
2. The tumors are large cell lymphomas of B cell origin and have identical features to those that develop after solid organ transplants. They are Epstein-Barr virus (EBV)-associated proliferations of donor B cells and can be either polyclonal or monoclonal.
3. Risk factors relate to severe immunosuppression and include:
   a. T-cell depletion.
   b. HLA-mismatched graft.
   c. Unrelated donor graft.
   d. Use of ATG during conditioning or after transplant.
   e. Conditioning regimens that include TBI.
   f. Allogeneic HSCT for congenital immune deficiency.
4. Clinical features include:
   a. Early onset after transplant, usually within 4 months of HSCT.
   b. Rapidly progressive and fulminant course with fever, malaise, and infiltration of one or more of the following organs: tonsils, nodes, skin, lungs, liver, GI tract, and CNS.
5. Therapeutic options may include:
   a. Reduction or cessation of immunosuppressive therapy.
   b. Conventional chemotherapy (although durable responses are generally not attained).
   c. Infusions of unirradiated donor lymphocytes that are thought to contain cytotoxic T cells presensitized to EBV.

      d. Treatment with antiviral drugs.
         i. Acyclovir or ganciclovir
         ii. α-Interferon
      e. Use of anti-B cell monoclonal antibodies.

C. Myelodysplasia/acute nonlymphoblastic leukemia
Myelodysplasia or leukemia usually develops at a later time than NHL but invariably within the first decade after HSCT; it occurs in recipients of autologous as well as allogeneic grafts.

1. Patients whose conditioning included radiation appear to be at higher risk than those conditioned with chemotherapy alone.
2. In autologous HSCT patients, prior treatment with agents known to induce secondary myelodysplasia/acute nonlymphoblastic leukemia appears to be a risk factor.
3. The outcome is generally poor.

D. Solid tumors
Various solid tumors of epithelial origin can occur many years after HSCT. Exposure to TBI or ATG appears to be a risk factor in their development.

1. Most common are various skin cancers, including basal cell carcinoma, squamous cell carcinoma, and malignant melanoma. Patients at greatest risk are those who develop cGVHD.
2. Brain tumors may develop (e.g., meningioma, or glioblastoma multiforme).
3. Bone tumors may occur, including osteosarcoma and malignant fibrous histiocytoma.

XI. WHEN TO REFER THE PATIENT BACK TO THE TRANSPLANT CENTER

A. Background
Many problems that develop after HSCT do not require the patient to return to the transplant center. However, it may be useful to have select biopsy specimens reviewed by a pathologist versed in HSCT pathology. This consultation can be particularly valuable when a diagnosis of GVHD is being entertained.

B. Patients who should be referred back to the transplant center include those with:

1. Newly diagnosed acute or chronic GVHD.
2. Severe aGVHD whose disease is refractory to conventional therapy and who are candidates for experimental therapy administered at the transplant center.
3. Severe cGVHD whose disease is refractory to conventional therapy and who are candidates for experimental therapy that must be initiated at the transplant center.
4. Graft failure.
5. Life-threatening viral infections that require adoptive immunotherapy with cells of donor origin.
6. Relapsed leukemia who are candidates for immunotherapy with donor-derived T-cells.
7. Post-transplant NHL who are candidates for adoptive immunotherapy with donor-derived T-cells.
8. A relapsed malignancy who are candidates for a second transplant using either the original source of HSCs or an alternate source of HSCs.
    a. Any regimen-related toxicity from the first transplant should have resolved.
    b. If TBI was used for conditioning before the first transplant, sufficient time (often up to 12 months) must have elapsed to permit recovery from radiation injury to normal tissues and allow the patient to undergo conditioning with a non-TBI based regimen without excessive regimen-related toxicity.
    c. If TBI was not used for the first transplant, the time interval before a second transplant can be performed may be considerably shorter.
    d. Ideally, patients who receive second transplants for disease recurrence should be in remission or in early relapse at the time of the second HSCT.

Bibliography

Bhatia S, Ramsay N, et al.: Malignant neoplasms following bone marrow transplantation. *Blood* 87:3633–39, 1996.

Deeg HJ: Follow-up after discharge from the transplant center. In Deeg HJ, Klingemann H-G, Phillips GL, eds.: *Bone Marrow Transplantation.* Berlin, Springer-Verlag; 1988. pp. 151–5.

Ferrara J, Deeg, H: Graft-versus-host disease. *N Engl J Med* 324:667–74, 1991.

Giri N, Davis EAC, Vowels MR: Long-term complications following bone marrow transplantation in children. *J Paediatr Child Health* 29:201–5, 1993.

Hoyle C, Goldman JM: Life-threatening infections occurring more than 3 months after BMT. *Bone Marrow Transplant* 14:247–52, 1994.

Moe GL: Low-microbial diets for patients with granulocytopenia. In Bloch AS, ed.: *Nutrition Management of the Cancer Patient.* Rockville, MD: Aspen Publishing; 1990. pp. 125–134.

Schultz K, Green G, et al.: Obstructive lung disease in children after allogeneic bone marrow transplantation. *Blood* 84:3212–20, 1994.

Smedler AC, Ringden K, Bergman H, et al.: Sensory-motor and cognitive functioning in children who have undergone bone marrow transplantation. *Acta Paediatr Scand* 79:613–21, 1990.

Somani J, Larson R: Review: Reimmunization after allogeneic bone marrow transplantation. *Am J Med* 98:389, 1995.

Sullivan K, Witherspoon R, et al.: Alternating-day cyclosporin and prednisone for treatment of high-risk chronic graft-v-host disease. *Blood* 72:555–61, 1988.

18

Psychosocial Care

Robert B. Noll, Ph.D., and Anne Kazak, Ph.D.

Since the prognosis for children with cancer has improved dramatically during the past 30 years while therapies have become increasingly arduous, more attention is being paid to quality of life for these children and their families. Children receiving treatment for malignancies and their families (siblings, parents, grandparents, and friends) as well as professionals (teachers, nurses, physicians, psychosocial providers, etc.) who care for them are placed in numerous stressful situations. While these stressful life events can be overwhelming, they can be managed in positive ways that encourage families to continue to function in the best possible fashion and facilitate personal growth. To promote positive adaptations, we strongly recommend that one person be assigned to each child or family as a primary psychosocial professional so that continuity of services can be maintained throughout treatment. When continuity of care is provided, trust and rapport can be established and maintained. This professional should have expertise in behavioral medicine, with special training relevant to conducting comprehensive interviews with families (including children); the use of relaxation, distraction, and/or hypnosis; facilitating liaisons with other health care professionals; the impact of severe childhood chronic illness on the family; psychodiagnostic and psychotherapy skills; and knowledge of childhood cancer. Teams that lack individuals with the above expertise often find that the care described in this chapter is deficient or sporadic because responsibility is divided.

I. ESTABLISHING OPEN COMMUNICATION AT DIAGNOSIS

A. The presence of the primary psychosocial provider at the initial conference with the family and at every meeting where

critical medical information is provided to the family is necessary so that this provider:
1. Has knowledge of exactly what was said.
2. Has the opportunity to observe familial reactions to information.
3. Can ask questions of the physician when he or she thinks the family is not understanding or material is too complex.

B. Follow-up interviews (within the 1st week) by a professional with expertise in psychosocial issues related to childhood cancer are necessary.
1. Interviews should include parents, siblings, ill child, and grandparents.
2. Interviews should serve as a model for communication to show adults how to discuss very difficult health care issues with their children.
3. The following issues should be included.
   a. Disease, treatment, prognosis, side effects, invasive medical procedures (to ensure clarity of communication and reeducation as needed)
   b. Insurance, financial concerns, social support resources (e.g., babysitting for siblings), transportation to the medical center, religious needs, any special social or economic issues
   c. Adjustment difficulties that are antecedent to the diagnosis of cancer and that may interfere with the child's care
      i. Marital dysfunction
      ii. Parental psychopathology
      iii. Children's behavioral/emotional/academic problems
4. Primary psychosocial professionals should have diagnostic skills to identify difficulties in the above domains.
5. Impressions from family meetings must be reviewed with the treatment team to facilitate the development of a comprehensive care plan.
6. Several follow-up interviews during the 1st week or two are almost always required.

C. Follow-up interviews must be completed again about 1–2 months after diagnosis and regularly thereafter throughout the illness to review issues and evaluate the child's and family's adjustment to cancer.

1. After the shock of the initial diagnosis and treatment has subsided, a better assessment of the patient and family is possible.
2. Consider including siblings, grandparents, and other meaningful supportive individuals in these meetings so that their questions can be addressed.

D. The team should immediately discuss parents' refusal to participate in these meetings.

1. Determine the reasons for resistance.
   a. Cultural issues
   b. Timing
   c. Discomfort with the specific provider
   d. Other
2. This is a team problem that requires a team solution.

II. ADAPTATION OF CHILDREN

A. Distinct social, emotional, and behavioral challenges are associated with the specific developmental phase of the child.

1. Infants, toddlers, and preschoolers are sensitive to separation from caregivers and prone to angry outbursts (tantrums).
2. Preschoolers have a difficult time with pain management related to medical procedures and may demonstrate regressive or aggressive behavior (tantrums).
3. School-aged children have anticipatory worries about medical procedures, separation anxieties, and concerns about reentry to school.
4. Adolescent issues are reviewed in Section III.

B. Depression and/or anxiety are the most common psychological/psychiatric concerns during treatment.

1. Find out what has been helpful in the past if the child has a history of being anxious and depressed when placed in stressful situations.
2. In the majority of instances where the youngster appears excessively depressed or anxious, these responses are normal reactions to feeling physically ill or experiencing acute life circumstances such as:

    a. Brief reactions to hospitalization.

    b. Side effects of therapy.

    c. Missing meaningful activities.

3. The treatment of choice is psychotherapy with the family or the child alone.

4. The use of antidepressant medications in children/adolescents has not demonstrated efficacy in a double-blind study. Therefore, their use is not generally recommended.

    a. Limit the use of medication to the following instances.

        i. Strong family history of problems with depression is present.

        ii. Difficulties were present premorbidly.

        iii. Current problems are chronic, unremitting, and interfere with day-to-day functioning.

        iv. Primary psychotherapeutic interventions have not been successful.

    b. Antidepressant medications are less effective for adjustment reactions.

III. ADAPTATION OF ADOLESCENTS

A. Special attention is required for adolescents because of the documented difficulties they encounter with adverse reactions to chemotherapy and well-substantiated noncompliance. Adolescents tend to be more reactive, do not show discomfort to medical staff, and are more difficult to treat than younger patients.

B. Signs of distress (such as excessive anxiety, moodiness, undue passivity, undesirable changes in behavior, academic difficulty, or more conflict at home) require attention.

C. Take special care to monitor nausea and vomiting and the adolescents' experience with chemotherapy.

D. The noncompliant teenager is a significant challenge.

1. Documented rates of noncompliance with oral medications are 60% without the medical team's knowledge.

2. Psychosocial management of the teenager might include:

    a. Primary prevention, where the parents are strongly encouraged at diagnosis to observe the teenager taking every oral medication.

    b. Providing regular psychosocial services.

    c. A team approach that integrates information from the medical team with input from parents, grandparents, teachers, peers, and other outside resources that are meaningful to the teenager.

    d. Early referral for psychotherapy when signs of atypical emotional distress occur.

IV. SIBLINGS

A. Monitoring the siblings' reactions to the diagnosis and helping parents deal with those reactions are essential.

    1. If concerns are raised, additional information should be obtained from the sibling, teachers, grandparents, etc., to ascertain the full extent of difficulties.

    2. Indications that siblings are having difficulties are:

        a. Extreme anxiousness.

        b. Apparent unconcern.

B. Siblings of children with cancer commonly feel distressed. These difficulties are not associated with long-term adjustment problems, but they are significant challenges that occur regularly.

C. Some common sibling concerns are:

    1. The desire for more information about the sibling's illness.

    2. Jealousy about the extra attention the ill sibling is receiving.

    3. Fears that the sibling is dying.

D. Visits to the hospital and outpatient clinic are strongly recommended but can be stressful. Take special care to prepare healthy siblings before visits.

    1. The initial visit should occur as soon as possible after diagnosis.

    2. The psychosocial professional should make certain that visits are not overwhelming.

        a. Preparation about technical medical equipment is helpful.

        b. Preparation about how ill their sibling looks is helpful.

            i. Verbal descriptions

            ii. Photographs

E. Siblings of children with cancer commonly report social or academic difficulties at school. Routinely ask parents about sibling functioning at school, and address problems immediately.

1. School-focused interventions with collaboration from the medical treatment team are recommended.
2. Education of teachers and peers regarding what is occurring for the ill sibling is often useful.

F. Major worries of many siblings are related to the illness and not having accurate information. With increasing age, siblings will benefit from knowing more details about:
1. The specific illness (e.g., leukemia).
2. A description of the illness (cancer of the blood).
3. Side effects of treatment (especially those that can be observed).
4. Length of treatment.
5. The ill child's prognosis.
   a. Many siblings are specifically concerned about whether their ill brother or sister will die, but are afraid to ask adults.
   b. Psychosocial professionals need to take a leadership role for the family.

V. COPING AND ADJUSTMENT BY PARENTS AND FAMILY

A. Parents of children with cancer have difficulties with excessive worry, depressed moods, somatic complaints, and challenges maintaining intimate relationships.
1. Findings are stronger for mothers, but fathers are known to have significant reactions.
2. Careful monitoring of parental mental health is a necessary component of cancer care for children.
   a. There is an association between maternal distress and the children's adjustment.
   b. Knowledge of premorbid adjustment and previous reactions to stress is helpful in predicting how parents will cope.

B. Parents will profit from regular contact with the psychosocial professional. These meetings, which should be a model for open communication, should focus on coping with stress, with special attention to:
1. Family functioning.
2. Parental distress.
3. Siblings.

 4. Grandparents.

 5. Problems with misinformation from outside sources.

C. Most parents will report having symptoms of anxiety, depression, and feeling overwhelmed. Problems with day-to-day functioning are not typical; immediately refer people with such problems for regular psychotherapy.

 1. Psychotropic medications for dealing with the stress of childhood cancer and its treatment should be limited to parents who do not respond to talk therapies or parents with preexisting psychiatric difficulties.

 2. Psychotropic medications are less effective for adjustment reactions.

D. Monitor family coping during treatment.

 1. The stress associated with childhood cancer can be especially challenging when parents have different styles of coping.

  a. Mothers report benefit from talking about what is happening, while fathers may use different strategies.

  b. Facilitating parental appreciation for varying coping styles is generally beneficial.

 2. Treatment of childhood cancer demands considerable parental time, and parents often must reallocate available resources and redefine roles within the family. Assistance with these processes can be very helpful.

E. Despite the many strains that childhood cancer places on the marriage, cancer in a child is not associated with long-term marital conflicts or increased divorce rates. It is a myth that should not be supported. Refer couples with serious marital problems for psychotherapy.

F. Parents commonly experience chronic distressing symptoms related to their child's cancer such as unexpected intrusive thoughts about cancer, difficulties making hospital visits, heightened concerns over minor health problems for all of their children, or recurrent dreams.

 1. Post-traumatic stress symptoms are common but rarely interfere with daily activity.

 2. When symptoms are so severe that they adversely affect day-to-day functioning, immediately refer the person for psychotherapy.

VI. GRANDPARENTS

A. While little research has been done on the reactions of grandparents to the diagnosis of childhood cancer, clinical observations suggest that grandparents are at high risk for excessive worry, depressed mood, and somatic complaints.

B. Grandparents are in double jeopardy as they observe the pain of their adult child coping with their grandchild's cancer and they observe the difficulties for their grandchild.

C. When grandparents live in the vicinity, they commonly play a key role with child care, daily living tasks, and care of the child with cancer.

D. Help for grandparents can be accomplished by specifically including them in family meetings to provide accurate information about the disease, prognosis, and treatment plans.

VII. RE-ENTRY TO SCHOOL

A. After obtaining parental permission, contact school personnel as soon as possible to let them know about the child's disease. Peers should also be informed what is happening, to preclude misinformation.
1. Contacting the school with specific medical information stops the rumors.
2. Children, teachers, and principals will associate childhood cancer with immediate death, so they need to be educated about the child's disease; treatment, side effects, anticipated days of school to be missed, and length; prognosis; and special issues (e.g., emergency catheter care).
3. Obtain information about how the child has done (academically and socially) in the past.

B. If an extended absence from school is inevitable, encourage school personnel to maintain contact with the patient and family via homebound teachers, letters, tapes, etc.
1. Videotapes from classmates are especially helpful for morale.
2. Peers should be encouraged to sustain contact during hospitalizations.
3. Homework should be completed insofar as it is medically feasible.

C. As soon as possible after initial diagnosis and treatment, within the limits of medical care, encourage children to return to school.
1. Before the patient returns to school, the primary psychosocial professional or an educational liaison specialist should talk with the child and parents about concerns they have about the child's return to school. Common concerns are:
   a. Changes in the child's physical characteristics.
   b. Ways the child can talk with peers about the illness.
   c. Misconceptions that childhood cancer is contagious.
2. Attending school signals the return to normal routines and provides parents and children reassurance regarding improving health and the need to reestablish normal expectations and routines for the child.
3. Maintaining friendships and routine interactions with peers is essential to normal psychological development and is at least as important as academic issues.
4. The social component of the school experience is extremely important. Homebound teaching is not sufficient and should be used only when the option to attend school does not exist.
5. Attending school even for short periods of time is preferable to permanent homebound education.
   a. Combinations of homebound instruction with limited school attendance when the child is feeling better are common solutions.
   b. Flexibility based on the child's changing health status is critical.

D. Children with brain tumors or malignancies that can compromise central nervous system (CNS) integrity through their therapies (acute lymphoblastic leukemia with CNS disease) have special problems related to school reentry. These patients commonly experience difficulties with intellectual abilities and academic achievement that are not detected unless explored.
1. Neuropsychological evaluations should be completed by a professional with experience working with children with malignancies and the cognitive sequelae of their diseases. Clinical and school psychologists are often not trained in this area.

    a. Facilitate appropriate classroom placements and the development of appropriate education programs.

    b. Carefully review the results with parents and school professionals to ensure their understanding of the child's cognitive abilities.

  2. The recommended scheduling of neuropsychological evaluations is as follows.

    a. Before reentry to school: neuropsychological screening

    b. Within 6 months of diagnosis: comprehensive neuropsychological assessment

    c. 1–2 years after diagnosis: comprehensive neuropsychological assessment (earlier if problems are being reported)

    d. 3–5 years after diagnosis: comprehensive neuropsychological assessment

      i. To fully appreciate the extent and nature of late effects

      ii. Especially necessary for patients treated with whole-brain radiation therapy

  3. Direct comparisons with earlier test results are critical to understanding the neuropsychological impact of the disease and treatment.

E. School intervention programs are exceptionally valuable for maintaining liaison between the family, medical staff, and school professionals. Their routine use is strongly encouraged.

VIII. RELAPSE

A. After a patient has a relapse, the psychosocial provider must meet with the entire family, including healthy siblings and grandparents, to ensure their understanding of what occurred and what will happen. Parents are generally overwhelmed by the relapse, so professional guidance is typically necessary.

  1. Families have greater emotional challenges at relapse.

  2. Fear of death becomes more prominent and should be explored if at all possible.

  3. Parents may decline to discuss this issue with their family, but professional guidance should be offered, as the majority of parents are not able to lead these discussions.

B. See Chapter 21 for more information.

Bibliography

Antonuccio DO, Danton WG, DeNelsky GY: Psychotherapy versus medication for depression: Challenging the conventional wisdom with data. *Prof Psychol Res Pract* 26:574–85, 1995.

Bennett DS: Depression among children with chronic medical problems: A meta-analysis. *J Pediatr Psychol* 19:149–70, 1994.

Gadow KD: Pediatric psychopharmacotherapy: A review of recent research. *J Child Psychol Psychiatry* 33:153–95, 1992.

Kazak AE, Blackall G, Himelstein B, et al.: Producing systemic change in pediatric practice: An intervention protocol for reducing distress during painful procedures. *Fam Syst Med* 13:173–86, 1995.

Kazak AE, Meadows AT: Families of young adolescents who have survived cancer: Social-emotional adjustment, adaptability, and social support. *J Pediatr Psychol* 14:175–91, 1989.

Kupst MJ, Natta MB, Richardson CC, et al.: Family coping with pediatric leukemia: Ten years after treatment. *J Pediatr Psychol* 20:601–17, 1995.

Larcombe IJ, Walker J, Charlton A, et al.: Impact of childhood cancer on return to normal schooling. *Br Med J* 301:169–71, 1991.

Mulhern RK, Wasserman AL, Friedman AG, et al.: Social competence and behavioral adjustment of children who are long-term survivors of cancer. *Pediatrics* 83:18–25, 1989.

Noll RB, Gartstein MA, Hawkins A, et al.: Comparing parental distress for families with children who have cancer and matched comparison families without children with cancer. *Fam Syst Med* 13:11–28, 1995.

Powers SW, Vannatta K, Noll RB, Cool VA, and Stehbens JA. (1995). Cancer and leukemia. In M Roberts (Ed.), *Handbook of pediatric psychology* (2nd ed.; pp. 310–26). NY: Guilford.

Ris MD, Noll RB: Long term neurobehavioral outcome in pediatric brain tumor patients: Review and ethodological critique. *J Clin Exp Neuropsychol* 16:21–42, 1994.

Sanger MS, Copeland D, Davidson ER: Psychosocial adjustment among pediatric cancer patients. *J Pediatr Psychol* 16:463–74, 1991.

Sawyer MG, Antiniou G, Nguyen A-MT, et al.: A prospective study of the psychological adjustment of children with cancer. *Am J Pediatr Hematol Oncol* 17:39–45, 1995.

Stehbens J, Kaleita, Noll RB, et al.: CNS prophylaxis of pediatric leukemia: What are the long-term neurological, neuropsychological, and behavioral effects? *Neuropsychol Rev* 2:147–77, 1991.

19

Alternative Medicine in Pediatric Oncology

Susan F. Sencer, M.D., and John J. Iacuone, M.D.

Increasingly, the families of children with cancer are pursuing alternative forms of cancer therapy This chapter introduces some popular alternative medicine therapies and shares ideas on how families may be helped to make informed and, it is to be hoped, rational decisions regarding them.

I. UNCONVENTIONAL OR ALTERNATIVE MEDICINE

A. Glossary of alternative medicine terms
  1. Synonyms are *unconventional* and *unorthodox* medicine. *Complementary* and *integrative medicine* imply combining alternative medicine and conventional treatments.
  2. Chiropractic: manipulation of the spinal column to correct nerve compressions believed to cause bodily dysfunctions
  3. Homeopathic: treating disease using infinitesimal dilutions of natural substances.
     Substances that cause symptoms similar to the disease are able to cure the disease. Each patient is so distinct that research into methodology is felt to be pointless. The term is often used to mean "holistic" medicine. Homeopaths generally oppose childhood immunizations.
  4. Naturopathy: treating disorders using diet, herbal medicine, and environmental modifications

B. Prevalence of alternative medicine
  1. Ten to 60% of adult cancer patients have used alternative

medicines. One-quarter of these use them while on conventional therapy, but half will not tell their physicians about the alternative medicine.
2. Few pediatric studies have been done.
   a. Australia (1994): 46% of the pediatric oncology population had used at least one alternative medicine. Less than 50% had discussed this use with their physician.
   b. Quebec (1995): 11% of children in a general pediatric outpatient clinic had used some type of alternative medicine. Patients tended to be older, mothers tended to be better educated, and parents themselves used alternative medicine.
   c. Vancouver (1996): 41% of pediatric cancer patients used either alternative or complementary therapies.

II. TRADITIONAL MEDICINES OF THE WORLD

A. The World Health Organization has urged the creation of a "new world medicine" combining the wisdom of indigenous cultures with Western scientific techniques.

B. Many cancer patients use unconventional cancer therapy as part of their traditional medical systems stemming from their ethnic cultures (e.g., Hmong and Native American healers). European countries, especially Germany and France, rely heavily on alternative medicine, and it is seen as an adjunct to Western medicine.

C. Traditional Chinese medicine is used by many patients. Practitioners tend to make relatively modest claims. Therapies are often compatible with conventional cancer therapy and are often used to counteract side effects. A massive body of research exists, although the studies are poorly designed by Western standards. Most Chinese medicine relies on the concept of *qi,* or energy. *Qi* is a physical entity and therefore can be measured and manipulated in an effort to control disease.
1. Acupuncture
   a. Acupuncture restores "energy balance" through the use of needles placed at vital points in the body along energy pathways, or "meridians."
   b. At Beijing Neurological Institute 90% of all head and neck surgeries and more than 70% of abdominal, gyne-

cologic, and chest surgeries are performed successfully under acupuncture analgesia.

c. Acupuncture's mechanism of action is unclear; it stimulates endorphin production in the brain and probably influences the production and distribution of many neuromodulators and neurotransmitters, thereby altering the perception of pain.

d. Pediatric uses include chronic pain (e.g., sickle cell disease), postanesthesia pain, and nausea associated with chemotherapy. Children, however, tend to be phobic about needles, limiting acupuncture's usefulness.

2. Acupressure
Massage or pressure at acupuncture sites for both diagnostic and treatment purposes.

a. Acupressure is less effective than acupuncture, but may be more long lasting. It can prolong the effects of acupuncture.

b. Pressure at the wrist at the P6 or neignan point can prevent nausea during chemotherapy and can significantly reduce the use of antiemetics. Elasticized wrist acupressure bands (Sea Bands) used for motion sickness are helpful.

3. Moxibustion
Burning of herbs at acupuncture sites.
The heat is felt to restore energy balance.

4. Qi Gong (energy medicine)
Similar to martial arts, with emphasis on centering physical balance and meditation

5. Herbal therapy
The principal mode of intervention of Chinese medicine. Many traditional herbal combinations include agents active against cancer; all drugs in current use are derived from plants. In the United States, herbs are generally bought at health food stores. Listed below are common herbs you may see in your practice, with information derived from controlled studies or medical case reports.

a. Herbs that can harm

i. Chaparall: sold as cancer cure, blood purifier, and natural antioxidant.
It has been traced to at least six cases of acute non-viral hepatitis, and one patient needed a liver transplant.

    ii. Comfrey
       It has caused obstructed blood flow in liver, cirrhosis, and newborn liver disease.
   iii. Ephedra: "energy-booster"
       It contains epitonin, ephedrine, and pseudoephedrine and can cause palpitations, nerve damage, psychosis. At least two deaths have been reported.
   iv. Lobelia: stimulant
       It can cause hypoventilation, hypotension, coma, and death.
  b. Herbs that may help
    i. Garlic: antibiotic qualities, lowers cholesterol; anticoagulant properties
    ii. Feverfew: effective against migraine headaches.
       It may cause mouth sores if chewed.
   iii. Ginger: nausea, especially chemotherapy or pregnancy related, motion sickness; anticoagulant properties.
   iv. Ginkgo: increased circulation
    v. Ginseng: inhibits the growth of neoplastic cell lines; stimulates normal protein synthesis and causes cancer cells to differentiate in vitro.
       It contains steroids, pectin, B vitamins, zinc, manganese, and calcium, among others.
   vi. Echinacea: "immunity booster,"
       For this reason it is popular among acquired immunodeficiency syndrome (AIDS) and cancer patients. It may increase resistance to upper respiratory infections when taken as soon as illness begins, but benefits may be lost with continued use. Benefits or risks for cancer patients are unknown.

III. UNPROVEN TREATMENTS FOR CANCER

  A. Dimension of the problem
    Billions of dollars of personal and family resources are expended yearly for alternative therapies. Four times more money is spent on unproven methods worldwide than on cancer research. Patients who use alternative medicine tend to be well-educated, symptomatic, and in early stages of the disease. All parents of children with cancer want to believe in miracles; those who seek alternative medicine have a strong

desire to find the individual with a "magic bullet," preferably with a semblance of scientific rationale.

B. Role of the National Institutes of Health (NIH) Office of Alternative Medicine

1. This office was established by the NIH to evaluate unconventional therapies and provide assistance to investigators.
2. NIH was under pressure from Congress to address issues of alternative medicine.
3. Proponents of unconventional therapies may have their proposals evaluated by preparation of a "best-case series" followed by a pilot clinical trial.
4. A best-case series involves retrospective identification of patients believed to have benefited from therapy and must be of sufficient detail and clarity to allow independently conducted clinical trials.

C. Alternative therapies: pharmacologic

Pharmacologic therapies (as opposed to lifestyle therapies) are associated with high rates of cancer quackery. The profit potential is very high for a "magic bullet" therapy. Secret mystery properties of the therapy are enhanced, although most have some degree of "plausibility factor" that gives them their strong lay appeal. This type of therapy does, however, lend itself to easier evaluation by randomized, controlled trials than do lifestyle change therapies.

1. For-profit alternative medicine clinics

   These are often in Mexico or the Caribbean, where they are not under U.S. Food and Drug Administration jurisdiction. Practitioners claim they can cure cancer, and denigrate conventional treatments, while conducting little scientific research into their very expensive therapies.

2. Antineoplastons

   a. Stanislaw Burzynski, M.D., Ph.D. (originally at Baylor, now at a private clinic in Houston), is perhaps the best-known alternative for-profit clinician.

   b. Burzynski believes cancer patients are deficient in "peptides" or neoplastons (small chains of amino acids). His treatment replaces "antineoplastons," which originally were derived from human urine, but more recently have been synthesized. Previous phase II trials in brain tumor patients have been suspended.

Although Burzynski has been indicted by the state of Texas numerous times, he has been the subject of very positive media attention, and remains a martyred hero to many of his patients. Some researchers believe than antineoplastons are primarily phenylacetate, which is currently being investigated as a potential active agent against brain tumors.

3. Colonics

At least seven clinics in the Tijuana area treat cancer using enema therapy. Coffee enemas are believed to open the bile ducts of the liver, improving detoxification.

4. Shark cartilage

a. Sharks, which have all-cartilage skeletons, rarely get cancer.

b. Shark cartilage contains an antiangiogenetic factor that, when implanted directly into tumors, does inhibit tumor capillary growth.

c. Significant research has been done, little of it suggesting that ingested shark cartilage actually will work as an effective antitumor agent.

d. The treatment is expensive. The suggested daily dose is much lower than those used in published reports.

e. Shark cartilage probably not absorbed well, nor as biologically active, in the oral form as the implanted form.

f. Other antiangiogenic agents are currently being studied for use in the treatment of hemangiomas as well as cancer.

5. Cancell/Entelev

This was eveloped in the 1930s by Jim Sheridan, a chemist, who said it, "Pushes cancer cell down the oxidation-reduction ladder toward a more primitive state." Sheridan claimed conspiracy by the FDA and American Cancer Society to supress his treatment. The National Cancer Institute (NCI) tested Cancell in 1990 and found it to have no significant biological effect. Since the 1980s, Sheridan's collaborator, Ed Sopack, has made up to 100 bottles per week in his garage and has given it away, keeping the ingredients secret. It turns teeth black, and is associated with liver failure.

6. Essiac

This herbal treatment was developed by Canadian nurse Renee Caisie from the formula of a Native American healer.

It was tested by Memorial Sloan-Kettering Cancer Center and the NCI in the 1970s and found to have no anticancer activity in animal systems, although some of its major ingredients have shown anticancer properties. It contains burdock, sorrel, and slippery elm.

D. Alternative therapies: lifestyle
Many alternative therapies rely on lifestyle changes as an adjunct to cancer therapy. These are too numerous to enumerate and include techniques that many clinicians use routinely in practice already, such as hypnosis and guided imagery. Some of the more popular forms of lifestyle therapies are the following.
1. Spiritual: primarily prayer
2. Psychological: group and individual psychotherapy, and support groups
3. Nutritional
   a. Macrobiotic diet, consisting primarily of whole grains, beans, and vegetables, which has spiritual and social connotations as well
   b. Megavitamins, which may have serious side-effects, including renal calculi and rebound scurvy with high-dose vitamin C, liver damage and pseudotumor cerebri with hypervitamin A, and irreversible calcifications of the soft tissues with vitamin D
   c. β-Carotene, which may have a chemopreventative role in the development of certain types of cancers
4. Mind-body medicine: includes hypnosis, imagery, relaxation, biofeedback, exercise, tai chi, and yoga
5. Body work: massage, acupuncture, acupressure, and therapeutic touch

IV. HELPING FAMILIES MAKE DECISIONS ABOUT ALTERNATIVE MEDICINE

A. Some suggestions for discussing alternative medicine with families
1. Avoid taking an authoritarian approach.
2. Use common English, avoid "medicalese."
3. Be open about discussing diet and vitamins.
4. Do not abandon your own convictions, but be open.
5. Offer to look into treatments with which you are unfamiliar.

B. Resources to give to families
1. American Cancer Society: 1-800-ACS-2345
2. National Institutes of Health, Office of Alternative Medicine: phone: 1-888-644-6226; fax: 301-402-4741; e-mail: Jacqui@helix.nih.gov
3. Cancer Information Service (NCI): 1-800-4-CANCER

C. Quick quack check
Unscrupulous promoters of unproven cancer therapies tend to have certain characteristics in common. Key aspects or behaviors to be wary of include:
1. Broad general claims. The substance can cure not only cancer, but also arthritis, diabetes, chronic fatigue, etc.
2. Offering of a "plausible" scientific rationale.
3. Emphasis on how controversial the therapy is, claiming persecution from the standard medical and legal communities.
4. Seeking of testimonials and publicity, but avoidance of peer review with high media profiles, especially in alternative and New Age presses.
5. Sressing the "natural" nontoxic aspect of their cure.
6. Using words such as *cut* for surgery, *burn* for radiation, and *poison* for chemotherapy.
7. Perpetuating the myth that there is a high-level conspiracy by the mainstream medical community to suppress alternative cancer cures because they threaten to undercut the profits of the cancer industry.

V. CONCLUSIONS

The amazing improvements in childhood cancer survival in the last 30 years are unprecedented. Nonetheless, there is a common misperception that cancer remains an untreatable disease. In addition, some people gravely mistrust "the medical establishment." Our primary goal must be to treat patients with the most up-to-date standard of care; therefore, we must keep lines of communication open with parents who seek alternative medicine, thereby assuring that they will allow their children to be treated with proven therapies. We run the risk of alienating patients and their families, and thus driving them away from standard therapy, if we rigidly refuse to consider alternative therapies. While no forms of alternative medicine have been shown scientifically to systematically cure cancer, several may indeed have a role in the quality of life and supportive care arenas.

Acknowledgments

The authors wish to thank Mary Jo Cleaveland, R.N., for her input in the preparation of this manuscript.

Bibliography

Burton Goldberg Group: *Alternative Medicine, the Definitive Guide.* Puyallup, WA: Future Medicine Publishing, Inc., 1993.

Cassileth BR, Brown H: Unorthodox cancer medicine. *CA Cancer J Clin* 38:176–85, 1988.

Eisenberg DM, Kessler RC, Foster C, et al.: Unconventional medicine in the United States: Prevalence, costs, and patterns of use. *N Engl J Med* 328:246–52, 1993.

Fernandez CV, Stutzer C, MacWilliam L, et al.: Prevalence and reasons for use and non-use of alternative/complementary therapies in pediatric oncology patients. *Proc Am Soc Pediatr Hematol Oncol* 5:16, 1996.

Lerner IJ, Kennedy BJ: The prevalence of questionable methods of cancer treatment in the United States. *CA Cancer J Clin* 42:181–91, 1992.

Lerner, M: *Choices in Healing.* Cambridge, MA: MIT Press, 1994.

Sawyer MG, Gannoni AF, Toogood IR, Antoniou G, Rice M: The use of alternative therapies by children with cancer. *Med J of Aust* 160:320–22, 1994.

Spigelblatt L, Laine-Ammara G, Pless B, Guyver A: The use of alternative medicine by children. *Pediatrics* 94:811–14, 1994.

U.S. Congress, Offfice of Technology Assessment: *Unconventional Cancer Treatments.* Washington, DC: Office of Technology Assessment; 1990. US Congress Publication OTA-H-405.

Zand J, Walton R, Rountree B: *Smart Medicine for a Healthier Child.* Garden City Park, NY: Avery Publishing, 1994.

20

Home Care for Children with Cancer

Pamelyn Close, M.D., M.P.H., Patricia Danz, R.N., B.S.N., and Jean Wadman, R.N., M.S.N., C.R.N.P.

Home care for children with cancer has become an increasingly popular adjunct to outpatient clinic- and hospital-based care. A limited number of studies have demonstrated that moving intravenous chemotherapy, antibiotics, nutrition, and hospice care from the inpatient and clinic settings to the home can be safe and efficient and can provide multiple economic and psychosocial benefits to patients and their families.

I. BACKGROUND: WHY MOVE THERAPY INTO THE HOME?

A. Pioneer efforts to move hospital care to the home began with the care of infants requiring long-term ventilator therapy, children with short bowel syndrome requiring hyperalimentation, children with osteomyelitis requiring weeks of intravenous antibiotic therapy, and hospice care for children dying of chronic or progressive diseases.

B. Pediatric oncology teams cite the following reasons for developing home care programs:
1. Increased intensity of therapies, resulting in increased hospital days and significant disruption of patients' families' lives
2. Improved technologies for intravenous therapy in the home, such as ambulatory infusion pumps and the wide use of central venous access devices
3. Rising costs of acute care pediatric beds

   4. Seasonal shortages of inpatient beds, resulting in chemotherapy delays
   5. Managed care/capitation issues

II. GOALS OF HOME CARE

A. To provide safe opportunities for children with cancer and their families to spend less time in the hospital or clinic using a quality controlled, coordinated home care team approach
B. To reduce the cost of care, but not at the expense of safety for children with complex diseases who require highly specialized treatment
C. To establish the standards of care for our unique patients as we develop new methods to deliver that care

III. BASIC PRINCIPLES OF HOME CARE FOR CHILDREN WITH CANCER

A. Collaborative group studies have demonstrated that children treated for cancer in an appropriate tertiary setting, under the direction of a qualified pediatric oncology team, have better outcomes.
B. The team concept in the provision of home care is of singular importance.
C. The multidisciplinary pediatric care team often includes the following people:
   1. Adult caregiver/parent and the patient
   2. Pediatric oncologist/fellow/resident/and local pediatrician or family practitioner
   3. Nurse (staff/clinical nurse specialist/pediatric nurse practitioner)
   4. Discharge planning coordinator/hospital case manager
   5. Social worker
   6. Ancillary health professionals (occupational therapist/physical therapist/nutritionist)
   7. Case manager from insurance company
   8. Home care provider team
      a. Pediatric oncologist on 24-hour call to the home care team
      b. Nursing coordinator
      c. Pharmacist
      d. Durable medical equipment supplier
      e. Reimbursement specialist

D. Each team member should have a defined role and clear accountabilities.
1. Practice structures at different institutions will change the accountabilities of various team members.
2. Within a given institution, however, consistency of team member responsibilities enhances the overall quality and reproducibility of a good home care plan.
3. Typical accountabilities for team members are presented in Table 20.1.
   a. Responsibilities involving assessments of the family, the source of payment, etc., are often performed by multiple team members.
   b. The physician, discharge planning coordinator, and home care nursing coordinator have final responsibility for the soundness and execution of a home care plan.

IV. CRITERIA FOR ELIGIBILITY

Criteria for eligibility are the initial screening tools used to help assure safety and quality control in the provision of home care. The choice of therapy, the patient's clinical situation, the family's psycho-educational profile, the resource profile for the home and community setting, and the characteristics of the home care provider must each withstand the application of a consistent set of standards. Furthermore, the realities of fiscal eligibility (or noneligibility) can contribute in a make-or-break fashion to the list of home care therapies that are considered for patients.

A. Characteristics of patients and parents that determine eligibility for home infusion therapy
1. Voluntary participation
2. Motivated family willing and able to learn how to manage an intravenous line and pump
3. Safe, suitably equipped home (see section B)
4. Trained adult available at the time of infusion (other than nurse)
5. Adequate venous access.
   Some but not all infusions require a central venous catheter.
6. Successful, uneventful completion of at least one course of the same therapy in the hospital
7. Medical staff evaluation that caretakers are adequate

    a. The medical team must feel confident that the caretakers are able to carry out the prescribed treatment plan.

    b. For patients who have multiple sets of parents, it must be clear who is the responsible party.

    c. In assessing families for home care, put aside stereotypical thinking. Lack of fiscal resources and formal education does not equal lack of motivation or ability to carry out a treatment plan. Likewise, abundant fiscal resources and formal education do not always bring to bear the requisite family skills to carry out a home care plan.

B. Home assessment

The following resources should be available:

1. Electricity
2. Telephone
3. A refrigerator to maintain medicines at the proper temperature
4. Reliable transportation to a hospital or emergency facility
5. Clean home

Ideally the home should have a space dedicated to the supplies necessary for home care, which is out of the reach of children.

C. Home chemotherapy

The therapies that lend themselves best to home administration:

1. Are highly repetitive (i.e., VP-16, ifosfamide $\times$ 5 days).
2. Save several days of hospitalization (i.e., VP-16, ifosfamide).
3. Require short nursing times each day (less than 4 hours).
4. Have had few or no complications for the patient during a first trial course in the hospital.
5. Are amenable to good control of emesis.
6. Use drugs that do not have a large cost discrepancy if purchased by the home care infusion company compared to the hospital.

D. Home antibiotic therapy

1. Non-neutropenic patients

Gram-positive and gram-negative organisms, including catheter infections, can be treated with one or two antibiotics in the home. Clinical criteria for moving therapy to the home include the following.

TABLE 20.1.
Responsibilities Matrix

Group	Personnel	Assess Medical Appropriateness of Therapy	Assess Patient Stability/Eligibility	Assess Caregiver/Ability/Skills	Assess Payment Source	Identify Agency	Assess Agency Ability to Provide Appr. Care	Family Psychosocial Assessment
Home	Community Resource					●	●	●
	Parent/Caregiver		●	●	●	●	●	●
	Patient		●	●	●	●	●	●
Home Care Agency	Field Nurse		●	●	●	●	●	●
	Patient Service Rep.							
	Respiratory Therapist		●	●	●		●	●
	Pharmacist	●	●	●	●		●	
	Home Care Coord.	●	●	■	●		●	●
Insurance Personnel	D/C Planner Dept.		●	●	●	●	●	
	Insurance Case Manager		●	●	■	■	■	●
Hospital Personnel	Child Life Team			●				●
	Nutritionist		●		●		●	
	Hospital Case Manager (1)		●	●	■	●	■	●
	Hospital Utilization Manager			●	■			●
	Discharge Hospital Planner		●	■	■	●	■	■
	Social Worker		●	●	●	●	●	■
	Staff R.N.		●	●		●	●	●
	PNP	●	●	●	●	●	●	●
	Resident/Fellow	●	●	●	●	●	●	●
	Attending Oncologist	■	■	●	●	■	■	●

	Home Assessment	Homecare Plan Responsibility/Goal Assessment	Communication with Patient/Family	Education of Patient/Caregiver	Develop Research & Assessment	Directing Care	Signing Orders	Generating Orders	Choosing Infusion Devices	Ordering Supplies	Evaluating Competency of Agency	Assessing Response to Therapy	Problem Solve When Patient at Home
	■	●	●	●■	■	■	■	●			■	■	●
		●	●	■	●	●		●	●		●	●	●
		●	●	●	●	●					●	●	●
	●	●	●	●	●			●	●		●	●	●
	●	●	●	●					●				●
	●		●	●	●					●			●
	●	■	■	■	●	●		●	■	●	●	■	■
				■									
	●	■	●	●	●			●	●	●	●		
	●		●					●					
	●	●	●	●				●			●		
	●	■	■	■	●	■		●	●	■	●		
												●	
	●	■	■	■	●	■		●	●	■	●		
	●		●	●	●				●		●		●

Key:
■ Primary Responsibility or Responsibility to Delegate to a ●
● Could Have Responsibility Based on Institution

    a. The patient is afebrile, is clinically stable, and feels well.

    b. All sites of infection and initially positive cultures have become negative on antibiotic therapy.

    c. Therapeutic drug levels have been established before discharge.

2. Neutropenic patients

Consider patients with fever and neutropenia initially treated in the hospital for continuation of treatment in the home with intravenous monotherapy (i.e., ceftazidime) if they meet the following "low risk" criteria.

    a. Age: noninfants

    b. Diagnosis: *not* acute nonlymphoblastic leukemia or acute lymphoblasic leukemia in induction

    c. Presentation: fever without signs of shock or localizing symptoms

    d. Clinical course: early defervescence, negative cultures, looks and feels "well"

3. Antifungal therapy

    a. Clinical criteria are similar to those for other home antibiotic therapy.

    b. Potassium loss is controllable by home supplements (oral or intravenous).

    c. Serum potassium levels and renal function can be checked frequently and addressed in a timely fashion.

V. HOSPITAL AND CLINIC THERAPIES THAT CAN BE MOVED INTO THE HOME

The therapies listed below have been reported as amenable for home treatment. Carefully consider the eligibility criteria for each therapy before choosing the treatment for use at home.

A. Chemotherapy program that meet the criteria noted in Section IVC

B. Antibiotic and antifungal therapy

1. Non-neutropenic patients

One- and two-drug standard antibiotic therapy for gram-positive and gram-negative organisms can be moved from the hospital to the home after initial diagnosis and stabilization of the infection.

2. Neutropenic patients

a. A randomized, controlled trial of home antibiotics in pediatric cancer patients with fever and neutropenia has not yet been performed to document the safety of this use of home care.

b. Smaller studies and anecdotal reports have suggested that there may be a group of low-risk patients who could be treated at home after an appropriate initial workup and observation in the hospital.

3. Amphotericin for documented or presumed fungal infections

a. Amphotericin B every day or every other day can be provided in the home for non-neutropenic patients for extended periods of time (see Section IVD-3).

b. Frequent, timely laboratory evaluations of renal function and serum potassium levels are required.

C. Home nutritional support (total parenteral nutrition, nasojejeunal and nasogastric feeds)

Nutritional support, especially for the immediate postchemotherapy patient, is often an important adjunct to primary treatment of a child's cancer (see Chapter 13).

1. Intermittent, cycled, or continuous nasojejeunal, nasogastric, or gastrostomy tube feedings can be done using home pumps.

2. For those patients who cannot tolerate nasojejeunal or nasogastric feedings, intravenous parenteral nutrition can be done in the home.

D. Hospice services and pain management

1. The development of small, efficient home infusion pumps used in combination with central venous catheter devices has advanced the art of pediatric hospice care immeasurably.

2. Dying children can now receive most supportive care therapies at home in their last weeks and days.

3. These therapies often include continuous intravenous pain medicines, hydration/total parenteral nutrition, palliative chemotherapy and antibiotics, and, in some locations, transfusions (see Chapter 21).

VI. CHARACTERISTICS OF HOME CARE AGENCY PROVIDERS

Many general home care companies state that they provide care for children. It is imperative to ascertain that a home care agency providing care for a child with cancer can provide experienced, good-quality nursing staff and pharmacy support in a timely fashion. Below are criteria to consider when identifying an agency as a care provider.

A. Experience in providing hands-on care for children with cancer
   1. Employment of pediatric nurses.
      Request resumes.
   2. Employment of pediatric oncology nurses with experience
   3. Agency's experience with the therapy ordered
      Provide theoretical problems and ask for solutions.
   4. Employment of pediatric case manager to promote continuity
   5. Identification of similar experience-based qualifications of characteristics about pharmacists

B. Accreditation status (Joint Commission on Accreditation of Hospitals, Medicare, Medicaid, Home Health certification)

C. Written standards of care are available for review.

D. Satisfactory contracting arrangements with third-party payers

E. For medical assistance patients, documentation that the agency accepts them for home care

F. Adequate scope of services provided: nursing, pharmacy, occupational/physical therapists, durable medical equipment.

G. Adequate on-call coverage, patient's home area serviced, and reasonable response times for daytime and off-hours calls

H. Mechanism for generating a signed plan of care and for obtaining orders and documenting communication pathway for hospital staff and for agency

I. Receptiveness of agency to inservicing opportunities provided by the hospital or clinic pediatric oncology staff

VII. FISCAL REALITIES

With the wholesale shifts in health care toward managed care and capitation, the pediatric oncology team options for home-based therapies are often limited or tightly proscribed. Some general guidelines to develop the best home care program for a new patient include the following.

A. Identify the payer source, home care benefits, and home care referral agencies immediately upon the child's diagnosis.

B. Before offering home therapy to the patient and family, be sure that the available home care referral agencies have the appropriate expertise to handle the desired home therapy.

C. The team must accept the truth that no home care would probably be better for the patient than bad home care.

Bibliography

Bendorf K, Meehan J: Home parenteral nutrition for the child with cancer. *Issues Comp Pediatr Nurs* 12:178–86, 1989.

Cambers EJ, Oakhill A, Comish JM, Cumick S: Terminal care at home for children with cancer. *Br Med J* 298:937–40, 1989.

Close P, Burkey E, Kazak A, Danz P, Lange B: A prospective, controlled evaluation of home chemotherapy of children with cancer. *Pediatric* 95:896–900, 1995.

Close P, Danz P, Burkey E, Kazak A, Lange BJ: Organization and evaluation of a high technology home care program for children with cancer. *Proc Soc Pediatr Res* 29:000, 1991.

Holdsworth MT, Raisch DW, Chavez C, Duncan MN, Parasuraman TV, Cox FU: Evaluation of economic impact with home delivery of chemotherapy to pediatric oncology patients. *Ann Pharmacother* (in press).

Jayabose S, Escobedo V, Tugal O, et al.: Home chemotherapy for children with cancer. *Cancer* 69:574–79, 1992.

Lange B, Burroughs B, Meadows A, Burkey E: Home care involving methotrexate infusions for children with acute lymphoblastic leukemia. *J Pediatr* 112:492–95, 1988.

Lange BJ, Close P, Danz P, et al.: *Home Infusion Therapy for the Child with Cancer: A Practical Manual for Parents and Providers.* Philadelphia: Children's Hospital of Philadelphia; 1991.

Wiemikows WJT, Rothney M, Dawson S, Andrew M: Evaluation of a home intravenous antibiotic program in pediatric oncology. *Am J Pediatr Hematol Oncol* 13:10147, 1991.

21

Terminal Care for Children with Cancer

Rita S. Meek, M.D., Jean B. Belasco, M.D., and
Robert B. Noll, Ph.D.

I. INTRODUCTION AND DEFINITIONS

   A. In the Western world, 30–40% of children with cancer die of
   their disease. In undeveloped countries, 70–80% of children
   with cancer may die.

   B. When relapses occur, the focus of therapy may change from
   the original one of cure to palliation and then to terminal care.
   Quality of life rather than prolongation of life is emphasized.
   1. Palliative care may be defined as the period when cure is
      no longer possible; treatments offered during this period
      are designed to prolong meaningful life. Extremely aggres-
      sive interventions are usually avoided. This period usual-
      ly lasts months and may last even more than a year.
   2. Terminal care may be defined as the period when treat-
      ments are provided for comfort without the goal of pro-
      longing life. This period may last weeks or months. It is
      never a time of "nothing to do," but is a time of providing
      intensive comfort measures, of increased personal
      involvement by health care providers, and of encouraging
      communication between members of the family.

II. MEMBERS OF THE TERMINAL CARE TEAM

   A. Members of the terminal care team include a core group of physicians, nurses, and psychosocial professionals who will continue to provide care in the hospital or in the home and/or will provide expertise and support to community care providers. Included are professionals from the patient's personal physician's office, the hospital, and hospice.

B. The child's family is an equal member of the team, bringing its individual strengths and weaknesses, ethics, and culture. The professional team must attempt to understand the family background, work within their philosophical and religious beliefs, and exploit areas of strength and support areas of weakness.

C. Clergy and volunteers are often part of the community resources.

D. Duties of the terminal care team include:
1. Making an assessment of the psychosocial strengths and needs of the family, their potential community supports, as well as their financial and insurance issues.
2. Being an advocate for the child with third-party insurance providers to assure that critical services, such as highly technical care or additional nursing hours, will be provided.
3. Arranging for additional services for the family so they can maintain their own health and continue to function.
4. Addressing immediate psychosocial needs of the family, including siblings, grandparents, and friends, and ensuring that bereavement services will be provided.

III. GOALS OF CARE TO BE AGREED ON BY THE FAMILY AND OTHER MEMBERS OF THE TERMINAL CARE TEAM

A. Provide comfort measures for problems that cannot be eliminated.

B. Anticipate events and train caregivers to handle potential problems.

C. Interventions should maximize the quality of life rather than the quantity of life.

D. Interventions may change as the child's condition changes.

E. There are few emergencies during the terminal phase of the child's illness that cannot be cared for at least as well at home as in the hospital, if the family is able and willing.

IV. LOCATION OF CARE

Terminal care can be provided in the home, a free-standing hospice, or the hospital, since it is a philosophy of care rather than precise interventions.

A. Issues to consider when deciding location of care
   1. The family's desire and commitment to have the child at home and their abilities to cope with the stresses, support each other, and share tasks
   2. The child's desire to be at home
   3. Siblings' needs to be part of caregiving process, according to their abilities to do so
   4. Parents' needs to provide attention and support for the siblings
   5. Parents' needs to be able to continue to function and work
   6. Community resources, such as home care agencies, which can provide the level of technology necessary for symptom control and respite care when needed
   7. The availability of the primary team to provide continuity of medical care and psychosocial support
   8. The type of medical problems that may arise and how manageable they would be at home or hospice

B. Benefits of terminal care at home
   1. Enhanced communication between the dying patient and the family
   2. Decreased isolation for the dying child
   3. Increased control and involvement for the patient, parents, and siblings
   4. "Normalization" of family life
   5. Increased participation by community-based health care professionals

C. Hospitalization
   Hospitalization, if later felt to be necessary, should be viewed as respite care and an opportunity to provide structured support for the family, and should provide the same level of services being provided in the home.

V. ISSUES TO ADDRESS IN TERMINAL CARE

A. Extent of support and intervention to control symptoms
   1. The family and medical staff should discuss, in advance,

the type and extent of medical intervention to be used to control symptoms, focusing on the goal of maintaining quality of life, through the use of comfort measures. Issues to address include:
  a. Transfusion support.
  b. Treatment of fever with antibiotics.
  c. Chemotherapy.
  d. Radiation therapy.
  e. Surgical interventions.
  2. Make a psychosocial assessment of social and emotional resources available to the family, so plans made by the medical team are feasible.

B. "Do Not Resuscitate" Order
  1. The "Do Not Resuscitate" order is part of the evolutionary process from palliative care to terminal care.
  2. Introducing this topic early in the process allows time for meaningful discussions.
  3. Discussion focusing on what will be done to prevent suffering, if and when the child is dying, may make "withholding of heroic measures" more understandable and acceptable.
  4. Emphasize that everything will continue to be done to keep the child comfortable and that palliative treatment will be given for problems that cannot be eliminated.
  5. Decisions such as these should be made by the family and medical staff working closely together.

C. Request for autopsy
  1. When appropriate, a discussion of the role and importance of autopsy is best done by the child's principal physician before the child's death.
  2. Introducing this topic early in the process allows time for meaningful discussions, but permission to perform an autopsy may not be obtained premortem.
  3. The person who is requesting permission for autopsy needs to explain
    a. What is involved in the procedure.
    b. That it will not interfere with the funeral service that is planned.
    c. That it will not disfigure the child (although a wig may be necessary if a craniotomy is performed).
    d. That it will not delay the funeral services significantly.

    e. That it is provided by the hospital without charge to the family (although there may be costs of transportation to the hospital if the child died at home).

4. The autopsy will provide information to the family and the medical staff regarding disease symptoms, toxicities of therapy, and extent of disease, which may be helpful to:
   a. The family in answering questions they may have regarding their child's illness.
   b. The medical staff in the management of future patients.
   c. Other pediatric oncologists, if the child has participated in a cooperative clinical trial.
5. Some families will refuse an autopsy, for personal or religious reasons; always respect their decision.

D. Funeral issues
1. The psychosocial professional can be helpful:
   a. In facilitating arrangements with the funeral home.
   b. In identifying funds that may be available through community or charitable resources to help defray funeral costs.
   c. In explaining that siblings of all ages routinely attend viewings and funerals without adverse psychosocial consequences.
   d. In helping the family decide what will be most satisfactory for their children.
2. Families generally welcome attendance by the medical staff at the child's funeral, since they perceive this as something the staff "wants to do" because the child and family are important to the medical team rather than something they "have to do." Obviously, respect the family's wishes if they wish the funeral to be private.
3. Personal letters to the family from the staff are particularly meaningful to the family.

E. Pronouncement of death
1. If it is anticipated that the child will die at home, give clear guidelines to the family about what they should do if they think their child is dying or has died, so the family does not panic and call 911 for emergency services.
2. Having a written "Do Not Resuscitate" order in the home may prevent unwanted resuscitative efforts made by medical personnel if the family does call 911.
3. It is important to clarify, in advance, who will make the pronouncement of death.

    a. In many states, nurses can pronounce the death of children who die at home in terminal care services such as hospice.

    b. In some states, a physician may need to make a home visit to pronounce the death.

    c. If it is anticipated that the child may die at home, the physician can notify the local coroner that this will be an anticipated death, to eliminate any unnecessary delays in removing the child's body.

4. If the child dies in the hospital, death is usually pronounced by the house staff or by an oncology physician. The oncology physician, other professional staff who have worked with the family and referring physician should, of course, be notified.

VI. CONTROLLING SYMPTOMS FOR THE CHILD IN THE TERMINAL PHASE OF CANCER

The following suggestions are applicable for a child receiving terminal care at home or in the hospital and are meant to be guidelines for care but are not intended to be exhaustive in scope. They must be adapted for the individual child and circumstances. When weighing the risks and benefits of managing symptoms in terminal care, strive for comfort for the child and the family.

A. Pain

1. Children frequently need significant amounts of narcotics to achieve adequate analgesia in the terminal phase of their illness.

2. Physicians caring for children in this phase of their illness must become knowledgeable about the use of a variety of analgesic approaches.

3. Prescribe adequate doses of analgesics to achieve freedom from suffering. No dose of pain medicine is "too high" or carries "too great a risk."

4. Pain may be complicated by feelings of grief, loss, anxiety, and depression. Psychosocial intervention and behavioral approaches to pain management may be effective in conjunction with analgesics.

5. If a child is in severe pain, consider use of:

    a. Continuous-infusion narcotics intravenously or subcutaneously with as needed bolus by patient/parent-controlled analgesia.

b. A fentanyl patch, which can last up to 72 hours, for patients weighing >50 kg. Erratic dosing may occur in patients who are febrile or hypermetabolic.

c. Methotrimeprazine (Levoprome) 0.2–0.3 mg/kg intramuscular (IM) q3–6h. Used in addition to opioids in patients with refractory pain, if the patient is vomiting and needs sedation, or if the patient has a headache related to a brain tumor. It may cause orthostatic hypotension and has a high incidence of extrapyramidal reactions.

6. If hyperalgesia occurs in patients treated with opioids, decrease the opioid dose and add methotrimeprazine and/or fentanyl.

7. If the above measures are inadequate, consultation with a pediatric anesthesiologist may be helpful.

a. If severe terminal agitation or pain refractory to high doses of analgesics develops, bifuse either of the following into opioid infusion.

i. Lorazepam (Ativan) 0.025 mg/kg/h or a calculated hourly rate based on previous dosage requirement

ii. Midazolam (Versed) 0.05–0.1 mg/kg/h

b. Pentobarbital coma can be achieved by using pentobarbital (Nembutal) 10–15 mg/kg IV over 1–2 hours or 3–4 mg/kg as bolus, followed by 1 mg/kg/h with titration for effect.

8 . See Chapter 11 for an overview of pain management.

B. Hypoxia

1. The major symptom from hypoxia is anxiety. Oxygen and opiates in whatever amounts necessary to relieve anxiety are the treatments of choice.

a. Opioids

i. Morphine 0.3 mg/kg per dose PO q3–4h, with no top dose,

ii. Morphine 0.1 mg/kg per dose IV q2–4h in narcotic-naive patient

iii. Titration in a narcotic-tolerant child, with no top dose

b. Other drugs to consider

i. Benzodiazepines

(1) Diazepam (Valium) 0.12–0.8 mg/kg/day in 3–4 divided doses PO

(2) Lorazepam (Ativan) 0.03–0.04 mg/kg/day in 3–4 divided doses PO/IV

      ii. Barbiturates, such as pentobarbital 2–6 mg/kg/day in 3 divided doses PO/IV/per rectum (PR)

2. As part of an end-stage state, excessive secretions may cause symptomatic distress. Medications may include:
   a. Sublingual atropine 0.02 mg/kg per dose (maximum dose 0.4 mg).
   b. Glycopyrrolate (Robinul) 40–100 µg/kg per dose PO 3–4 times/day, or 4–10 µg/kg per dose IV/IM 3–4 times/day.

C. Bowel obstruction
   1. Partial or intermittent bowel obstruction may cause severe symptoms of pain and vomiting.
   2. Symptoms may improve with:
      a. Sublingual atropine 0.02 mg/kg per dose (maximum dose 0.4 mg).
      b. Glycopyrrolate (Robinul) 40–100 µg/kg per dose PO given 3–4 times/day.
      c. Aggressive laxative and enema regimen.
      d. Histamine H_2 receptor blockers.
      e. Lower–dose morphine.
      f. Antiemetics.
      g. Dietary changes.
      h. Belladonna and opium suppositories ($\frac{1}{4}$ to $\frac{1}{2}$ suppository for children, and 1 suppository for adolescents and adults up to 4 times/day) for painful or tenesmic states caused by tumor obstructing the bowel or urinary tract.
   3. Some children may still require nasogastric suction for decompression.

D. Infections
   1. Avoid uncomfortable diagnostic workups for fever.
   2. Treat local infections that are causing symptoms, such as a urinary tract infection, only to reduce discomfort.
   3. If a child's quality of life is irreversibly deteriorating, antibiotics are usually not appropriate for serious infections such as pneumonia or sepsis.

E. Nutritional support
   1. Anorexia may result from progressive cancer. Cachexia may be part of the dying process and may be irreversible.
   2. Aggressive hydration and nutrition may not increase the patient's sense of well-being during the end-stages of dis-

ease. Malnutrition and dehydration are usually more unpleasant for the family than the patient, and families often respond well to the reassurance that the child is not uncomfortable. However, giving and withdrawing of nutritional support is usually determined by parental, cultural, and religious needs; the oncology team should understand it in that context.

F. Seizures
 1. Discuss the possibility of seizures, advising that most are self-liming, and educate caregivers about first aid care.
 2. If seizures are likely, have appropriate medications with previously determined dosages available and train caregivers in its use.
 3. Treatment of status epilepticus may include:
    a. Lorazepam (Ativan) 0.1 mg/kg IV in infants and children (maximum 4 mg per dose) or 0.07 mg/kg IV in adolescents (maximum 4 mg per dose) at not more than 2 mg/min.
    b. Phenobarbital 15–18 mg/kg/day IV in 1 or 2 doses over 2–3 minutes each.
    c. Phenytoin (Dilantin) 15–20 mg/kg IV over a period of 15–20 minutes.
    d. Phenytoin (Dilantin) 15–20 mg/kg nasogastric or per gastrostomy in 3 divided doses over 2–4 hours to minimize GI side effects (oral route may not be optimal).
    g. Diazepam (injectable) (Valium) 0.3 mg/kg per dose IV in 2–3 min; may repeat dose of 0.2 mg/kg prn.
 4. The physician should consider ordering maintenance anticonvulsant therapy to avoid recurrence of seizures

G. Anxiety and depression
 1. Children and adolescents in the terminal phase of their illness may be anxious and/or depressed.
 2. The psychosocial professional with whom the child or adolescent has established rapport should work with the family to understand the issues and should offer emotional support. Counseling with families is helpful, and, as relevant issues are clarified, anxiety and depression will frequently lessen.
 3. Preschool and school-aged children commonly have a fear of being alone or in pain, and frequently react to parental distress.

4. Teenagers have similar concerns and also worry about what will happen to their significant others if they die. Occasionally, teenagers have existential concerns about death.

5. The diagnosis of depression in children and teenagers with cancer is complex and requires a knowledge of psychopathology development, and experience with childhood cancer.

   a. Young children with depression may have a more depressed appearance, somatic complaints, psychomotor agitation, phobias, separation anxiety, and hallucinations.

   b. Adolescents may exhibit hypersomnia and hopelessness.

   c. Antidepressant medications can be tried, although they may be no more effective than placebos. These medicines are usually well tolerated by young patients, are inexpensive, and may have some efficacy in pain management. Medications include:

      i. Amitriptyline (Elavil) 0.25–2 mg/kg per dose PO or 25–50 mg in adolescents.

      ii. Nortriptyline (Pamelor) 1–3 mg/kg per dose PO or 25–50 mg in 3–4 divided doses in adolescents.

      iii. Imipramine (Tofranil) 1.5–5 mg/kg/day PO (maximum 5 µg/kg/day, maximum 150 mg/day).

   d. If tricyclic antidepressants are not tolerated, consider serotonin reuptake inhibitors, such as sertraline (Zoloft) 50–200 mg/day or fluoxetine (Prozac) 20–80 mg/day.

   e. In anxiety disorders, as needed use of benzodiazepines, such as alprazolam (Xanax), may be helpful.

H. Sleep disturbances

   1. Sleep disturbances are very common in the terminal phase of illness.

   2. If caused by a specific etiology, such as anxiety, depression, pain, central nervous system disease, or side effects of medications, treat accordingly.

   3. Nonpharmacologic techniques such as relaxation, guided imagery, and distraction are often beneficial for insomnia.

   4. Medications that may be helpful include:

      a. Hydroxyzine (Vistaril) 0.5–2.0 mg/kg PO at bedtime.

   b. Diphenhydramine (Benadryl) 0.5–1.0 mg/kg PO at bedtime.
   c. Chloral hydrate 50–75 mg/kg PO at bedtime.
   d. Benzodiazepines, e.g., diazepam (Valium) 0.5 mg/kg PO at bedtime.
   e. Barbiturates, e.g., pentobarbital (Nembutal) 2–6 mg/kg PO at bedtime.
   5. If the insomnia results in part from depression, amitriptyline (Elavil) 0.5–2 mg/kg PO at bedtime or nortriptyline (Pamelor) 1–3 mg/kg/day may be helpful.
   6. If excessive sleepiness occurs secondary to chronic opioids, methylphenidate (Ritalin) 0.3 mg/kg per dose up to 10–15 mg PO 2–3 times/day may be helpful.
I. Mucositis (see Chapter 14-II)

VII. FAMILY STRENGTHS AND NEEDS DURING TERMINAL CARE

A. Anticipatory grieving is associated with better long-term outcomes for survivors of loss.
   1. The prevention of long-term devastation for the grieving but surviving parents and siblings can often be accomplished when the professional members of the team deal with these anticipatory issues.
   2. Physicians, nurses, or psychosocial professionals can facilitate discussions about death and dying between parents, siblings, grandparents, and the ill child, since families typically need assistance talking about these issues.

B. The professional team members can help parents of a dying child communicate with each other.
   1. Parents frequently have different coping mechanisms and achieve different levels of accepting their child's impending death.
   2. Parents can be helped to focus on their child and their shared loss, rather than focusing on their differences and feeling angry with each other.
   3. Encourage the parents to share their concerns about death and dying and to affirm their relationships with each other and with the other members of the family.

C. Team members can help the parents communicate with their other children.

1. Parents often need to be encouraged to be honest with their children and to avoid euphemisms that create new fears. While parents may want to "protect" their other children from the knowledge that the ill child is dying, considerable literature has shown that the children already know.
2. Siblings have an easier time with their grief after the death of a brother or sister if communication is open and the sibling is involved and present during the terminal illness.

VIII. BEREAVEMENT

A. A bereavement meeting should be scheduled after the child's death.
   1. Many parents can benefit from one or more meetings with members of the oncology team in the first years after the death of their child. The appropriate timing for such meeting(s) should be determined by the families.
   2. The details of the child's illness, the medical aspects of the terminal event, and the results of the autopsy can be discussed.
   3. The staff can use this as an opportunity to provide emotional support, explore with the family whether additional bereavement services would be helpful, and assess for symptoms of anxiety and depression in the family members, so that appropriate referrals for support can be made if necessary. Siblings and nonparent relatives can be invited.
   4. The medical staff can convey to the family how much their child meant to the team.

B. Parents and siblings of a child who dies from cancer are at risk for psychosocial morbidity.

C. During the initial year after the death of a child, telephone contact with a member of the oncology team may be helpful in assessing whether excessive psychosocial morbidity is present, so that an appropriate referral can be made.

D. Many families benefit from grief support groups, which may be available in local communities.

IX. STRESSES ON HEALTH PROFESSIONALS

A. Professionals who work with children with cancer are often in the midst of human tragedy that results in personal emotional pain for the health care professional.
   1. Common immediate reactions to this type of stress include anxiety, frustration, irritability, helplessness, and anger.
   2. Delayed stress reactions include lingering sadness, grief, and guilt.
   3. Failure to address these issues openly increases the professionals' risk of emotional distress.

B. Numerous strategies exist for professionals to lessen the burden of distressing events and accelerate recovery, including:
   1. A well-balanced family and emotional life outside of work.
   2. Psychosocial debriefings with the oncology team to discuss critical incidents.
   3. Informal or formal support groups that meet regularly to focus on these complex issues.
   4. Physical exercise to reduce stress reactions.
   5. Use of relaxation techniques, such as guided imagery or self-hypnosis.

Bibliography

Ambrosini PJ, Bianchi MD, Rabinovich H, Elia J: Antidepressant treatments in children andadolescents. Affective disorders. *J Am Acad Child Adolesc Psychiatry* 32:1–6, 1993.

Antonuccio DO, Danton WG, DeNelsky GY: Psychotherapy versus medication for depression: Challenging the conventional wisdom with data. *Prof Psychol: Res Practi* 26:574–85, 1995.

Aring D: Intimations of mortality: An appreciation of death and dying. *Ann Intern Med* 69:137–52, 1968.

August DA, Faubion WC, Rynn ML, Haggerty RH, Wesley RJ: A clinician driven home care delivery system. *Cancer* 72:3542–47, 1993.

Berde C, Ablin A, Glazer S, et al.: Report of the subcommittee on disease-related pain in childhood cancer. *Pediatrics* 86:818–25, 1990.

Bluebond-Langner M: *The Private Worlds of Dying Children.* Princeton, NJ: Princeton University Press; 1978.

Brewer EJ, McPherson M, Magrab PR, Hutchins VL: Family-centered, community-based, coordinated care for children with special health care needs. *Pediatrics* 83:105–6, 1989.

Burish TG, Redd WH: Symptom control in psychosocial oncology. *Cancer* 74:1438–44, 1994.

Committee on Children with Disabilities: *Guidelines for Home Care of Infants, Children, and Adolescents with Chronic Disease. Pediatrics* 96:161–64, 1995.

Glazer HR, Landreth GL. A developmental concept of dying in a child's life. *J Hum Ed Dev* 31:98–105, 1993.

Lauer ME, Mulhern RK, Hoffman RG, Camitta BM: Utilization of hospice/home care in pediatric oncology: A national survey. *Cancer Nurs* 9 (3):102–7, 1986.

Rolland JS: Anticipating loss: A family systems developmental framework. *Fam Pract* 29:229–44, 1990.

Whittam EH: Terminal care of the dying: Psychosocial implication of care. *Cancer* 72:3450–62, 1993.

Index

Page numbers in *italics* denote figures; those followed by "t" denote tables.

Jossey-Bass Teacher

Jossey-Bass Teacher provides K–12 teachers with essential knowledge and tools to create a positive and lifelong impact on student learning. Trusted and experienced educational mentors offer practical classroom-tested and theory-based teaching resources for improving teaching practice in a broad range of grade levels and subject areas. From one educator to another, we want to be your first source to make every day your best day in teaching. *Jossey-Bass Teacher* resources serve two types of informational needs—essential knowledge and essential tools.

Essential knowledge resources provide the foundation, strategies, and methods from which teachers may design curriculum and instruction to challenge and excite their students. Connecting theory to practice, essential knowledge books rely on a solid research base and time-tested methods, offering the best ideas and guidance from many of the most experienced and well-respected experts in the field.

Essential tools save teachers time and effort by offering proven, ready-to-use materials for in-class use. Our publications include activities, assessments, exercises, instruments, games, ready reference, and more. They enhance an entire course of study, a weekly lesson, or a daily plan. These essential tools provide insightful, practical, and comprehensive materials on topics that matter most to K–12 teachers.

JB JOSSEY-BASS

Teaching Writing in the Inclusive Classroom

Strategies and Skills for All Students

Roger Passman, Ed.D.
Katherine S. McKnight, Ph.D.

BICENTENNIAL
1807
WILEY
2007
BICENTENNIAL

John Wiley & Sons, Inc.

About the Authors

Roger Passman, an educator for over twenty years, is currently an associate professor in secondary education at Northeastern Illinois University, where he also coordinates the graduate program in secondary education. His classroom experience includes nearly ten years as a middle-level social studies and language arts teacher in Chicago public schools. Passman is a regular contributor to scholarly journals in the areas of curriculum and instruction, literacy, social studies methods, and educational policy, with an emphasis on inclusion of all children in regular education programs. A tireless teacher educator, he regularly presents at professional conferences, including those of the National Council of Teachers of English and the American Education Research Association. He received his B.S. degree from Bradley University in Peoria, Illinois, his M.Ed. from Northeastern Illinois University, and his Ed.D. from National-Louis University in Evanston, Illinois.

Katherine S. McKnight has been a literacy educator for over sixteen years. For over ten years she taught in a Chicago public high school where many of the lessons featured in this book were developed. She is passionate about creating curricula that engage all students in the regular education classroom. Currently an associate professor in secondary education at Northeastern Illinois University, she also serves as chair of the Teacher Education Department. She teaches courses in English education, literacy, and secondary education curriculum and instruction. In addition, she consults and works with Chicago public school teachers on professional development and team teaching. She regularly publishes in professional journals and is a frequent presenter at professional conferences, including those of the National Council of Teachers of English. She received her B.A. degree from George Washington University, her M.Ed. from Northeastern Illinois University, and her Ph.D. from the University of Illinois at Chicago.

To Susan, Ben, Andrew, and Leah or Becki
they know who they are.
—Roger Passman

For Jim, Ellie, and Colin, who bring joy to my life.
—Katherine S. McKnight

This book is also dedicated to our students,
past and present, who are the reasons why we teach.

Contents

Chapter Three: Developing Mini Lessons

Chapter Four: Discovering Organization

Contents

Acknowledgments

Since we assert that writing is a "solitary social activity," we must acknowledge that our efforts would not have been realized in this book if it had not been for some key individuals who pushed along the process.

Steve Thompson, former editor for Jossey-Bass, provided initial feedback and was our original guide on this project. He is a teacher in the truest sense. We would like to thank Kate Gagnon and Lesley Iura, also at Jossey-Bass, for their editorial wisdom and support. We are grateful to Barbara Fuller for her diligent and meticulous edit during the development phase of this book. Margie McAnneny and Elizabeth Forsaith also need to be recognized for their support and guidance during this project. Finally, Bradley Berlage, our graduate student assistant extraordinaire, helped us during the final stages of the book.

Chicago, Illinois
September 2006

Roger Passman
Katherine S. McKnight

W h y
W r i T e V
W A n y h o i o i
A y h o c e
? w T h A d
e o r y n
r v a n d

Chapter One

Why Write, Anyhow?

Understanding Voice, Theory, and Standards in Contemporary Classrooms

Teachers often cry out in desperation when a special education student is placed in their regular education classroom. "I have no training in skills to cope with the needs of the exceptional child!" they scream.

We simply do not believe that this kind of fear and prejudice is justified. Inclusion is a fact of life in most schools, precisely as it should be. We argue that when teachers adopt the writing approach known as TIP—*T*each, *I*ntroduce, *P*ractice—they are well equipped to create needed accommodations for their special education students without much additional effort (see Figure 1.1).

What Is the TIP Writing Process?

The TIP Writing Process individualizes teaching, focusing on the needs of each student in the classroom. Blending aspects of strategic writing and mechanics with a pure workshop approach, it may be described as an extension of the workshop approach that is more appropriate for classroom use, especially in underserved and inclusive classrooms. Because of its workshop approach, it allows students

Figure 1.1. The TIP Writing Process.

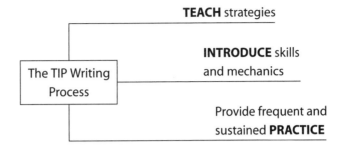

to write at their own level and pace. They are never made to feel less than their peers; rather, everyone shares in the process of creating with words and ideas.

We think this idea is best illustrated by three individual narratives that are part of our teaching experience. The stories of Jane, Jamie, and Debbie (pseudonyms are used for all people and places described) help lay bare the false assumption that regular education teachers are not fully equipped to handle the needs and requirements of their exceptional students.

Jane's Story: Learning to Participate Through an Ice Cream Social

Jane has cerebral palsy. When Roger was first introduced to Jane she was eight years old and in third grade. She was confined to a wheelchair, wore diapers, and never spoke. Roger was told by the school principal that Jane was unable to fully participate in class and he might better spend time working with those children who would, indeed, actively engage in the writing process. He had been hired as a consultant in Lawrenceville, Texas, working with teachers and students to improve the writing scores in the elementary division of the Unified Lawrenceville Independent School District. One of his responsibilities as a consultant to the district was to model various approaches to inclusion. After his conversation with the school's principal he realized he had his work cut out for him.

All he had heard about Jane was true. She was wheeled into the classroom by her full-time aide, who quickly disappeared from view. Jane was left in a rear corner of the third-grade room pointed toward the windows. She didn't speak or move from the position in which she was left. All of the fourteen other students in the room ignored her, as did the teacher. Jane was alone, confined to the limits of her chair, a chair she could not move by her own means. Looking out the window into a beautiful, blue October Texas sky, Jane appeared sadly isolated and abandoned.

Roger walked over to Jane and asked, "Are you going to write with us today?" She barely shook her head, moving it from left to right only two times before she resumed staring out the window into space. He moved back to the front of the

class and resumed his modeling of "better" writing practice with Ms. Applewood's students. This routine was repeated twice a week for nearly three months. He never failed to ask Jane if she was going to write with the rest of the class and she never failed to shake her head no, making no sounds to acknowledge her response.

One day—it was early February on a nice West Texas winter day—one of Ms. Applewood's students asked, "Dr. Passman, what's your first name?" He replied, "Doctor." To which she insisted, "No, Dr. Passman, what's your real first name?" He made a deal with the class. It was Tuesday and he would be back in the school on Thursday. "If," he told the group, "you can find out my first name without asking any of your teachers by the time I get back on Thursday, I will throw an ice cream party for your class." At the end of the class period Jane motioned him back to her chair. For the first time she spoke to him. "Can I have ice cream?" she asked very softly. These were the first words he ever heard her speak.

"Sure, Jane," he offered, "but only if you write with us on Thursday."

"OK, I'll do it." And she smiled.

He arrived on Thursday to a gaggle of third-grade students all anxious to share that they had learned his first name was Roger. An ice cream party it was, and they scheduled it for the following Tuesday. When he arrived, Jane was already in the back of the room—only this time she was facing in toward the class. She held a pencil in her hand and a board shaped in the form of a writing desk was secured to the handles of her chair. He gave the class their assignment and went back to visit Jane. She struggled to write her name on the paper but she did it, and she smiled a proud, toothy smile. He told her that he would write anything she told him to write, that he would be her hands. Dictation seemed to be an accommodation that made sense. For the next fifteen minutes, while the other students were writing, Jane dictated a wondrous story of how she and her mom and sister went to Lujack for pizza, where she ate three whole slices of pepperoni and drank a whole Coke. She told about the drive to and from Lujack, how her wheelchair was secured to her mom's van, how nice the people were in the Pizza Hut where they ate. She included details, humor, and in the end, displayed a clear and focused voice in her writing.

Students shared their writing in what was called the Author's Chair. Jane volunteered to read but was so shy that she whispered to Roger, "Could one of my friends read for me?" They decided that Cassie would serve as Jane's voice. At the end of Cassie's reading of Jane's dictation Jane was beaming. Joyful tears were running down both cheeks as every child in the room stood and applauded.

The following Tuesday Jane gorged herself on ice cream and chocolate cake. When Roger saw her in the hallway in the morning she smiled and told her aide to push her chair over to him. When she was close enough for him to hear she shouted, "I showed my mom my writing and she was so proud she gave me a dollar!" Jane never stopped writing after that day. Roger taught her teachers and her aide how to take dictation from Jane. Her stories grew and became more sophisticated. Her voice came through. She began to participate in group

prewriting work. In short, Jane became a writer, and it began to affect everything else she did for the rest of the school year.

The next school year began and Jane was out of diapers. She had a motorized wheelchair, and she had a walker. She spent at least half of every school day out of the chair walking around the school. In fourth grade she participated in the TIP writing sessions as a full participant. Her peers learned to take dictation, serving as her hands. She struggled to sign every piece she wrote. Jane still participated in occupational therapy and continued to receive special services for her math and reading skills, but she became a writer.

Jane's story is extreme but not unusual. She had been told so often that she couldn't that finally she simply wouldn't participate. It took Roger three months to break through the shell of isolation. The fact that it took her love of ice cream and desire to participate in the social side of the classroom was a bonus. But what really turned the tide was that he never stopped asking her if she wanted to participate. He didn't push or force her. That would have been counterproductive. He simply asked her to join in. When she did he made an accommodation that ensured her participation. **The lesson is simple: never give up on a child. Even when you feel overwhelmed and undertrained, never give up.** Look for the motivator, the one thing that will engage a child. In Jane's case it appeared to be the fact that Roger paid some attention to her, that he was interested in having her join the group and participate as an author in a community of authors.

Jamie's Story: Patience and Creativity Pay Off

The most important lesson that Katie has learned—which is probably true of all writing teachers—is how far patience and creativity can take you. This lesson came to light when Katie worked with Jamie, a seventh-grade student. Jamie lacked the confidence to write. She would tell Katie, "I don't write. I don't like it, and besides, I don't write really well."

As Katie worked together with Jamie on writing, she discovered that the child had received negative feedback about her writing and very few opportunities to practice and explore writing. After many months of positive reinforcement and practice, practice, practice, Jamie had a breakthrough. A story she wrote about getting ready for school on Labor Day weekend was filled with details and her wicked sense of humor. This was a turning point.

Jamie continued to gain confidence as a writer because she knew that she could tell stories. Through her storytelling and personal narratives she developed her writing skills, and they began to trickle into her school writing. Her reports were filled with details and her own commentary. Jamie found her voice as a writer.

It has been our experience that when students are in environments where they are expected to write, as Jamie was, they eventually do find their own voice. They may find their voice quickly, or it can take weeks, even months. But it does

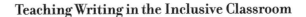

happen when the writing lessons and learning environment embody patience, creativity, and the expectation to write, write, write.

Debbie's Story: Labels Create the "Can't"

Roger met Debbie in seventh grade, when he was giving writers' workshops to classes at her school. She was diagnosed as severely learning disabled, was far behind what one might expect of a seventh-grade reader and writer, and appeared quite unwilling to put forth the effort to succeed. Her special education resource teacher told him, "Debbie cannot put two English words together to make a sentence, so please don't make her write." Roger said nothing.

The first day of their writers' workshop Debbie approached his desk with a timidity that he had never seen before. "Mr. Passman," she whispered. "I can't write." She simply hung her head waiting for his response. He did not tell her what she wanted to hear. "Debbie," he retorted. "What are the rules of the writers' workshop?"

"Well, we can write about anything we want?" she responded, questioning the veracity of the whole idea.

"So, what's the problem? All I want you to do is try and write to the best of your ability. Just try, Debbie, that's all."

"OK," she whispered, but he sensed disbelief.

Well, it was true. Debbie could not put two words together to make a sentence at first. Her writing was immature, tortured, and frankly, not very good. But Roger was patient. In October his patience was rewarded when Debbie came to him and asked if she could write poetry. He asked her what the rules of the workshop were.

"I can write anything I want in any format I want," she said. Her voice was louder than it had been when he first met her.

Debbie began to write poetry. He learned how she hated her big sister, little brother, and mother's boyfriend. He learned how she had an aunt who made her laugh and a cousin who didn't. While her poetry was mainly dominated by the rantings of a twelve-year-old seeking to carve out a place in a hostile world, it was improving on a regular basis.

By the time eighth grade started she argued that she no longer needed special education pullout services and would rather stay in the room with her friends. A conference including Mrs. Cane, the special ed resource teacher, Debbie's mother, Debbie, and Roger was held in which it was decided that Debbie could stay full-time with her peers. However, she agreed that if she felt the need for additional help she could always count on Mrs. Cane's assistance.

It is important to mention that Debbie had a condition in which fatty tumors grew on her brain stem and had to be surgically removed from time to time. One of her surgeries occurred during her eighth-grade year. At the end of the year a schoolwide project requiring all eighth-grade students to write an autobiography was announced, and in the end, Debbie produced a twenty-one-page

typewritten document that spoke of her illness, her surgeries, and her prognosis. She even included a medical glossary at the end so readers would know what words like *brain, surgery, hospital,* and *tumor* meant. Debbie became an author. Her writing was maturing. She was developing voice.

Debbie graduated eighth grade and went on to high school. In her third year in high school she shared an essay with Roger that her junior-year English teacher entered in a contest. Debbie won second prize for her essay entitled "The Incredible Mr. Passman." It opened this way:

> Do you think that reading and writing are dull? Boring? A waste of your good time and effort? I am here to tell you that you are wrong! You see, I used to think this myself but then I met the incredible Mr. Passman.

Her piece went on to describe how patience and letting her find her own way had been the key factor in her learning to write. In the end, she vowed never to let any disability stand in her way.

Debbie is not an exceptional case. We have had many exceptional children in our classrooms during our years of teaching. We made the choice to learn to work with rather than complain about the students we taught. Debbie was, however, a primary inspiration in the development of the TIP Writing Process.

A Word About Our Goals

Just because students have a disability does not mean we can ignore their needs. No, we were never trained as special education teachers, but we were *educated to be teachers.* Our obligation as teachers is to reach out to every child in the classroom, to find ways to approach every child in order to affect that child's perception of self. We could no more ignore Jamie's needs than we could dismiss Jane's isolation or Debbie's learning-disabled label. To have done so would have been to "other"—to marginalize students in order to somehow fix them, to make them *normal.*

We reject "othering" and marginalization. We support differentiated instruction that is inclusive of the needs and interests of all students in the classroom, although we affirm that their needs and interests must be focused in a larger notion of curriculum and standards. We like to think of teaching as building a "curriculum box" that defines the parameters for classroom inquiry, providing students with the needed tools and strategies to wander through it in both a rigorous and focused manner.

This book is about individualizing writing instruction and how through the very act of doing so, a teacher can find accommodations for every student in the classroom. It is about helping to provide students with the tools and strategies they need to become authentic writers while drawing on their needs and interests for learning.

The TIP Writing Process is inclusive; it is designed to embrace everyone. The great paradox is that while focusing on individualizing the delivery of instruction for students, we are, in fact, building effective learning communities where all learning styles and differences are honored by all participants. In sum, *we teach the students who are placed in front of us—not those we wish were in front of us.*

It Ain't All Theory—But a Little Bit Helps

This book is about authentic writing in all classrooms with all children. Teaching authentic writing is, to a large extent, about helping students develop strategies to find their own voice. But first, in the next few paragraphs, we concentrate on some theoretical background to help teachers think about the foundations of writing.

Let us begin by stating unequivocally that we believe sound practice rests on a bedrock of sound theoretical understanding. There is an old country song entitled "If You Don't Stand for Something, You'll Fall for Anything." Although the cynical interpretation of the title suggests notions of unquestioned loyalty, a concept we reject, there is something to the idea that knowledgeable and informed opinion is a shield against unwarranted imposition of external solutions to internal problems. Indeed, a baseline knowledge is required in order for teachers to claim the title of professional. Without the theoretical underpinnings that make our practice transparent we are highly susceptible to the *fix de jour* that promises instant success in the classroom, often without credible evidence to support its claims. Without a strong foundation in theoretical constructions one can never be completely sure of one's practice in the classroom. This is especially true when teaching writing. It is important to understand both the historical and theoretical posturing that permeates the field.

We break down our exploration of theoretical and historical contexts by looking first at *product approaches* to writing. Next we explore *process approaches,* including linear process models. Finally, we look at workshop models. We argue that neither product, process, nor workshop models fully explain either how writers work or how teachers can best teach writing in the classroom. Our solution to the problem is the *balanced approach* that we call TIP. Blending both workshop and direct teaching approaches, TIP emphasizes the development of authentic approaches to writing.

Product Approaches: Understanding Writing As a Sum of Its Parts

Product approaches to teaching writing take two principal forms: development of *mechanical skills,* such as competence in spelling, punctuation, and grammar, and development of competence in the use of appropriate *rhetorical formulas* in order to narrate, compare, and contrast, argue persuasively, and closely describe a process, among others. Although there is much overlap between the

two forms it is easiest to think of them as separate entities. Both have to do with dividing the writing task into constituent parts, teaching those parts, and then expecting students to be able to write effectively when asked to. We believe that product approaches generally ignore the creative aspects of writing, the aspects that help students identify the task of writing itself as important and authentic, precisely because they concentrate on the parts rather than identifying the whole. In addition, we argue that product approaches leave the writer frustrated and often without the tools needed to develop a clear and personally identifiable voice.

Skills Approaches

As noted, skills approaches to writing concentrate on issues of form and mechanics, such as spelling and grammar. Teaching skills is not a trivial matter. In order to develop coherent internal arguments so that their writing confidently represents their thinking process, students must have a grounding in and competence with the appropriate mechanical tools. They must have a sense of how to correctly identify problems and issues and find appropriate and warranted solutions to the problems being posed in order to construct meaning through the act of writing. Furthermore, in order to fulfill the secondary purpose of writing—to communicate effectively—students must know how to organize their writing in a coherent and sequenced manner, form sentences, and punctuate those sentences for maximum effectiveness. They also need to correctly spell words on the page. But students do not seem to profit from *skilling drills,* designed to make the skills of writing second nature and fully transferable to the composition process. Hillocks (1986), for example, demonstrated that the pure teaching of grammar does not have a significant impact on student writing quality or production.

Indeed, it appears that, counter to common wisdom, teaching skills does not significantly enhance student appreciation of writing at any level. Often the skills approach is designed to "fix" that which is wrong in student writing. Perl (1979) points out that with novice writers the skills approach tends to cut off any creativity and dampen enthusiasm for continuing to write.

The skills approach manifests itself in the English language arts classroom in two ways. The first are the previously mentioned worksheets in which students must complete dry and uninspiring exercises designed to drill specific skills into their heads. While easy to grade, these worksheets have a destructive impact on student engagement with and joy in the writing process. The red pencil marks on a piece of student writing that purport to point out the error of students' ways are a second example of the skills approach. Both forms are devastating to students identifying themselves as writers. Both tend to discourage students from developing writing competency. It is problematic that both approaches remain prevalent in K–12 classrooms to this day.

Rhetorical Approaches

Since the late 1970s much discussion of writing process has filled the pages of books and journals devoted to literacy. Although this discussion has had some impact on how writing is taught, it has not dramatically changed what occurs in

the classroom. One change has been to add a discourse about rhetorical form to the overall discourse about writing in K–12 classrooms. But the discussion of rhetorical forms remains a skills-based argument that is superimposed on a discussion of process writing in the classroom.

The most popular form of the rhetorical approach is the ubiquitous five-paragraph essay or some iteration of it, such as the "hamburger model." Using this ever-popular structure, writers craft a first paragraph in which they introduce the topic of the essay in the first sentence—the topic sentence—write three additional sentences addressing the main points of the essay, and finally, write a last sentence summarizing the points made and transitioning to the next paragraph. They then compose an introductory sentence in each of the next three paragraphs closely resembling the main points of the first paragraph. Then they write three sentences supporting the main points in each paragraph. Finally, each paragraph receives a summary and transition sentence to the next paragraph. The fifth paragraph is essentially a summation of the arguments made in the first four paragraphs. The first sentence is written to emphasize the main point. The next three sentences summarize the main arguments of the paper. And the final sentence summarizes and concludes the essay. (The hamburger visually represents the five-paragraph essay. The top and bottom halves of the bun represent the opening and closing paragraphs, while the lettuce, onion, and meat represent the three internal paragraphs.) Note that each paragraph is designed to be a mini essay, each consisting of five sentences.

The five-paragraph essay has even found its way into narrative text, when writers are told to write an introduction, tell what happened next, then next, and then next, and finally tell the reader what happened last, bringing the story to a nice, neat conclusion.

Yet although the five-paragraph essay is taught as an appropriate rhetorical form in American schools, nowhere can one find examples of such essays in the real world. Real writers do not write that way. The five-paragraph essay, then, cannot be understood as *authentic* simply because it offers no value to a student beyond the four walls of the classroom. We believe that teaching the five-paragraph essay form is an immoral and unethical use of adult power in the school building and must be abandoned to permit teachers to engage students in the real work that writers actually do.

We are not saying that rhetorical problems do not have prototypical forms attached to them. In fact, the purpose of rhetorical forms is both to internalize and to focus the writing process on the organization of the thinking process as well as make the product of the writing process meaningful to the unknown reader. Without form, a piece of writing may not communicate anything either to the author engaged in the process of constructing meaning through writing or to the reader engaged in the process of constructing meaning through transactions with the text produced by the author. Instead, we find fault with the notion that rhetorical form can be reduced to formula without extinguishing the underlying internal thinking and external communicative goal of writing—to come to know and to potentially communicate meaning and vision to a reader.

Process Approaches: Movement Toward Authenticity

Writing is a messy, recursive process. It turns in on itself, imposing composing, revising, editing, and audience concerns on the writer at every step. Authors who take the process approach include Flower and Hayes, and Murray.

In an early description, Flower and Hayes (1997) proposed a cognitive process theory of writing that includes three main points:

1. The writing process—which includes prewriting, drafting, revising, editing, and publishing—is a recursive process and a unique thinking process.
2. Writing is developmental. Students acquire skills and experiences that develop writing ability.
3. Once students develop confidence, or voice, in their writing, they are able to develop a sense of authorship. In other words, they see themselves as writers.

Flower and Hayes (1997) refer to the act of composing as *translating* because it engages so many processes at once—from spelling and grammatical issues, to structural issues, to the physical act of creating letters and words, to the more sophisticated levels of composing such as creative solutions to rhetorical problems. The more automatic the mechanical processes of writing become, the better able the writer is to engage in creative thinking and writing. Finally, they argue that the writer alone sets rhetorical goals in the process of writing.

Murray (1997) makes a distinction between formal training and experiential knowledge in writing. He comes down on the side of experience, arguing that formal critical training in writing is not relevant to the teaching of writing. In Murray's view, all writing is experimental. The writer, Murray argues, "doesn't test his words by a rule book, but by life. He uses language to reveal the truth to himself so he can tell it to others. It is an exciting, eventful, evolving process" (1997, p. 4). Murray proposes that as soon as a teacher has a basic understanding of the writing process and feels comfortable with the basic implications of teaching that process, she or he should start teaching process writing to students. He supports the notion of knowledge-in-action (Ryle, 1949; Schön, 1982) by debunking the idea that in order to teach writing effectively a great deal of expertise is required.

For Murray, writing begins with a community of learners in the classroom supported by a caring teacher in which every member is in a position of learning and teaching through doing. According to Murray, the writing process consists of three stages:

Prewriting: Everything before the first draft (thinking)
Writing: The first draft (draft writing, including revision)
Rewriting: Reconsideration of subject, form, and audience (discourse-rhetoric, including editing and publishing)

Teaching Writing in the Inclusive Classroom

In the next sections, we will take a look at two process approaches for teaching writing: the linear model and the workshop model.

The Linear Model

The linear model divides the writing process into four or five parts. The main parts are *prewriting, first draft writing, peer editing or conferencing, revising,* and often *publishing or sharing.* This model is quite elegant in the sense that it divides the process into segments that may be practiced in successive daily lessons. Monday is devoted to prewriting, while Tuesday is set aside for first draft writing, and so on. However, the problem with this model is that it does not represent the way in which writers actually work. Murray (1991, 1997), in contrast, describes the writing process as one that begins in fits and starts and is recursive, folding in on itself before the writer can begin to think of finishing. It is not a five-day process that fits neatly into the school calendar. It is unrealistic to demand one finished essay per week without undermining the authentic process in which writers are engaged.

The Workshop Model

Originally made popular by Calkins (1994), and later, specifically in the middle schools by Atwell (1987), the workshop model recognizes the underlying recursive nature of the writing process by acknowledging that students may not be at the same place at the same time on any given piece of writing. The workshop model rests on the idea that writing is highly personal, requires doing rather than talking about it, and in the end, students will find all of the mechanical aspects of writing they need for producing appropriate pieces, writing that mirrors their thinking processes as they develop a working sense of authorship and voice.

Our main argument against using the workshop model exclusively is that it fails to address authentic notions of academic rigor, mainly because rhetorical choices are left entirely up to the student. Although we agree that rhetorical goals should be set by the writer (Flower & Hayes, 1997) and that effective writing tends to be a messy, recursive practice (Murray, 1997), we also believe that writing instruction must be both balanced and authentic for students to find voice and a sense of authorship. In short, effective writing instruction must include aspects of process, product, and workshop models if students are to profit from the experience.

The TIP Writing Process: A Balanced, Authentic Approach

The TIP Writing Process balances the needs of writers by addressing writing as an authentic classroom activity. As noted earlier, TIP is an acronym:

- *Teach* appropriate rhetorical strategies while modeling rhetorical problems. Full-blown strategy lessons are included in Chapter Two of this book.
- *Introduce* skills and mechanics through mini lessons and conferences without assessing these skills or mechanics. Cleaning up and correcting mechanics are left for the final draft. During conferences—meetings between teacher and one to three students to discuss the students' writing—the teacher may suggest strategies or teach a relevant writing skill. Students may also have peer conferences, in which they discuss each other's writing; we have witnessed students sharing their writing skills and strategies.
- *Practice, practice, practice.* Provide frequent and sustained practice both in and outside of the classroom.

During each phase of the TIP Writing Process students are exposed to authentic writing activities that, in turn, lead to significant success in writing (Passman, 2001, 2003, 2004).

Authenticity and Effective Practice

So far we have frequently used the term *authentic.* We think it is about time we defined it so that what we are talking about becomes clear. In brief, teaching authentic writing means developing the students' voice as authors and preparing them to risk extraordinarily personal insights with potential strangers.

We understand authenticity or authentic teaching and learning from two perspectives. The first perspective is based on the work of Newmann and his colleagues (Newmann, Byrk, & Nagaoka, 2001; Newmann, Marks, & Gamoran, 1995a; Newmann, Secada, & Wehlage, 1995b; Newmann & Wehlage, 1993). They define authenticity or authentic practice as a three-part whole:

1. Assignments and assessments must have value for the student beyond the classroom.
2. Assignments and assessments must be academically rigorous or challenging.
3. All work produced must have an audience beyond the teacher.

Pure workshop approaches satisfy Points 1 and 3 but fail at Point 2 because students make all assignment decisions. Product models fulfill Point 2 but fail to fulfill Points 1 and 3. Process models generally fit into the same rubric as workshop models. By adding the notion of academic rigor to the mix in writing pedagogy as well as making up for the shortcomings of Points 1 and 3 in the process or workshop models, the TIP Writing Process balances the need to focus on the writing process while also developing skills.

Flow and Optimal Experience

Closely related to Newmann's concept of authenticity is Csikszentmihalyi's (1990) notion of *flow*. *Flow* is an integrated system including seven key components that make up an optimal experience. An *optimal experience* can be understood as something like a Zen moment, being in "the zone," or simply being fully and authentically connected to an activity or enterprise. *Flow* contains the following components:

1. Activities must be challenging and require skills.
2. Activities must merge action and awareness.
3. Activities must provide clear goals and immediate feedback.
4. When engaged in optimal activities one must concentrate on the task at hand.
5. Optimal activities present the engaged participant with a paradox of control.
6. Participants in optimal activities experience a loss of self-consciousness.
7. Participants in optimal activities experience a transformation of time.

Looking at both the Newmann and Csikszentmihalyi constructions, what becomes clear is that an engaged student is more likely to perform well in school than one who is not engaged. While this may appear too obvious to commit to paper, it is our experience that students are not so engaged in the great majority of schools across the country.

We want to elaborate on both perspectives and then discuss how they merge into a unified system for engaging students in writing activities that, in turn, can have a significant impact on all other school activities and interests. In the Newmann (Newmann et al., 2001; Newmann et al., 1995a; Newmann et al., 1995b; Newmann & Wehlage, 1993) perspective, which we will call the *pedagogical model of authenticity*, the emphasis is on how teachers design activities for student engagement. Teachers have the responsibility to develop lessons that are meaningful to students on many levels. Teachers cannot rely on worksheets or mindless, dronelike activities to occupy students' time. By creating lessons that are academically rigorous, teachers challenge their students to perform beyond even their wildest dreams. Academic rigor is all about teacher expectations. Finally, teachers are responsible for finding and developing an audience beyond themselves. The audience becomes the capstone of authentic pedagogy in the sense that it shifts responsibility for performance in the student's mind. Performing for the teacher alone allows students to play the "real school" (Metz, 1990) guessing game of how to please (or distract) their teacher. By removing the teacher from the mix—although never entirely—students become aware of their responsibility to communicate their ideas to a broad audience, one they cannot simply outsmart.

In the flow concept (Csikszentmihalyi, 1990), in contrast, the emphasis is placed on the engaged performer rather than on the teacher. In order to engage

the participant in optimal performance the activity must provide a challenge to the participant. If there is no challenge, whether that challenge is competitive—as in a game—or intellectually stimulating, the experience itself will feel like drudgery. While engaged in optimal activity, participants tend to merge action and awareness in the sense that their actions become more or less automatic. But this does not occur overnight. Participants engaged in optimal activities go up a learning curve in which the skills of the activity are internalized over time. As less active memory is devoted to the skills aspects of the optimal activity, memory is available for creative solutions to externally presented problems. In short, as processes become automatic, awareness of the experience becomes optimized. In flow, participants must have clear goals and receive immediate, or nearly immediate, feedback. In early learning stages feedback is important to help participants develop an automatic response to routine events. As expertise is developed, however, feedback affects the meaning of participation, providing pleasure for the participant, perhaps for a job well done. If given feedback and goals, participants are more likely to concentrate on the task at hand in order to achieve what might be called *clarity*.

So far, the idea of flow is pretty straightforward. The next three aspects of it help participants reach truly optimal experiences. Optimal activities present engaged participants with the *paradox of control*—that is, they feel totally in control of their efforts and the external aspects to which they direct their efforts. Feelings of ease and enjoyment characterize this level of participation. While they feel like they own the world, the paradox is that they only really control their own efforts. Participants experience a loss of self-consciousness while engaged in optimal experiences. They are so fully engrossed in doing what they are doing simply for the sake of doing it that they have no time to be self-conscious. Finally, participants reaching flow find time transformed. Participation is not dependent on clock time; rather, pace is established as a by-product of intense concentration.

By combining the notions of the pedagogical model of authenticity and flow we are able to create a model of authenticity that addresses both teachers and students and their roles in authentic engagement. When teachers design their lessons using guidelines established by the pedagogical model of authenticity they generate a context for learning that leads their students into optimal experience or flow. Students engaged in optimal experience, in turn, demand from their teachers a context that is engaging.

What We Believe About Writing

But enough of theories. Our goal in this book is to provide practical and useful strategies to help teachers develop strong classroom practice in teaching writing to help students develop voice. As we move away from theory, it is important to clarify the lens we look through. Writing is relatively easy—good writing is very difficult. Writing is a learned language process, similar to reading and repre-

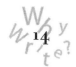

senting. Writing engages the author in tasks that appear on the surface to resemble speaking, or oral language, but that is not the case. Spoken and written languages have things in common, to be sure, but they do not represent the same cognitive process. In this section of the chapter we address what we believe to be true about writing and how these ideas have shaped our view of writing instruction in all classrooms.

What Writing Is Not

First let's take a look at what writing is not.

Isolated Skills Developed Through Drill-and-Kill Worksheets

Ask most students what they think about writing and they are apt to respond, "Writing is boring, a waste of time." Roger notes that when he first heard students refer to writing as boring he was scandalized to think that they did not hold the act of placing pen to paper with proper respect. But the fact is that students who are taught to write from a set of mechanical and rhetorical rules find the process difficult and unmanageable. When worksheets and isolated skills are emphasized in the classroom students cannot embrace writing as anything but difficult and meaningless, and hence, boring.

A Set of Mindless Writing Exercises

Like drill-and-kill worksheets, mindless writing exercises have no place in the writing classroom. Asking students to write about "what I did last summer" is neither inspiring nor meaningful to either them or their teachers. You know the topics we are referring to: "My Best Friend," "My Hero," "My Trip to the Zoo" (or the museum, farm, hospital, Los Angeles, and so forth). These topics do little to inspire students and make for horrendous reading by their teachers. How many nights do you want to sit up reading dull papers that result from dull, mindless writing activities?

All About Assessment

The testing movement has it all wrong (Kohn, 1999). Writing can be and is always assessed by an audience of readers. But the preposterous notion that forcing a student to write to a mindless—oops, there we go again—writing prompt that derives from some state committee's writing question for an assessment exam is foolhardy and disadvantageous to the practice of good writing instruction. Writing tests lead to the preceding two evils of writing instruction and force good teachers to engage in the classroom pedagogical iniquity that fails to engage students in any authentic manner: the teaching of writing formulas.

All About Rhetorical Formulas

Many writing formulas are bantered about classrooms. There is the base formula for the five-paragraph essay—introduction, detail, detail, detail, and conclusion—and its many adaptations. One that we've already discussed is the hamburger

model. Power writing and others are designed to engage students in formulaic approaches to the writing task. The problem with all of these formulas is that they remove the creativity from the writing process, leaving only the rhetorical form.

Other formulas have streamlined the writing process—which, as already noted, researchers in writing generally agree is a messy and recursive process—into a linear approach. Yet, the writing process is neither linear nor timely. It is difficult, creative, recursive, and subject to fits and starts with drafting overlapping revision, and prewriting interfering with completion.

What Writing Is

The preceding paragraphs explained all the things that writing *is not*. We may sound petulant but we believe it is important to emphasize that good teaching of writing includes none of these elements. Quite the contrary, writing is first about making thinking visible and then, and only then, about communication with a broader audience. Just an aside: it is conceivable that the audience may consist of only the author and no one else, especially if the writing represents initial efforts at solving a problem. This section will deal with all of the things that writing *is*.

Related to the Other Language Arts

Six processes are often considered to be connected in the English language arts: listening, speaking, reading, writing, and more recently, observing and representing (see Figure 1.2).

These skills are paired into innate and learned phases. For example, listening, the innate skill, is paired with reading, the learned skill, because both require the recipient to process the words of others in order to make meaning. Speak-

Figure 1.2. The English Language Arts.

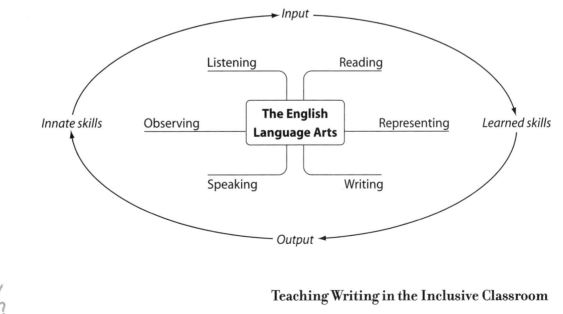

Teaching Writing in the Inclusive Classroom

ing and writing are paired in much the same way because both require the production of language for the communicative benefit of others. Finally, observing and representing employ the ability to see and reproduce the world in graphic or visual terms. Each skill is related to its counterpart as well as to all the other skills attributed to language production and reception, but none is quite the same as another and especially not the same as its immediate counterpart.

In the case of writing, we can safely say that it is not spoken language transferred to print. Different rules apply to spoken English and written English. Vocabulary differs in spoken and written English. Grammar, in the form of the mechanics of punctuation, only applies to written language. This is not to say that syntactical and grammatical relationships do not apply to spoken language—but the rules are different. Oral language, for example, is structured in phrases that, when combined, form coherent thoughts. In contrast, written language relies on sentence structure and paragraph structure for conveying meaning. Oral language uses punctuation in the form of such words as *like, um, uh, y'know,* and *sort of,* as some prime examples. Speakers often punctuate thoughts with these or other apparently useless words. In contrast, writers must monitor punctuation in the form of periods, commas, semicolons and colons, question and exclamation marks, quotation marks, and so on in order to help readers make sense of what they are reading. Thus, there are punctuation rules in both spoken and written English, but they are different. Many teachers tell their students to "write it just like you say it" as they try to help struggling writers through a difficult passage in their writing. The problem is that this does not work very well. If students follow this advice, the only punctuation mark they'd include might be the word *and.* We are sure you have seen papers like this one (you may have even written some along the way):

> First I woke up and then I went to the bathroom to brush my teeth and then I had breakfast and then I met Billy and we went out to play and we played baseball and I hit a home run and then we went to the park to swing and I went home and I ate dinner and I went to bed. The End

Now, it seems that the author of this piece was writing exactly the way he spoke. While this is an uninspired piece, think about how much better it would read if the "ands" were eliminated in favor of periods and some capitalization. But such language is perfectly acceptable in spoken English, because "and" serves as a punctuation marker separating complete thoughts.

One of us actually learned this lesson the hard way. When Roger decided to purchase a voice-activated software package designed to help write long papers, what he found was that, in trying to vocalize what really is a different thinking process, his papers were no better, certainly no easier to write, and in many ways, worse. Rather than correcting the problem, the software exacerbated it.

Janet Emig (1977) argued that writing is a unique way of thinking. One key feature of Emig's argument is that writing is far more responsible than speaking. The mere fact that the author of a written piece does not have to let anyone see

it until he or she is completely satisfied with it makes it very different from speech. Once uttered, spoken words cannot be taken back. Neither can writing be retrieved, but the author has the luxury of not making public his or her every thought. In this sense writing is a responsible form of communication, further differentiating it from speaking.

A Solitary Social Activity

No, this is not an oxymoron! Writers need solitary time to think, to read, and to write. This is time without interruption, solitary time in which they are engaged with themselves in creative production. Writers crave isolation. They need frequent and sustained periods of time to plan, think, and create. No telephones, radios, or television sets to distract. Writing is done in solitary conditions.

But isolation is only appropriate for the thinking and drafting stages of writing. Once satisfactorily drafted, writers need an audience with whom to bounce ideas around. Editors who help writers identify what they really want to say to others are an integral part of the social function of the writing activity. Revision and editing are not solitary events. Quite the contrary, as ideas are forming the writer requires the social interplay of another voice, sometimes as a guide, often as a critic, in order to polish the work into something publishable.

And then there is the audience, the readers of the piece, those with whom the author is communicating once it is clear that the act of writing has come to an end. Without the social construction of the audience there would be fewer reasons to write anything at all, ever. Beyond the process of thinking through a problem, of coming to know what one thinks, of making one's thoughts visible— all good reasons in themselves for taking pencil to paper—why write if no one will read what you have written, challenge your thinking, and perhaps benefit from your thinking process?

An Effort in the Context of Fun

Remember *flow!* A few years ago Roger was working with teachers in West Texas on developing authentic writing practice in K–12 classrooms. He was returning to a small rural school in Heavenly, Texas (again, place name is pseudonymous), that he had visited two times before. It was a sultry mid-April morning. The sun was just over the horizon, the temperature already nearly 90 degrees, and there was not a cloud in the sky. As he approached the front entrance to the school two sixth-grade boys were sitting on the stairs. One turned to the other and exclaimed, "Oh, here comes the guy that makes writin' fun!!!" Both boys rose to greet him, and as one held open the door, he asked, "Are y'all comin' to our class today?" He could not contain the excitement in his voice. Now, who ever can recall a student that excited about writing?

The simple truth is that Roger had engaged these two boys in the act of writing—he had made writing fun. This does not mean that he presented the "lite" version of writing to the students. Quite the contrary, he established high expectations and demanded rigorous adherence to those expectations. Good writing is difficult, and difficult tasks are satisfying.

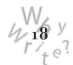

Teaching Writing in the Inclusive Classroom

Flow teaches us that optimal experiences are ones that embody both goals and skills. Flow also instructs us that skills are not developed overnight. Writing begins by thinking through ideas and then communicating constructed ideas to an audience. The act of writing becomes fun when it becomes clear that one is actually thinking responsibly and has something to say and it is important to communicate those ideas to an audience. Skills, in turn, become important when an author feels the need to communicate his or her thinking to an audience.

Something That Can Be Taught

Finally, we believe that writing can be taught. The TIP Writing Process is a way to engage students in authentic activities that lead to their experience of flow. The process is interrelated. It depends on caring teachers engaging students in activities of worth. It depends on teachers focused on high expectations, demanding more than their students ever thought themselves capable of achieving. Teaching writing is an enterprise that encourages and emancipates; it empowers students with language and voice and expression.

The TIP Weekly Schedule

Table 1.1 shows a typical week's writing schedule using the TIP approach.

Table 1.1. Typical TIP Schedule.

Monday	Teach strategy.
Tuesday	Practice writing.
Wednesday	Introduce skills, generally through mini lessons.
Thursday	Reteach strategy.
Friday	Practice writing.

A Few Words About Standards

Our position on standards in American education is simple and complex. In an ideal world where every teacher is well prepared, participates willingly in meaningful professional development, and practices engaging pedagogy with students who come to school ready and willing to engage in school-based teaching and learning, there would be no need to have a professional conversation about standards in education. In the practical world, however, that conversation is unavoidable.

As we begin our discussion of standards we follow Applebee's (1996) position that standards, in order to contribute meaningfully to any discourse on teaching and learning, must serve as the beginning of a professional conversation about the curriculum rather than define the curriculum itself. In other

words, conversations about what is important to teach and learn should be broad-based and then contextualized to meet the needs, both practical and political, of local school settings. We develop our position in the next paragraphs.

Our goal is not to thoroughly explore each aspect of thought that goes into our position, but rather to succinctly clarify how we understand the place of standards in American education.

The Principled Argument

Stanley Fish (1999) asserts that arguments made from principle are doomed to fail primarily because they are forced to compromise on all points. This compromise leads to a blurring of boundaries and a denial of what Derrida (1999, 2002) has referred to as *vision* or *horizon,* a concept closely allied to notion of grounded selfhood. A clear example of what Fish is talking about may be seen in the Illinois State Board of Education document justifying standards in Illinois (*Illinois Learning Standards,* 1997):

> Maintaining high expectations for all students is a component of fairness in education. *All students* include those who choose college and those who choose more technical career preparation directly from high school; those for whom English is a second language; those with learning disabilities and those who are gifted and talented; those who are returning to education for completion of a diploma, even as adults; and those from advantaged and disadvantaged socioeconomic backgrounds.
>
> For most special needs students, their Individualized Educational Programs (IEPs) will be linked to the standards, with accommodations and individualized approaches to the depth and timetables for achievement. For individuals with severe disabilities, few of these standards may apply in terms of achievement.
>
> While the task of helping virtually all students achieve the standards may seem daunting, the alternative is not acceptable. Different expectations for different groups of students lead students to demand less of themselves—and unfortunately allow them to deliver on these lower expectations.

The clear principle embodied in this justification statement for the Illinois standards is that by setting high standards for all and making those standards readily available for all to see, all students, as well as their parents and their teachers, will know exactly what is expected of them. The clear implication is that students will, in turn, achieve at the same high level of performance no matter what their circumstance as they approach school and schooling. By lumping together the college bound with those bound for a technical career and those with learning disabilities and those gifted and talented as well, the absurdity of the principled argument becomes clear on its face. To lump together polar opposites one must deny real differences that exist, differences that arise from race, class, gender, culture, historical accidents, and so on.

This folly is further heightened by the statistical barrier of the norm or mean, the fiftieth percentile, which half of any given population must exceed while the other half must fall below. This is simply a mathematical certainty. We like to think of this approach as the Lake Wobegon paradox. It is statistically impossible for all the men to be strong, all the women good-looking, and all the children above average. No matter how hard we wish it to be, no place like Lake Wobegon can, does, or even should exist. The weak disclaimer at the end of the Illinois statement, which appears to recognize the difficulty of its position by asserting that "a daunting task" has been placed before us, is not enough to overcome the flawed approach taken in the first place; it is not enough to sweep away the differences that arise because of race, class, culture, or historical circumstance.

The argument made by the state of Illinois is, at its core, assimilative and fictive in the sense that it is designed to preserve a nonexistent world. It seeks to dismiss difference in favor of a monistic view of society and culture. Thus, standards tend to sweep differences under the rug where they are covered up and out of the way. There is no room in this discourse for acculturation, for incorporating diverse elements into an amalgam of cultures that is inclusive and exclusive at the same time.

Barbara Tuchman (1978) pointed out that the knights and bishops of the mid- to late 1300s were unable to get past their traditional roles in a changing society. "Chivalry was not aware of its decadence, or if it was, clung ever more passionately to outward forms and brilliant rites to convince itself that the fiction was still the reality" (p. 438). By hanging on to what was already lost, the nobles and clergy of Europe set out to standardize cultural awareness as a preserving, conservative force. It had the opposite effect, giving rise to the middle class and the ultimate demise of the feudal system. It can be argued that the standards movement, in all its pomp and glory, calling for ever more detailed levels of accountability, is the chivalry of the late twentieth and early twenty-first centuries. It is hanging on to what is already lost, or perhaps, never really existed in the first place, in the false hope that past perceived glory will somehow be retrieved and the world will once again be set right.

The Assimilationist Stance

Tuchman's distant mirror seems to be clearly reflecting our own times. To be sure, there is a movement to return to the "good old days" in schooling as in many other walks of life. Across college campuses today culturally conservative faculty bemoan the fact that students simply do not read the way they used to or ought to (Bloom, 1987) or that youth cultures disallow the very forces of liberal education by disrupting commonly accepted cultural practices of decency and morality (D'Souza, 1991). Still others claim to have the functional answer to the problem of cultural decadence. The only way to be culturally literate, E. D. Hirsch (1987) claims, is to remain true to a Western canon that defines what it

means to be civilized. Harold Bloom (1987) and Dinish D'Souza (1991) also claim that the abandonment of the Western canon to multicultural influences lowers the intellectual response of students to academic problems and opportunities, forcing a disintegration of what is otherwise known as civilization.

The problem, as we see it, is that standards in the sense imposed by Bloom, Hirsch, and D'Souza also focus on assimilation as a way to preserve a fictional past. These authors, as well as others of a similar outlook (for example, see Ravitch & Finn, 1987; Schlesinger, 1998), argue that it is paramount that schools teach a single American culture to diverse bodies of students. These "cultural literacists" subsume all contributing forces into a single, monistic, monolithic American cultural reality. Much like the proponents of principled positions, the cultural literacists deny differences in race, culture, class, and gender while creating fictions about what is and is not American.

In this case, however, the denial does not result merely from a principled stance. For the cultural literacists, the problem is much deeper. It is, in fact, a denial embedded deeply in the task of sorting that accompanies the privileging of one set of values over all others. Cultural literacy proponents define who does and does not belong in their fictive American narrative. Cultural literacy presents us with standards that co-opt alternative narratives, sort by class, culture, and race and otherwise separate performance into "acceptable" and "unacceptable" categories. In order to belong, to be culturally literate, one must deny one's own cultural horizons. Those who do not choose to take this stance are relegated to a position of perpetual outsider. In a pluralistic democratic society we find this stance deplorable.

A Simple Fact: Too Many Standards

Marzano and Kendall (1998) examined the standards guidelines prepared by all of the organizations that represent the various content areas of education nationally. Groups writing standards included organizations such as the National Council of Teachers of English/International Reading Association acting in tandem, the National Council for the Social Studies/American Historical Association also acting in tandem, the National Council of Teachers of Mathematics, the National Science Teachers Association, and many others. The authors simply counted the number of standards, their associated benchmarks and outcomes, and then, through a reasonably simple calculation, determined that a child who entered school and was taught all of the extant standards would have to remain there from kindergarten through grade 22 to complete all of the work demanded by the standards writers.

Marzano and Kendall (1998) present arguments that speak to the pollution of the standards movement by bureaucratic tendencies to overanalyze and micromanage just about anything. Their point is that the micromanagement of standards places impossible burdens on teachers and students, burdens that tend to deny access to well over 40 percent of this nation's school-age children because

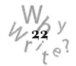

of the emphasis on assimilation through the narratives of dead white men. We believe that the tendency to micromanage removes standards from active discussion by setting the curriculum in stone so that it is perceived merely as a strategy for teachers to implement rather than allowing for meaningful and productive discourse about the process of teaching and learning.

Acculturation Instead of Assimilation

Thus far, this discussion has focused on notions of assimilation rather than acculturation. As noted, Derrida (1999, 2002) speaks of horizon, or vision, as a foundational element of identity. The idea of horizon is fixed in cultural identity and can only be maintained through an acute sense of cultural awareness. The failure to directly relate to one's horizon because of imposed reconfiguration of vision intended to assimilate marginalized cultures into a dominant cultural entity have been seen as disruptive to foundational social organization (Street, 1995).

Street (1995) argues that the imposition of one group's culture on another has a significant impact on language and language usage when the dominant language is imposed either through conquest or colonization. Street maintains that before a redefinition of balance in social relationships is accomplished, a time frame measured in centuries is appropriate, not months or years.

DuBois ([1903]1989) explains this phenomenon in terms of the worlds within and without the veil: one world accommodates the dominant cultural influence while the other remains culturally coherent by retaining all that is meaningful for survival. The notion of observing the world through twin lenses and being able to switch between worlds for purposes of survival is critical for DuBois.

Brodkin (1998) tells a different tale. In her insightful work *How Jews Become White Folks & What That Says About Race in America,* she outlines a history of the failure of assimilation and a renewed focus on acculturation as a means of retaining cultural identity in the face of ever increasing loss of horizon. In Brodkin's narrative the drive toward assimilation was fueled by the desire to become one with the new land, a place where *pogroms* and violent discrimination were things of the past. In becoming white folks, or Americans, Brodkin argues, Jews lost what made them distinct, they lost horizon or vision. In third- and fourth-generation American Jewish families today there is a movement to reclaim that lost vision by reaffirming some distinctiveness while remaining Americans. Jews, Brodkin argues, have largely rejected assimilation in recent years in favor of acculturation without rejecting what makes them Americans.

That is how acculturation works. Vision and horizon are maintained while shared cultural values are balanced within the vision created by diverse cultural affiliation. Race, gender, class, and culture are not denied but rather celebrated. One group finds no need to dominate another. Quite the contrary, through the component pieces constructed of diverse interests and ideas whole-cloth societies are built. We might add that none of this occurs without meaningful discourse about what counts among shared and sharing communities.

A Place for Standards

And so we return to the beginning. We believe that standards in education serve an important, albeit limited, function. Standards must be painted in broad-brush strokes, stating what might generally be important in developing a curriculum. In this role, standards become conversation-starters. Educators at all levels can—indeed must—find some common ground on which to develop conversations about the curriculum. We emphasize that these conversations should be local and contextualized, deeply embedded in the community served by the school. Issues of race, gender, culture, class, and so on must be a part of this ongoing conversation—they must be made a part of the conversation and not kept separate from any meaningful discussion.

Unfortunately, standards have become something else. Bureaucratic pressures have intervened to create volumes of micromanaged approaches to educational standards. Standards are developed nationally by content area governing bodies and by most state boards of education too, and many large local districts have developed their own, competing standards documents as well. Some states, like Texas, have chosen to codify educational standards as a matter of state law; others, such as Illinois, have made standards a function of administrative regulation. In some extreme cases, boards of education have or are in the process of adopting scripted lessons for all subjects in all grades. In all cases, however, standards are dissected into smaller units called *benchmarks* and then again into even smaller units called *objectives*. With this kind of curriculum management, professionals are not given reasonable options for developing local responses to the larger question of what needs to be taught.

Yet all children are not cut out of the same cloth. We strongly believe that standardization, although fine for interchangeable parts in automobiles produced on assembly lines, is inappropriate for education. Our position on standards, then, is to pay close attention to professionally adopted broad statements about teaching and learning in order to stimulate meaningful, authentic dialogue about how best to achieve the larger goals without giving up cultural vision or horizon. We reject wholly the movement to micromanage education in favor of an open and vibrant, intellectually viable schoolhouse. We believe that good teaching takes care of bad testing and bad standards—yet, while arguing against the notion of standards, we also realize the *realpolitik* of the American classroom in the first years of the twenty-first century.

The fact is that standards have become an integral part of the American education system. Furthermore, when properly aligned with assessment instruments, they can prove valuable. Standards and their resulting assessments can provide teachers and administrators with important information about what and how to teach. Therefore, we highlight which NCTE/IRA (National Council of Teachers of English/International Reading Association) standard or standards each lesson in this book helps students meet. This should help teachers integrate the strategies we are advocating with their district or school requirements. The Appendix at the back of the book provides the text of all of the standards in full.

Teaching Writing in the Inclusive Classroom

Who Will Benefit From the TIP Approach?

This book is written for teachers, primarily those working in grades 6 to 12. It is directed at all teachers: those exclusively teaching writing, those teaching in the content areas, and those teaching in classrooms in which students of differing learning styles gather to learn. Although the book targets teachers of adolescents, we believe that the strategies and ideas contained herein are appropriate for teachers in all grades; see, for example, the earlier section "Jane's Story." In younger grades care must be taken to adjust the mini lessons and strategies to the appropriate instructional level, so as not to cause students to reach a level of frustration that impairs learning. But other than that bit of warning, this book is good for everyone.

Chapter Two

Developing Voice and Authority

A number of years ago one of Roger's students—let's call him Colorado since that's not his real name—made a formal request of Roger. "Mr. P.," he pleaded. "You gots to show me where the periods goes!!" After a year and a half of intensive direct instruction in rhetorical strategies, mini lessons introducing grammar, skills, and mechanics, and hours upon hours of frequent and sustained practice in a writer's workshop format, Colorado became aware that he had something important to say—something he could write meaningfully about. Unfortunately for Roger, Colorado's main pubescent interests involved low-rider cars. That's all that he wrote about. Roger learned about shock absorbers, sound systems, and how to make cars bounce. But the long and the short of this student writer–teacher story is that Colorado grew as a student and wound up in his last quarter of eighth grade with straight A's on his final report card. This is, of course, the point of teaching strategies for writing in an engaging and authentic way. Strategic rhetorical approaches to writing help students develop a sense of authorship— they cultivate the notion of voice. Colorado certainly provides a prime example.

It is clear that writers generally do not write well if they believe they have nothing to say (Daniels & Zemelman, 1985; Emig, 1977;

Murray, 1997). Helping students find the voice with which to express what is most important to them has the additional benefit of improving their writing across all genres in addition to developing the personal narrative that is the core of all writing (Murray, 1991).

The TIP approach to writing individualizes and differentiates according to the needs and talents of all students in the inclusive classroom. When we teach effective writing strategies we expose all students to focused approaches for solving rhetorical problems. Not every strategy taught will be effective with all students. However, teaching many strategies opens up the door for students to find the approaches that work well for them.

Another anecdote will illustrate. When Roger was in eighth grade, his English teacher insisted on students outlining each and every paper they were assigned to write before she would allow them to commence with the actual writing of the paper. Roger, unfortunately, never got outlining prior to the fact. Oh, he could outline quite well from an already completed text, but to try and organize his thinking in so linear a manner didn't fit his learning style. He is a *lister*. He makes lists, constructs webs, and draws pictures as he plans his writing. In fact, sometimes he skips that phase and simply begins to write. Revision and editing follow. In eighth grade, because he was required to turn in an outline, he had to write the paper first and then outline what he had written. Our point is that Roger's teacher was far too limited in her approach to strategies, offering her students one and only one way to solve a rhetorical problem.

We advocate providing students with a virtual buffet of strategies—what we often refer to as the "Old Country Buffet" or "Luby's Cafeteria" pedagogy. Give students choices of approaches to solve similar problems and do so in an engaging and authentic manner and they will thrive. In West Texas, the phrase "Fellers, there's more 'n one way to get to the roof!" is often heard. We take that quite seriously and insist that we provide students with many ways to "get to the roof." Working with strategies in this way allows students at all levels to meet their personal expectations as writers and fulfill the external curricular needs of both the school and the district.

Lessons for Developing Voice and Authority

This chapter presents full-period strategy lessons, as well as some mini lessons (a concept covered in more depth in the next chapter), designed to help students develop voice.

Lists of Ten

Young writers often complain that they have no idea what to write about when they are asked to write freely about anything they care to. Writing can be so intimidating. But it doesn't have to be. Here is a quick scaffolding idea to help your students find topics to write about. The activity should be done early in the semester.

Materials

You will need one manila folder or large sheet of construction paper for each student and an assortment of markers.

Procedure

Step 1. Have students create writing folders. Have them decorate the manila folders or create their own folders from the sheets of construction paper and then decorate them.

Step 2. Tell your students that the writing folders are there to hold any and all writing that they do during the year. Good stuff, bad stuff, ideas, partly finished pieces, finished work—in sum, any writing at all. Explain too that the writing folder is a personal and private file for the student's eyes only.

Step 3. Assign the following homework. Ask your students to make a list of ten items for each of five categories. Here are some category suggestions:

Ten people I'd really like to have dinner with
Ten favorite songs
Ten favorite foods
Ten places I'd like to visit
Ten favorite books
Ten favorite games
Ten important goals for the future
Ten important things I'd like to learn about

You get the idea.

Step 4. When the students return with their lists in hand, have them staple or glue the lists on the inside of their writing folder's front cover.

Step 5. The next time students say they have nothing to write about, refer them to their List of Ten, where they will find at least fifty fresh ideas to write about.

NCTE/IRA Standard

12. Students use spoken, written, and visual language to accomplish their own purposes (e.g., for learning, enjoyment, persuasion, and the exchange of information).

Basic Description

Before students can master the requisite skills for effective writing in any genre, they must develop a sense of voice or authorship that only comes through extensive practice in telling their own story. To help them do that, we have created three simple writing strategies that rely heavily on both description and personal narrative. Our goal is to help students develop voice, storytelling ability, and ways to richly describe a scene or an action that's an intimate part of the narrative being told. This activity should be done in two parts, with each taking about five to ten minutes.

Setup Activities

Have students prepare for this writing assignment by completing one or more of the following setup activities.

Setup 1. Ask students to make a list of from ten to twenty specific sensory experiences (visual, oral, tactile, olfactory) that can be identified as integral to the telling of their story. Once they complete their lists, instruct them to choose about half of the experiences listed and identify specific words or phrases that help describe those experiences. For example, a list of terms to use in describing a walk home might include the following: *oak tree.* Additional words or phrases that help describe the oak tree may include such terms as *landmark, turn left, welcome shade,* and the like.

Setup 2. Ask students to close their eyes and imagine vividly the narrative they are going to write. While their eyes are closed, remind them in soft tones that they should picture in their mind's eye the sounds, the smells, the feel of every item, of every space in their story. After giving them adequate time to visualize their story, give them sheets of paper divided into six or eight blocks. The sheets serve as storyboards on which students can draw the details of their story in some graphic form. At this point, emphasize that students will not be evaluated on their drawings in any way. Quite the contrary, the storyboard will simply allow them to brainstorm ideas, to prewrite. In other words, the storyboard will serve to improve their writing and is only a tool to that end.

Setup 3. Have students refer back either to their preliminary list (Setup 1) or their visualization (Setup 2). Then have them select a partner and share their story orally. In the beginning, instruct the listeners to ask the storytellers for more and more details. When students become used to the idea of telling stories and listening to stories closely, this instruction will no longer be necessary. Allow adequate time for the tellers to develop all of the details in their story and for the listeners to press critically for more details as the story develops.

Procedure

After completing any of the three setup procedures, have students write their narratives. Writing times will vary, depending on a number of variables:

Teaching Writing in the Inclusive Classroom

Moment in time during the school year. During the earlier part of the academic year, writing time segments will be shorter. They will get longer as you progress through the course of the year.

Teacher discretion. You can vary the amount of time devoted to this activity after considering the classroom context and the students involved.

Length of time devoted to writing in the school's daily schedule.

NCTE/IRA Standards

4. Students adjust their use of spoken, written, and visual language (e.g., conventions, style, vocabulary) to communicate effectively with a variety of audiences and for different purposes.

5. Students employ a wide range of strategies as they write and use different writing process elements appropriately to communicate with different audiences for a variety of purposes.

11. Students participate as knowledgeable, reflective, creative, and critical members of a variety of literacy communities.

12. Students use spoken, written, and visual language to accomplish their own purposes (e.g., for learning, enjoyment, persuasion, and the exchange of information).

Rich Description

Learning to be descriptive means more than merely learning about adjectives, adverbs, and other modifiers. Rather, students must discover ways to enrich language and text by adding imagery, description, and other levels of richness to their writing. The following exercises can be mixed and matched to nurture students as they begin to see multiple ways of prewriting, sharing, and thinking.

Because they are concentrating on narrative structure in familiar contexts, they have the opportunity to develop voice or a sense of authorship in their writing. Because they must provide rich description, they develop a larger vocabulary, as well as add depth to their writing.

Procedure

Option 1. The Walk Home. Ask students to write a descriptive story about their walk home from school (or, for students who don't walk, their bus ride home or their trip home with the parent or caregiver who picks them up). Emphasize that the story should contain references to people, places, and things they encounter along the way. They need to write about the things they see, the people they run into, or anything special that might occur along the way. For example, if they walk home with a friend, that friend should become an important part of the narrative. Also emphasize that their narrative should begin as they leave the classroom and only finish when they enter their home.

Option 2. My Favorite Room. Have students focus on their favorite room in their home. Emphasize that the story they tell about this room should include a sense of purpose, why this room was chosen from the others. What is special about this space, about this place? What happens there that can happen nowhere else but there?

Option 3. My Favorite Food. Ask students to place a favorite food in the context of a story that includes other characters. For example, ask them to write about the last time they ate their favorite food, who they were with, what the occasion was, what happened during the meal, and how they felt about the whole situation.

NCTE/IRA Standards

4. Students adjust their use of spoken, written, and visual language (e.g., conventions, style, vocabulary) to communicate effectively with a variety of audiences and for different purposes.
5. Students employ a wide range of strategies as they write and use different writing process elements appropriately to communicate with different audiences for a variety of purposes.
11. Students participate as knowledgeable, reflective, creative, and critical members of a variety of literacy communities.
12. Students use spoken, written, and visual language to accomplish their own purposes (e.g., for learning, enjoyment, persuasion, and the exchange of information).

The Frame

When a frame is held at arm's length, it provides students with a field of vision similar to a telephoto lens (see Figure 2.1). When it's held close to the face, it mimics a wide-angle lens. Of course, when held midway between the face and the length of the arm, it acts like a normal lens on a camera. In this activity, students use a frame to help isolate segments of their environment.

This activity should take about forty-five minutes.

Figure 2.1. The Frame.

Materials

You will need black construction paper. Before beginning the activity with your students, create a frame of your own from the construction paper. Fold an 8½ x 11-inch sheet of paper in half. Then, with scissors, cut a narrow half-square out of the folded side. When you open the page, the frame will appear.

Procedure

Step 1. Use the frame to create a narrow field of view for students to describe. Ask students to focus through the lens. Have them focus on a fixed object or set of objects—something that they find visually interesting. Model how to use the frame.

Step 2. Have students draw what they described in the frame.

Step 3. Instruct students to create a narrative that helps tell the story of the picture they sketched. Create characters that live in the space they created. Make them real as they navigate through the space.

NCTE/IRA Standards

4. Students adjust their use of spoken, written, and visual language (e.g., conventions, style, vocabulary) to communicate effectively with a variety of audiences and for different purposes.

5. Students employ a wide range of strategies as they write and use different writing process elements appropriately to communicate with different audiences for a variety of purposes.

11. Students participate as knowledgeable, reflective, creative, and critical members of a variety of literacy communities.

12. Students use spoken, written, and visual language to accomplish their own purposes (e.g., for learning, enjoyment, persuasion, and the exchange of information).

Round Robin Theme Exchange

This exercise is useful in motivating reluctant writers and readers to develop topic and theme. We have both taught this writing strategy many times, but the story that comes to mind took place in an urban seventh-grade classroom. The class was relatively passive and the writing they produced lacked energy. Like many others, this group of prepubescents did not have a sense of authorship or an interest in telling stories. We were stumped but not discouraged. One day, we tried a Round Robin Theme Exchange. It should be noted that this was a diverse classroom in every sense of the term: English language learners, students of various socio-economic classes and ethnic groups, and finally, mainstreamed special education students. It was an amazing experience to see the students become animated and excited about their writing. At the end of the class period, after laughing to the point of tears, students begged us to do this exercise again. Needless to say we obliged, about a month later. It was an unforgettable experience: witnessing student writers of all levels finally "get" the notion that writing can be fun. They became storytellers for the first time.

This lesson takes at least thirty-five minutes and is a good activity to repeat often at the beginning of the year.

Procedure

Step 1. On the chalkboard, write a story starter that is general yet designed to capture the interest of your students. Following are some starters that have been used with great success:

> The night was cold and damp. There was a chill in the air as we huddled around the campfire singing and telling stories. A low cloud bank seemed to glow from the light of the fire as the wind whistled through the lush leaves of the trees above. An owl hooted in the distance. A coyote howled at the night. Suddenly, it became very quiet when. . . .

> Everyone was called to the square. We didn't know why. Up on the stage stood the mayor and the governor. They looked serious, as if something was amiss. The gathering crowd began to mumble as rumors spread like wildfire around the square. Suddenly, it was the mayor's turn to speak. . . .

Step 2. On the chalkboard, write the following phrase: "I have nothing to write about at this time."

Step 3. Tell your students that they will be writing to complete the story that has been started on the board. (They will ask if they have to copy what is on the board. Respond, "No.") Instruct your students that they are to begin writing when, and only when, you say "Go." They are to stop writing, even if they are in the middle of a sentence, when you say "Stop." During the time between Go and Stop, tell your students that they must be constantly writing. If they cannot think of anything to write, they must write the phrase "I have nothing to write about at this time" over and over until they can think of something to write about.

Step 4. When you are certain the students are ready, say "Go." Time them for anywhere from one and a half to two minutes, and then say "Stop."

Step 5. Ask your students to pass the story they have been working on to another student, someone at least three seats away from themselves. Once the papers have been exchanged and you are certain that everyone has a paper other than the one they began with, ask them to read the new story they have in their hands. When you say "Go" they are to continue the new story until you again say "Stop." Again, time them for one and a half to two minutes. Repeat this step two or three times.

Step 6. When you decide the last time has come, tell your students to conclude the story.

Step 7. Collect the writing and randomly select seven to ten pieces to read aloud. Of course, there are bound to be a few students who thought it was funny to write the filler phrase over and over. Make sure to read those aloud first. Get it over with without specifically acknowledging the author. This behavior will quickly stop. Read the papers anonymously so that students can learn from each other without egos getting in the way. If a student insists on being acknowledged as an author, make that student do something silly like jump up and down and yell, "I wrote that!!!"

Step 8. After reading each paper, ask students if it was a piece of writing that, as a first draft, hung together in a reasonably organized fashion. Only praise is appropriate at this point. As students begin to establish voice it is appropriate to add critique to the oral reviews of work shared with the class, but it is important to begin with praise at the start.

Extension Activity

As an optional last step, brainstorm the purpose of this exercise.

NCTE/IRA Standards

4. Students adjust their use of spoken, written, and visual language (e.g., conventions, style, vocabulary) to communicate effectively with a variety of audiences and for different purposes.
5. Students employ a wide range of strategies as they write and use different writing process elements appropriately to communicate with different audiences for a variety of purposes.
11. Students participate as knowledgeable, reflective, creative, and critical members of a variety of literacy communities.
12. Students use spoken, written, and visual language to accomplish their own purposes (e.g., for learning, enjoyment, persuasion, and the exchange of information).

Teaching Writing in the Inclusive Classroom

Sight, Smell, Taste-Touch, Sound (SST-TS)

Mature writers appeal to the five senses by telling what something looks like, what it smells like, how it might taste, what it feels like, and what it sounds like. Through this metacognitive awareness, writers rely on rhetorical metaphor to represent an image for their readers. The SST-TS acronym will help students develop a checklist for their own descriptive writing.

This lesson generally takes twenty to thirty minutes.

Materials

Photocopy Exhibit 2.1 and distribute it to your students.

Exhibit 2.1. SST-TS: Descriptive Writing Checklist.

Directions: Use this checklist to review and revise your writing. Use it for all your drafts and finished piece of writing.				
	First draft	*Revision*	*Revision*	*Finished piece*
1. Before I began writing, I brainstormed ways in which I could include each of the five senses in my piece.				
2. In the first sentence I appealed to one of the five senses to introduce my main topic.				
3. I described my topic by appealing to each of the five senses at least once.				
4. Each of my sentences contained at least one representation of a sense.				
5. My concluding sentence was descriptive.				
6. I used transitions to connect my ideas and create unity in my writing.				
7. I used complete sentences and checked my use of punctuation and capitalization.				
8. I asked one of my peers to review my writing and used suggestions to improve my writing.				
9. I wrote a final draft and am ready to publish my writing.				

Procedure

Step 1. Read aloud a descriptive paragraph to your students. The following, from *A Sound of Thunder,* by Ray Bradbury, is a good choice.

> It came on great oiled striding legs. It towered thirty feet above half the trees, a great evil god. Each lower leg was a piston, a thousand pounds of white bone and thick ropes of muscle. Each thigh was a ton of meat. And from the upper body two delicate arms dangled out front with hands that might pick up men like toys. The snake neck coiled. Its mouth hung open showing a row of teeth like daggers. Its eyes rolled. They showed nothing but hunger. It closed its mouth in a death grin.

Step 2. Dissect the paragraph with your students, identifying elements of SST-TS that are contained in the writing.

Step 3. Ask your students to write a descriptive paragraph in which they use each of the elements of SST-TS at least two times. Some suggested topics are as follows:

Elephants
Race cars
Kitchens
A party
A vivid sunset
A spring rainstorm

NCTE/IRA Standards

4. Students adjust their use of spoken, written, and visual language (e.g., conventions, style, vocabulary) to communicate effectively with a variety of audiences and for different purposes.
5. Students employ a wide range of strategies as they write and use different writing process elements appropriately to communicate with different audiences for a variety of purposes.
11. Students participate as knowledgeable, reflective, creative, and critical members of a variety of literacy communities.
12. Students use spoken, written, and visual language to accomplish their own purposes (e.g., for learning, enjoyment, persuasion, and the exchange of information).

Picture Writing

Picture Writing is a technique that encourages students to engage their visual knowledge as they prepare a story from a picture. Students are given a broad selection of pictures from which to choose those that most interest them. Picture writing allows the teacher to tap into students' visualization ability. By looking at details in their visual image and then converting those details into a narrative, students learn to focus on the details of their own story and the way in which they tell it. The procedure is quite simple.

We have found this technique to be especially appropriate for special needs students who otherwise have difficulty exploring details, identifying details, and expressing those details in their own writing. This strategy engages alternative intelligences that go beyond the intellectual act of writing words on a page. Picture writing, because of the broad selection and choices available to students, is a way for teachers to both individualize and differentiate instruction simultaneously.

This activity takes about thirty-five to forty-five minutes.

Materials

Provide students with a selection of images that you have already attached to sheets of writing paper.

Procedure

Step 1. Have each student choose one sheet of paper containing one image. Instruct the students to explore the picture, looking for a story embedded in it. Suggest that they come up with a story based on their own personal experience that they can relate to the image shown in the picture. Allow ample time, as much as five minutes, for this exploration.

Step 2. Ask students to share the stories they have discovered in the pictures orally with a partner. This step is, in fact, a rehearsal or form of prewriting that allows the students to more fully embed the narrative they have chosen to tell in their cognitive memory, making the act of writing more memorable and significantly more creative. Allow three to five minutes for sharing.

Step 3. Once students have shared their stories with each other, ask them to write it on the paper you supplied. Ask them to pay attention to the structure of the story they choose to tell, as well as to the form of the narrative itself.

NCTE/IRA Standards

4. Students adjust their use of spoken, written, and visual language (e.g., conventions, style, vocabulary) to communicate effectively with a variety of audiences and for different purposes.

5. Students employ a wide range of strategies as they write and use different writing process elements appropriately to communicate with different audiences for a variety of purposes.

11. Students participate as knowledgeable, reflective, creative, and critical members of a variety of literacy communities.

12. Students use spoken, written, and visual language to accomplish their own purposes (e.g., for learning, enjoyment, persuasion, and the exchange of information).

The Alien Encounter

Often young writers have a difficult time with description or elaboration in their writing. Part of the problem is one of vision—they have not been taught how to look for those ubiquitous details that we all take for granted. This is another simple exercise designed to help students become aware of the details around them. The point is to help them uncover what they take for granted, to focus on the everyday details, on the mundane, in order to include that level of description in their writing.

We often set up this activity by asking students to imagine that we have been abducted by an alien being named Farndwark from the Andromeda Galaxy. Farndwark threatens to destroy Earth unless he can receive an adequate explanation as to why Earthlings use chairs and desks. Once students have inspected their chairs and desks, and after they share their information with a partner, they are asked to write Farndwark a letter providing him with descriptions that are accurate, creative, and meaningful enough to persuade him not to destroy Earth.

This activity takes about forty-five minutes.

Materials

You will need blindfolds for half of your students.

Procedure

Step 1. Group your students in pairs. Have one member of the pair place a blindfold over his or her eyes. The other member of the pair will act as a scribe, writing down specific descriptions related by the blindfolded partner.

Step 2. Instruct the blindfolded partners to feel their desk and describe what they feel to their partner. Explain that they have to use their hands to "see" the desk in a new way. Elaborate instructions are in order. The students must "see" the desk in three dimensions, so they will have to feel the top, sides, edges, bottom, legs, and seat if one is attached—in fact, every part of the desk if they are to describe it accurately. Explain that their descriptions must be concise and specific. "The desk has a gouge on the side" is not as strong as "The desk has a gouge that feels like it is about an inch long on the left edge just below the writing surface that runs on an angle from front to back near the far corner."

Step 3. Once the partners have finished creating their list, you have several options available:

Ask each pair to collaborate on writing a description of the desk as if they were writing a novel. Their description must make the reader "see" or visualize the desk they are describing.

Have partners exchange their lists with another team and have them use the new list to describe the other desk.

Have students write individually to describe the desk and compare descriptions.

Extension Activity

Ask students to describe their walk home, their favorite room in their home, or what someone looks like.

NCTE/IRA Standards

4. Students adjust their use of spoken, written, and visual language (e.g., conventions, style, vocabulary) to communicate effectively with a variety of audiences and for different purposes.
5. Students employ a wide range of strategies as they write and use different writing process elements appropriately to communicate with different audiences for a variety of purposes.
11. Students participate as knowledgeable, reflective, creative, and critical members of a variety of literacy communities.
12. Students use spoken, written, and visual language to accomplish their own purposes (e.g., for learning, enjoyment, persuasion, and the exchange of information).

The Archaeologist

Helping students develop their observation skills leads to significant improvement in their ability to add description to both narrative and informational text. It is not enough to tell students to include detail in their writing; rather, we have to show them how to do it. The Archaeologist exercise provides a strategy for observation that is at once engaging and fun.

The Archaeologist has many benefits:

It increases observation of minute details.

It enhances note-taking skills.

It develops analytical skills.

It develops interpretive skills.

It improves critical selection skills.

Asking students to observe the most minute details, take notes on what they observe, and discuss and analyze their findings are powerful ways to engage them in authentic writing practices. And when you ask students to critically analyze the papers in their group in order to select one to represent them all, you help develop their editorial and revision skills.

Setup

The activity begins in a dramatic, almost shocking, manner. Without saying a word, the instructor walks into a classroom, moves directly to the wastepaper basket, and turning the basket upside down, empties its contents in the center of the room. Once the giggling stops, the instructor sets the stage.

Procedure

Step 1. The first question to ask is this: "What is an archaeologist? What exactly do they do?" Your goal is to get to the idea that archaeologists study trash, that much of their work actually takes place where people have discarded everyday items. Then ask students to activate their imaginations and pretend that they no longer live in the twenty-first century, but rather in the twenty-fourth. Then ask them to imagine that they are archaeologists engaged in a dig during which they have uncovered the very classroom we are sitting in.

Step 2. Divide the class into four groups, giving each group between five and seven minutes to examine the trash on the center of the floor. Instruct the groups to bring paper and pencil so they can take notes on their observations. While one group is closely examining the trash, tell the other three groups to observe the trash from afar if they have not yet done a close examination, or if they have, to begin to discuss and interpret what they have seen up close. When all four groups have had an opportunity to closely examine the trash (we make the last group responsible for returning the trash to the wastepaper basket), give them ten minutes to discuss their findings. During this time, instruct them to think about the people who inhabited the space they are studying and what they can learn about those people from the information found in the trash, and only from the information found in the trash.

Step 3. At the end of the ten-minute discussion, ask students to write individual reports, imagining that they will be presented to a prestigious group of archaeologists meeting to discuss the new findings. Give them another ten minutes to write, and then have the students reassemble in groups, share their papers, and select the one paper that will represent their group at the meeting. The first time we do this exercise we ask the students to suggest things to look out for that will help them select the best paper, the one that will represent their group. Students then share the four selected papers with the whole group.

NCTE/IRA Standards

4. Students adjust their use of spoken, written, and visual language (e.g., conventions, style, vocabulary) to communicate effectively with a variety of audiences and for different purposes.

5. Students employ a wide range of strategies as they write and use different writing process elements appropriately to communicate with different audiences for a variety of purposes.

11. Students participate as knowledgeable, reflective, creative, and critical members of a variety of literacy communities.

12. Students use spoken, written, and visual language to accomplish their own purposes (e.g., for learning, enjoyment, persuasion, and the exchange of information).

The Blueberry

Students find it difficult to elaborate when they write. The problem is that details are ubiquitous. They are all around us, yet unseen—taken for granted. The problem for teachers of writing is to find ways to help students examine what they take for granted and open their eyes to new ways of seeing.

This exercise helps students uncover what they already know about a simple fruit and then write a deep, rich description of it. You may use this as a mini lesson in the classroom or assign it as homework. In either case it is useful for you to write your own description and share it with your students.

This activity takes about ten minutes.

Procedure

Step 1. Instruct your students to write an essay about a blueberry. Give them time to think about this for a few moments, then add—"Oh, by they way, in your essay you may not use the word *blue*, you may not use the word *berry*, and you may not use the word *blueberry*—not even in the title."

Step 2. Share the students' writing with the class, singing the praises of the writing and the description. Here's an example, written by Yolanda, a seventh-grader:

> Crunchy, melt in your mouth, just a little bit tart. Round, the size of a small marble. The color of azure lakes and cobalt skies. Complements sugar and cream, cereal and pancakes, muffins and waffles, and, oh yes, pies. Morning would not be the same without you!

Extension Activities

Have students describe a color without using the name of the color.

Have students describe a feeling without naming the feeling.

Turn this exercise into a contest by having students choose their own color or feeling and then see if their description is good enough for the other students to figure out what it is they are describing. Here's an example, written by a group of eighth-graders:

> The taste of spinach softly melting on my tongue. The stain of grass on my new blue jeans. Mint leaves, broccoli, and Granny Smiths, frogs and lizards, grasshoppers and, oh by the way, bleacher seats at Wrigley Field all sing to me of lush landscape and happy times. It says GO.

NCTE/IRA Standards

4. Students adjust their use of spoken, written, and visual language (e.g., conventions, style, vocabulary) to communicate effectively with a variety of audiences and for different purposes.

5. Students employ a wide range of strategies as they write and use different writing process elements appropriately to communicate with different audiences for a variety of purposes.

6. Students apply knowledge of language structure, language conventions (e.g., spelling and punctuation), media techniques, figurative language, and genre to create, critique, and discuss print and nonprint texts.

11. Students participate as knowledgeable, reflective, creative, and critical members of a variety of literacy communities.

12. Students use spoken, written, and visual language to accomplish their own purposes (e.g., for learning, enjoyment, persuasion, and the exchange of information).

The Hall Walk

The Hall Walk is closely related to The Archaeologist. In The Archaeologist, students examined the trash collected in a room—that is, they examined fine detail. The Hall Walk asks students to examine gross detail. Students imagine that they have newly arrived as representatives of some alien culture. Their task is to determine the climate and culture of the school building they are visiting.

The Hall Walk benefits students in a number of ways:

Observation of large or gross detail is enhanced.

Note-taking skills become analytical skills, and interpretive skills are enhanced.

Collaborative writing skills are developed.

This strategy is especially helpful with exceptional children because of the collaborative and multisensory elements that are required for its successful completion. This strategy is a living example of Vygotsky's Zone of Proximal Development.

This exercise takes about forty to fifty minutes.

Procedure

Step 1. Divide the class into four or five small groups.

Step 2. Instruct the students to take notebooks and pencils into the hall and look for "artifacts, signs, and symbols" that help define the climate and the culture of the school.

Step 3. Ask students to take notes on what they observe while they're in the hallway. We generally allow ten to fifteen minutes to gather information.

Step 4. On returning to the classroom, have students discuss in their small group the data they gathered. Make sure to remind students to talk about the artifacts, symbols, icons, and signs that help develop the sense of the place they are examining.

Step 5. Break the writing phase into two parts. During the first part have students write individually, constructing a picture with as much detail as possible describing the climate and culture of the school. Ask that they use only the evidence they collected during their walk through the hall. During the second part, ask the students to rejoin their small groups, this time sharing their individual papers in order to create a group piece.

Step 6. Have the students share the group pieces with the entire class.

Extension Activity

If the hallway is unavailable, divide the classroom into quadrants, and assign each group a quadrant to explore.

NCTE/IRA Standards

4. Students adjust their use of spoken, written, and visual language (e.g., conventions, style, vocabulary) to communicate effectively with a variety of audiences and for different purposes.

5. Students employ a wide range of strategies as they write and use different writing process elements appropriately to communicate with different audiences for a variety of purposes.

11. Students participate as knowledgeable, reflective, creative, and critical members of a variety of literacy communities.

12. Students use spoken, written, and visual language to accomplish their own purposes (e.g., for learning, enjoyment, persuasion, and the exchange of information).

The Reporter

The Reporter helps students combine strategies for gathering information, translating that information into meaningful detail, and writing an effective piece of informational text that both informs and engages the reader. This is not an exercise for novices. Quite the contrary, it requires that students have already developed a good sense of voice or authorship. Therefore, it should only be introduced in the later part of the school year.

In this exercise students get real-life experience because they research, interview, report, and take a stand on issues they've identified as important. They are given an opportunity to experience the same set of facts from more than one perspective. The exercise will help them understand the difference between informational writing and persuasive writing.

This lesson takes about forty-five to fifty minutes.

Procedure

Step 1. Brainstorm with your students to come up with significant current events or problems in the school or community.

Step 2. Once you have identified a substantial number of problems or events, arrange the students into pairs, or at most, groups of three. Then ask them to gather background information on one of the issues the class has identified as important.

Step 3. Once the students have adequate background information on the event or problem, have them interview two to three people who have a direct interest in the issue. Make it clear that the interviews should contain standard informational questions, eliciting the who, what, when, where, why, and how of the issue from the person being interviewed.

Step 4. At the close of the interviews have students write two pieces. The first should be purely informational, as if it were an article in a newspaper or a story on a television or radio news report. The second piece should take the form of an editorial in which the students express their own opinions or take a stand on the issue in question.

NCTE/IRA Standards

1. Students read a wide range of print and nonprint texts to build an understanding of texts, of themselves, and of the cultures of the United States and the world; to acquire new information; to respond to the needs and demands of society and the workplace; and for personal fulfillment. Among these texts are fiction and nonfiction, classic and contemporary works.

3. Students apply a wide range of strategies to comprehend, interpret, evaluate, and appreciate texts. They draw on their prior experience, their interactions with other readers and writers, their knowledge of word meaning and of other texts, their word identification strategies, and their understanding of textual features (e.g., sound-letter correspondence, sentence structure, context, graphics).

4. Students adjust their use of spoken, written, and visual language (e.g., conventions, style, vocabulary) to communicate effectively with a variety of audiences and for different purposes.

5. Students employ a wide range of strategies as they write and use different writing process elements appropriately to communicate with different audiences for a variety of purposes.

6. Students apply knowledge of language structure, language conventions (e.g., spelling and punctuation), media techniques, figurative language, and genre to create, critique, and discuss print and nonprint texts.

7. Students conduct research on issues and interests by generating ideas and questions, and by posing problems. They gather, evaluate, and synthesize data from a variety of sources (e.g., print and nonprint texts, artifacts, people) to communicate their discoveries in ways that suit their purpose and audience.

8. Students use a variety of technological and information resources (e.g., libraries, databases, computer networks, video) to gather and synthesize information and to create and communicate knowledge.

11. Students participate as knowledgeable, reflective, creative, and critical members of a variety of literacy communities.

12. Students use spoken, written, and visual language to accomplish their own purposes (e.g., for learning, enjoyment, persuasion, and the exchange of information).

Copyright © 2007 by John Wiley & Sons, Inc.

Transactional Writing

Writing expository or informational text is different from writing narrative text. Or is it? Informational writing assumes that the author has done some research, determined what the facts are, and focused on a point. Narrative writing assumes that the author has searched his or her memory or imagination for details that help support the story being told. It is very important for students to be able to compare and contrast their writing styles in informational and narrative approaches. You might have students compare a piece of their personal writing with the piece they create for this exercise.

This lesson takes about forty-five to fifty minutes.

Procedure

Step 1. Ask your students to write a partisan, persuasive report about their school building. Here's an example assignment:

> You have been appointed school reporter for the *Daily Gazette,* a paper read by over 100,000 people in our area. Your first assignment is to write an investigative report on the conditions of the _____ school.

Step 2. Explain that a persuasive report on a school like yours would likely cover the following (write these on the board):

Functionality	Noise control
Safety	Energy efficiency
Aesthetics	Security
Structural issues	Floor plan/layout
Durability	Facilities
Decor	Playgrounds
Athletics	Music
Integrity	Teachers

Step 3. Explain that students may not be able to cover each of these items, or may even think of some that you haven't listed. Tell them that you are only asking them to consider each of these items and then decide which ones are important to write about.

Step 4. Allow time for data gathering. Students should have a fixed amount of time to patrol the building for the sole purpose of gathering information and interviewing people that may help them in their quest.

Step 5. When students return to class, ask them to write their article for submission to their editorial board (a group of three students). The task of the editorial board is to nominate one article from their group for sharing with the class. Then have each group read the selected piece to the rest of the class.

Step 6. Begin a debriefing discussion about the assignment. You will want to discuss at least the following three questions with your students:

How did you feel about this assignment when you first heard about it? How do you feel now?

How was this writing task different from writing a story about your own experience? (Stress the fact that it was not personal and that the writing came from transactional encounters with the world and not from memory or imagination.)

How did this piece get written? What did you have to do in order to accomplish your task?

NCTE/IRA Standards

4. Students adjust their use of spoken, written, and visual language (e.g., conventions, style, vocabulary) to communicate effectively with a variety of audiences and for different purposes.
11. Students participate as knowledgeable, reflective, creative, and critical members of a variety of literacy communities.
12. Students use spoken, written, and visual language to accomplish their own purposes (e.g., for learning, enjoyment, persuasion, and the exchange of information).

Visualizing

When students learn to visualize a scene, they become better at describing it. But visualization does not come naturally for many children. This exercise is designed to help students learn to visualize and then describe a scene, either real or imaginary.

This lesson takes about forty-five to fifty minutes.

Procedure

Step 1. Give your students this loosely constructed introduction to help them search their memories for an accident they can work with:

> I'd like you to think of an accident that you can recall. Everyone's been in an accident at one time or another—or they've seen one or been affected by one. Most accidents, though not all, involve injuries. Sometimes accidents happen in cars, but not always. There are other kinds of accidents as well. In fact, some are "happy" accidents, like when people stumble on something good. Do you have an accident you'd like to write about? Do you have it clearly in your mind?

Step 2. Ask several students to share out loud accident experiences they have had. Do not move away from this phase until every student sincerely reports that they have an accident in mind that they would like to work with. Then say the following in a very matter-of-fact tone: "Now put down pens and pencils and close your eyes. I'm going to take you back to just one minute before the accident happened. Try and take yourself back to that place and time in your mind. The clock is stopped exactly one minute before your accident."

Step 3. Then, using long pauses, introduce the following questions into the silence, reminding the students to keep their eyes closed and only visualize.

> Take a long look around, a slow look. Where are you? What do you see?
>
> Turn and look to your left. What do you see?
>
> Turn and look to your right. What do you see?
>
> Look all the way behind you. What is there?
>
> What are you doing?
>
> What do you smell?
>
> How do you feel?
>
> Now the clock begins to tick again. The accident is happening. What do you see? Feel? Smell?

Step 4. Give the next instruction in a soft, almost hushed voice. Be very deliberate: "All right, you may open your eyes now. I'd like you to make a list of what you have just seen and felt. Words, phrases, images, colors, feelings, memories—include everything you have seen and felt. No need for sentences, just make a list. Don't worry about organization, just make a list."

Step 5. Allow students about five minutes to make their lists, longer if they seem to still be working. At the end of the allotted time, ask them to write an account of the accident, taking any approach they want to take. Remind them that this is a rough draft, so finished quality is not expected. Remind them too that they will be expected to share their drafts with two or three other students in editing groups. Allow twenty to twenty-five minutes for this part of the exercise. While your students are writing their accidents, write your own accident story (choose a fresh one every time).

Step 6. When students are finished with their drafts, assign them to groups of three writers and allow fifteen minutes for them to share what they have written. Make no specific requirements about the format for sharing other than to tell them that they should use this time to help each other improve their writing—that is, encourage them toward supportive sharing rather than critical sharing.

Step 7. When students return to the whole group at the end of fifteen minutes, ask for volunteers to share their drafts with the whole group. If you do not get many volunteers, read your story as the first participant. Or ask for nominations from each group to pick a story they feel should be shared without predetermining the criteria for choice.

Step 8. Finally, debrief the session. Ask your students:

How did you feel about the assignment at first?

How did the prewriting experience help? Why?

What problems did you run into getting the piece written?

How did it feel to share in the small group?

How did you feel as an audience for other writing?

NCTE/IRA Standards

4. Students adjust their use of spoken, written, and visual language (e.g., conventions, style, vocabulary) to communicate effectively with a variety of audiences and for different purposes.
5. Students employ a wide range of strategies as they write and use different writing process elements appropriately to communicate with different audiences for a variety of purposes.
6. Students apply knowledge of language structure, language conventions (e.g., spelling and punctuation), media techniques, figurative language, and genre to create, critique, and discuss print and nonprint texts.
11. Students participate as knowledgeable, reflective, creative, and critical members of a variety of literacy communities.
12. Students use spoken, written, and visual language to accomplish their own purposes (e.g., for learning, enjoyment, persuasion, and the exchange of information).

Writing Directions

Often, writers are plagued with imprecision. It is not enough for the instructor to say, "Be specific in your writing." We have to show students why being precise is important. This exercise is designed to do just that.

This activity takes about forty-five to fifty minutes.

Materials

You will need enough small magnetic compasses to hand out one to each pair of students in your class.

Procedure

Step 1. Divide the classroom into groups of two. Supply each group with a compass.

Step 2. Place each group at the threshold of the classroom door and instruct them to walk to the library (or lunchroom, gym, principal's office, or other location in the school), writing down the number of steps taken, the turns required, and the corresponding compass directions.

Step 3. Share this example: "Take three steps north, turn left or west, take twenty-five steps west. Turn right or north, take seven steps north to the top of the stairs, go down twelve steps to the landing. Turn right or east and take three steps. Turn right or south, go down twelve steps, and continue eight steps and turn right or west." And so on.

Step 4. Send teams off at thirty-second intervals, armed with their compasses and paper and pencil. Depending on the distance of the location the team is to describe, we generally allow from fifteen to twenty minutes before the teams return to the classroom.

Step 5. As the teams return to the classroom, ask team members to read and review their directions.

Step 6. When all teams have returned, ask them to exchange their directions with those written by another team. Then instruct the teams to follow the directions they have just been handed. In our experience, most teams don't get past the front door of the classroom!

Step 7. Ask students to do a "quick write," discussing what went wrong and what they could do to fix it in the future. Using the quick write as a prompt, lead the class in a discussion of precision in writing.

NCTE/IRA Standards

3. Students apply a wide range of strategies to comprehend, interpret, evaluate, and appreciate texts. They draw on their prior experience, their interactions with other readers and writers, their knowledge of word meaning and of other texts, their word identification strategies, and their understanding of textual features (e.g., sound-letter correspondence, sentence structure, context, graphics).

4. Students adjust their use of spoken, written, and visual language (e.g., conventions, style, vocabulary) to communicate effectively with a variety of audiences and for different purposes.

5. Students employ a wide range of strategies as they write and use different writing process elements appropriately to communicate with different audiences for a variety of purposes.

11. Students participate as knowledgeable, reflective, creative, and critical members of a variety of literacy communities.

12. Students use spoken, written, and visual language to accomplish their own purposes (e.g., for learning, enjoyment, persuasion, and the exchange of information).

Teaching Writing in the Inclusive Classroom

The Friday Essay

The Friday Essay is a simple activity designed to help students learn to write to a prompt. This is, of course, an important skill in our era of high-stakes testing, especially when those tests include writing samples. We have often found that the writing prompts provided on high-stakes tests do not match student experiences. The Friday Essay helps students learn how to write to a prompt even when the prompt makes no sense.

The Friday Essay is only written on Friday. It is not the Monday or the Thursday Essay. If there is no class on Friday, then no Friday Essay will be written. The Friday Essay was developed many years ago when students in Roger's class were provided with agenda books by the school. Each agenda book had a weekly motivational quotation and a handy study tip. On Friday, students were asked to write an essay in any genre, using either the motivational quotation or the study tip as a guide to their writing.

Students are never told that they are writing to a prompt. The only reference ever made to this assignment is that they are writing the Friday Essay. By focusing on the writing rather than on the prompt, students are able to learn the trick that every politician knows—answer the question you want to answer, no matter what question was asked in the first place. The qualifier is that the students, like politicians, must refer to the prompt or the question that was originally asked. The Friday Essay builds students' confidence in writing and is another tool for developing voice.

Here are some sample prompts:

"Never, ever quit."—Winston Churchill

"Any philosophy that can be put in a nutshell, belongs in one."—Hillary Putnam

"Try not to become a person of success but rather to become a person of value." —Albert Einstein

"Success isn't permanent, and failure isn't fatal."—Mike Ditka

"People grow through experience if they meet life honestly and courageously. This is how character is built."—Eleanor Roosevelt

"In the end, we will remember not the words of our enemies, but the silence of our friends."—Martin Luther King, Jr.

"He who knows does not speak. He who speaks does not know."—Lao-tzu

"Freedom is not worth having if it does not include the freedom to make mistakes." —Mahatma Gandhi

"Ill deeds are doubled with an evil word." —William Shakespeare

NCTE/IRA Standards

3. Students apply a wide range of strategies to comprehend, interpret, evaluate, and appreciate texts. They draw on their prior experience, their interactions with other readers and writers, their knowledge of word meaning and of other texts, their word identification strategies, and their understanding of textual features (e.g., sound-letter correspondence, sentence structure, context, graphics).

4. Students adjust their use of spoken, written, and visual language (e.g., conventions, style, vocabulary) to communicate effectively with a variety of audiences and for different purposes.

5. Students employ a wide range of strategies as they write and use different writing process elements appropriately to communicate with different audiences for a variety of purposes.

11. Students participate as knowledgeable, reflective, creative, and critical members of a variety of literacy communities.

12. Students use spoken, written, and visual language to accomplish their own purposes (e.g., for learning, enjoyment, persuasion, and the exchange of information).

Chapter Three

Developing Mini Lessons

Writing, like the other language arts, is developmental. Students learn language arts skills best through individualized, authentic experiences. A one-size-fits-all approach is not ideal, as a National Council of Teachers of English study indicated (Geuder, Harvey, & Loyd, 1974). This study determined that the curriculum and pedagogical strategies that successful writing teachers used varied, but they were all based on targeting what their student writers needed.

In this spirit, and in the spirit of John Dewey, the writing mini lesson builds on what students already know. It improves and develops students' writing through experience and discovery. Thus, the writing mini lesson is a proven strategy for individualizing writing instruction.

Using the Writing Workshop and Mini Lesson Approach

When we entered language arts teaching in the late 1980s, the writing workshop was not an established pedagogy in sixth- to twelfth-grade language arts or English classrooms. Katie recalls that many

of her colleagues were suspicious of her ninth-grade writing workshop. She was a novice teacher—age twenty-two at the time—and the writing workshop gurus, such as Lucy Calkins, Nancie Atwell, and Constance Weaver, were not familiar icons. Some of her fellow teachers argued that these students needed to learn writing through more teacher-directed and structured assignments. Writing workshops and mini lessons were too "loosey goosey" for the writing curriculum. Yet alongside the healthy doubters, Katie did encounter some other writing workshop teachers who argued with her that student-directed and engaging mini lessons that teach students how to manipulate and develop written text in personally meaningful ways was rigorous. With two of her colleagues, she found opportunities to collaborate as she constructed her writing workshop and mini lessons.

Today, the mini lesson is no longer an unfamiliar term in writing instruction. For the past two decades, mini lessons have become a cornerstone of the field. The pedagogical term has been popularized by several writing experts, including Lucy Calkins (1994), Nancie Atwell (1989), and Constance Weaver (1996).

Mini lessons are short lessons designed to teach specific writing skills to a whole class. Most often, writing mini lessons address a concern that the teacher has about the students' writing. Mini lessons can also introduce new skills or language and grammar. Finally, mini lessons create the opportunity for teachers to share their expertise with the students as they guide them through the writing workshop. The workshop model is student-directed, which means that students are given opportunities to make some decisions about different writing activities, but in the TIP approach the teacher creates the learning environment in which students can make those choices.

Developing Mini Lessons

When Katie teaches the writing pedagogy course to future middle and high school teachers—a course where secondary English teachers learn strategies for teaching writing—she often tells the following story:

It took me about one to three years as a new teacher to feel comfortable determining students' needs and making professional judgments about the students' skills. As I evaluated students' writing I would jot notes on legal pads as I graded the students' papers. My notes assisted me as I determined what writing skills were most essential for my students. Sometimes I had to teach the difference between *its* and *it's*. I looked for frequent errors and misunderstandings. From these legal pad lists, I developed a plan of action for the next series of mini lessons.

Determine Content Need

As writing teachers, we see patterns in student writing. Our students in our teacher education classes may think we're nuts sometimes, when we tell them

Teaching Writing in the Inclusive Classroom

that there are definite skills patterns that can determine mini lessons. However, when our teacher education students gain classroom experience, they often confide that we were right.

The writing mini lesson must always build on what the students already know and address a present need for them. Topics are determined by the students' writing, as the teacher reviews, reads, and evaluates. For example, we might realize as we read student papers that they need to learn about apostrophes or commas.

Keep Them Short

Mini lessons are generally five to twenty minutes long. Often when we teach strategies for developing mini lessons, our teacher education students and practicing teachers create lessons that become a full forty- to fifty-minute class period lesson.

Make Them Simple

It is also tempting to teach more than one writing morsel since so many of these skills are related and dependent on each other. The mini lesson format prompts writing teachers to be focused, reflective, and selective as they develop their content and instructional strategy. When teachers think reflectively about their lessons, it can lead to better teaching (Cochran-Smith & Lytle, 1993).

Mini lessons should be broken down to the barest components so that students can focus on the critical content of the lesson. For example, teaching all of the punctuation marks in one mini lesson may be too much. Teaching end mark punctuation in a mini lesson is a sufficient "chunk" to teach your student writers in a five- to twenty-minute session.

This point can't be stressed enough. We know from our classroom experiences that the first time we teach something like sentence fragments or run-ons, it won't "stick." It may take copious mini lessons for these complex concepts to stick with student writers. Think about it. How many skills are encompassed in understanding sentence fragments and run-ons?

Engage Students and Provide for Interaction

These too are important points to stress. Worksheets and exercises do not support the students' learning and retention of grammar and writing skills. There's enough research out there to back this assertion as fact. Excessive worksheets and skill and drill are not helpful. Instead, consider the students' experiences and what they already know about language. Language is all around us, and students must have opportunities to explore language actively.

In addition, use as many senses as possible as the students explore the subject of each lesson. The mini lessons provided in this volume employ the different senses at every opportunity.

Provide Practice Time

Once the students are exposed to the new skill or piece of information, they need meaningful opportunities to practice and use it. Again, this doesn't mean copious worksheets or overworking the photocopy machine. These practice and application opportunities must be designed to engage the students meaningfully.

Consider What's Next

One of our favorite questions to ask learners is this: "What did you learn and why is it important?" This question is also relevant for teachers as they consider their students and their learning. Once a mini lesson is completed, it's time to consider whether the students need even more experience and practice in that subject or if they are ready to learn another writing skill or grammatical point. Teachers may follow up with a debriefing. Or they may revisit a skill that is presented in a mini lesson, because many of these skills may need to be taught in more than one mini lesson. This may seem an obvious pedagogical point, but it is critical to the success of the writing workshop. We must remember that we need to teach the students we have, not the ones we wish were in front of us.

Get Students Comfortable

It is important to be consistent in delivering mini lessons. For many students, this is a very different teaching and learning experience from what they are accustomed to. They will need some experience with this model before they become comfortable with it. The opposite is true as well; many students have no difficulty in engaging in mini lessons.

Evaluate

The writing mini lesson is most successful when useful and relevant information is provided in the context of the students' own speaking, listening, writing, and reading experiences so they can see that their knowledge of grammar serves as a tool for producing clear and accurate communication. Exhibit 3.1 provides an evaluation form for assessing the effectiveness of a mini lesson.

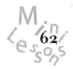

Exhibit 3.1. Mini Lessons Evaluation Form.

Mini lesson topic: _____

Mini lesson title: _____

Context: Does the lesson work as a direct response to a student need/writing concern?

Simplicity: Is the lesson simplified and does it still present the information effectively?

Practice/application: What opportunities do the students have to practice the new information or skill?

Active/engaging: Is the lesson active and engaging? What senses are you using in this lesson? How are the students actively involved in this lesson? How have you drawn the students into the lesson?

Follow-up: How did the lesson go? What did the students respond to in the lesson? What contributed to their success or frustration in this lesson? What will you need to do next? What will you need to review with the students?

Mini Lessons and Special Education Students

Mini lessons can meet the individual writing instruction needs of both special education and mainstream students. Mini lessons are especially valuable in classrooms where special education students have been mainstreamed because they allow for curriculum differentiation and the individual education plans of special education students.

By design, mini lessons are a result of a teacher's consideration of the individual needs of her students, and the instructional structure of mini lessons provides the flexibility for teachers to make changes based on their students' skill development. The Council for Exceptional Children (CEC) is an outstanding resource for both regular education and special education teachers in developing adaptations for special needs students who are mainstreamed into a regular education classroom. CEC recommends that mainstreamed students can meet the demands of this curriculum if appropriate adaptations are developed and implemented. In reference to mini lessons, special needs students can thrive in a regular education classroom when teachers recognize individual differences and create instruction where all students can meet the goals. Mini lessons allow for differences because they are a direct response to the developmental levels of students in a writing workshop setting.

Here are some general tips for writing workshop adaptations for special needs students who are mainstreamed into a regular education classroom:

1. The regular education and special education teacher need to complete a plan that will address the specific educational needs and necessary adaptations for the mainstreamed special needs students. They should be sure to communicate these adaptations to the parents, and when the adaptation is no longer needed, slowly remove it.
2. As with their regular education students, they should clearly articulate the goals and expectations for the students.
3. When creating mini lessons, teachers should incorporate Howard Gardner's theory of multiple intelligences. This volume offers many examples where more than one type of intelligence is included in the mini lesson design. It's important to do this for regular education students, but it's even more critical for special needs students.
4. Teachers can model their process in writing through think-alouds.
5. They can teach specific writing skills through mini lessons.
6. They can provide a motivating environment for writing for *all* students, including mainstreamed special needs students.
7. They can develop adaptations that encourage students to be independent learners.
8. Teachers should make sure that instructions are detailed and presented in additional modalities, other than orally. Directions must be clear and explicit.
9. They should provide multiple opportunities for students to demonstrate what they have learned.
10. Finally, it's important to be consistent in expectations for all students and support them in reaching those expectations.

In the next chapters, we present mini lessons targeted at specific skills necessary in the writing process: organization; sentence structure, punctuation, contractions, descriptive vocabulary, and more; and research.

Chapter Four

Discovering Organization

Teaching student writers how to organize their ideas is challenging. It is, perhaps, one of the greatest challenges for the writing teacher. Yet teaching students how to organize their writing is critical in developing coherence and clarity for the writer's audience. When Katie was in high school, during a time of product formulaic writing assignments, her ninth-grade English teacher would write *coherence* on her papers. She recalls:

I never understood what coherence actually meant. I thought that my writing made perfect sense. I would ask my teacher to help me with my writing and her response to me was, "You need to organize your writing better so that your reader can understand your main points." I tried to add more words, move words around, and became increasingly frustrated. My teacher didn't explain to me how to organize my writing, nor did I have opportunities to develop any writing skills that would help me to organize chunks of information into a coherent text.

When she became a writing teacher, Katie developed mini lessons that provided students with opportunities to actively chunk information so that they could organize their writing and thus develop coherence in their writing.

Developing Organizational Mini Lessons

Here are some points to consider when developing organizational mini lessons for student writers:

1. Make the lessons active and engaging.
2. Provide multiple strategies for organizing information.
3. Give students opportunities to "move" information around.
4. Make sure the mini lessons develop students' skills in outlining and organizing information *prior to* writing.
5. Incorporate multiple intelligences and design lessons so that more than one modality is applied by the students.

The mini lessons presented in this chapter are designed to help students develop their organizational skills.

Don't Spill the Topics

Don't Spill the Topics is designed to develop students' ability to focus their topics for writing and research. Students are often overwhelmed by topic selection. This mini lesson prompts them to visualize their topic and helps them narrow down a broader topic. It is also a hands-on activity that actively involves the student.

This mini lesson takes about ten minutes.

Materials

You will need sticky notes, several cups of different sizes (clear cups are especially good for this activity since it requires visualization), and pebbles, beans, seeds, or anything that can be poured and counted.

Direct the students to a table, desk, or counter where these materials are displayed. Explain to the students that you will demonstrate how to narrow a topic for writing.

Procedure

Step 1. Take the largest cup (twenty ounces is a good size) and fill it with beans. Label the cup with a topic—"Bugs," for example. Explain to the students that all of the beans in the cup represent all of the possible topics that you could write about that are related to the big topic, which is bugs. Explain that you could not possibly write about all of these topics since there must be over a hundred beans (or topics) in the cup! The next step is to narrow down the topic.

Step 2. Pour the beans from the twenty-ounce cup into the next cup (twelve ounces). Point out to the students that a good number of topics have been left behind. This new cup could be labeled this way: "Flying Bugs."

Step 3. Repeat Steps 1 and 2 by pouring the beans into the next cup (eight ounces). Again, more topics are left behind. Perhaps you can label this cup "Butterflies." Affix this label and proceed to the next cup, labeling each of them, until you reach the smallest cup (about four ounces).

Step 4. When you and the students have reached the final cup, the topic should be narrowed enough for writing.

Step 5. Review the activity with the students, using the following questions:

What happened to the beans when we poured them from cup to cup?

What did we have to do to the beans so that they could fit into the next cup?

What did we do with the leftover beans? What do the leftover beans represent?

What do the beans in the cup represent?

How can this activity help you as a writer?

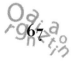

NCTE/IRA Standard

5. Students employ a wide range of strategies as they write and use different writing process elements appropriately to communicate with different audiences for a variety of purposes.

Teaching Writing in the Inclusive Classroom

Sweet Organization

Sweet Organization is an activity designed to help students develop organizational skills in their writing. Katie often finds that students need tangible models for the development of this abstract skill. Students are often overwhelmed by outlines and other organizational models. This activity engages them in a challenge that demands logic and organization. The resolution of the challenge can take many different forms, which is important for writers to witness because successful organization of ideas in writing can follow many different formats.

This activity takes about ten minutes. If the extension activities are included, it can take twenty to thirty minutes.

Materials

You will need paper lunch bags and a wide variety of prepackaged candy. For the extension activity, you will also need to make handouts (see Exhibit 4.1 and Figure 4.1). This activity also works well with items other than candy—try office supplies, pictures, or cosmetic or personal grooming items, for example.

Procedure

Step 1. Divide the students into groups of two or three. Direct them to a table, desk, or counter where several paper bags filled with a wide variety of candy await their attention. Tell the students that they are not allowed to open the bags until they are instructed to do so.

Step 2. Explain to the students that on your signal, each group is to dump the contents of their paper bag onto their table. Once the bags are emptied, the students must organize the contents in any way that they see fit as a group. They then need to give the contents of the bag a name. The students have five minutes to complete this task.

Step 3. After five minutes, ask the students to explain how they organized their paper bag contents. As the groups explain their organizational strategy, model an outline or web diagram on an overhead or chalkboard. It's important that the students observe that no two groups organized their paper bag contents in an identical manner. Discuss how this relates to writing. Prompt the students to answer questions like these: How are items emphasized in the organization that your group created? What happens if we take out _____ ? What happens to the organization? What happens if we add _____ ? What happens to the organization?

Step 4. Create a list of the students' realizations and observations about organization and outlining. To get started, ask this question: "What did you learn and why is it important?"

Step 5. The student-generated lists about organization and outlining should remain posted in the classroom. Through this activity, the students should gain a clear understanding of how to cluster ideas and information for writing.

Extension Activity

Distribute the models for a traditional outline (Exhibit 4.1) and a web diagram (Figure 4.1). Direct the students to change the organization of their paper bag contents. The idea is for the students to learn that they can organize the contents in more than one way. Once they reorganize the contents of the bag, show the sample outline and the sample web diagram. After modeling how to create both, have the students complete either the traditional outline or the web diagram so that it represents the new organization of the paper bag contents.

NCTE/IRA Standard

5. Students employ a wide range of strategies as they write and use different writing process elements appropriately to communicate with different audiences for a variety of purposes.

Exhibit 4.1. Candy: The New Brain Food: Outline.

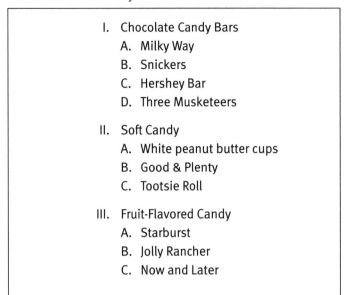

I. Chocolate Candy Bars
    A. Milky Way
    B. Snickers
    C. Hershey Bar
    D. Three Musketeers

II. Soft Candy
    A. White peanut butter cups
    B. Good & Plenty
    C. Tootsie Roll

III. Fruit-Flavored Candy
    A. Starburst
    B. Jolly Rancher
    C. Now and Later

Figure 4.1. Candy: The New Brain Food: Diagram.

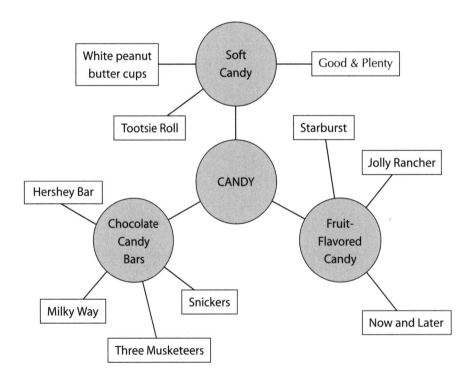

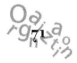

Paragraph Jigsaw

Paragraph Jigsaw is designed to develop students' knowledge of paragraph structure. This tangible model helps them recognize structural elements such as topic sentence, supporting sentences, and concluding summative paragraph sentences. Furthermore, this activity engages students in a challenge that demands logic and organizational skills. More than one organizational structure can solve a challenge, which is an important outcome for student writers to witness. Student writers need to envision multiple possibilities for their writing.

This activity takes about twenty minutes.

Materials

You will need envelopes, paper, pens or pencils, and index cards. Make an envelope for each student group that contains the sentences for one of the example paragraphs (following).

Procedure

Step 1. Divide the students into groups of three and instruct them to organize the sentence strips in the envelope into one logical paragraph. Instruct the students that they have five minutes to complete the task.

Step 2. When the five minutes are up, ask the students to explain how they organized their sentences. As the groups explain their organization strategy, write their answers on an overhead, chalkboard, or large sheet of paper. Here are some sample questions for the large-group discussion:

How do you know that the sentences should be in this order?

What sentence (the topic sentence) indicates to the reader the content of the paragraph?

What does the last sentence of the paragraph indicate? What information is included in this sentence?

How do you know that this is a paragraph?

What should a good paragraph contain?

The large-group discussion should be limited to ten minutes.

Step 3. Instruct the students to revise the paragraphs so that they are in their own words and contain more details and illustrations.

Step 4. Have students share their paragraphs with their classmates.

Example Paragraphs

Here are some sample paragraphs that can be used for this activity. The sentences are in order; cut them and mount them individually on index cards and place them unsorted into the paper bags.

Copyright © 2007 by John Wiley & Sons, Inc.

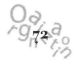

Example Paragraph 1

The Sun's activity influences the heliopause, a region of space that astronomers believe marks the boundary between the solar system and interstellar space.

The heliopause is a dynamic region that expands and contracts due to the constantly changing speed and pressure of the solar wind.

In November 2003 a team of astronomers reported that the spacecraft *Voyager 1* appeared to have encountered the outskirts of the heliopause at about 86 astronomical units (AUs), or 149,598,000,000 meters, from the Sun.

The astronomers based their report on data that indicated the solar wind had slowed from 1.1 million km/h (700,000 mph) to 160,000 km/h (100,000 mph).

This finding is consistent with the theory that when the solar wind meets interstellar space at a turbulent zone known as the termination shock boundary, it will slow abruptly.

However, another team of astronomers disputed the finding, saying that the spacecraft had neared but had not yet reached the heliopause.

Example Paragraph 2

A tornado becomes visible when a condensation funnel made of water vapor (a funnel cloud) forms in extreme low pressures, or when the tornado lofts dust, dirt, and debris upward from the ground.

A mature tornado may be columnar or tilted, narrow or broad—sometimes so broad that it appears as if the parent thundercloud itself had descended to ground level.

Some tornadoes resemble a swaying elephant's trunk.

Others, especially very violent ones, may break into several intense suction vortices—intense swirling masses of air—each of which rotates near the parent tornado.

A suction vortex may be only a few meters in diameter, and thus can destroy one house while leaving a neighboring house relatively unscathed.

NCTE/IRA Standard

5. Students employ a wide range of strategies as they write and use different writing process elements appropriately to communicate with different audiences for a variety of purposes.

Persuading Paragraphs

Persuading Paragraphs is designed to introduce persuasive writing elements through the contemporary genre of advertising. While working collaboratively, students identify and list characteristics of persuasive writing. This lesson was developed by Katie when she was teaching a tenth-grade English class about ten years ago. The infamous five-paragraph essay (see Chapter One) was an essential part of the curriculum, and the students had to successfully demonstrate on the state writing examination that they mastered persuasive writing skills.

The concept of persuasive writing is challenging for student writers to master. Students need a tangible connection rather than the more abstract literature-based examples that most are given in English class. Concrete examples, like advertisements, can facilitate their understanding of the persuasive writing concept. We have always found that more direct and concrete examples help student writers conceptualize the skills we are teaching. This lesson is particularly good for visual learners, as shown by the following example taken from Katie's class.

Lavita, who had been diagnosed with a learning disability, was assigned to Katie's "regular" tenth-grade English class. Lavita struggled when she was given persuasive writing prompts like "Explain why Huck Finn is a moral character." It was difficult for her to make connections between her writing and what she had already learned about Huck Finn.

One of Lavita's many talents was that she was a beautiful artist. Katie felt that there must be some way to connect Lavita's keen ability to express herself through visual art and her writing. As she flipped through some teen magazines one day, it hit her: she could take the visual images in advertisements and connect them to persuasive writing. In the advertisements and visual images, Lavita observed how these ads tried to convince her to buy certain products or services. She commented, "You know these ads are just word pictures. Word pictures have text, they just don't use actual words."

When Katie pioneered this lesson in that class over ten years ago, Lavita clearly picked up on the persuasive elements of the images that she observed in the advertisements. It was the first time that Katie was able to see some improvement in her writing. When she asked Lavita about the images and the persuasive paragraph that she wrote as a result of this mini lesson, she said, "I could see the words. That's why this was easier to do than the last one" (the previous essay assigned).

This activity takes about twenty to twenty-five minutes.

Materials

You will need chart paper, markers, magazine or other print advertisements, entrance slips (make handouts from Exhibit 4.2), and an envelope for each group. Each envelope will contain one or two print advertisements that you have selected from magazines or other print media and another handout (made from Exhibit 4.3). You will also need a projector and a transparency (made from Figure 4.2).

Procedure

Step 1. When the students enter the classroom, give them five minutes to complete the entrance slip (Exhibit 4.2). Discuss their answers in a whole-class discussion and record them on chart paper.

Step 2. Divide the class into groups of three to five students. Use the responses to Step 1 as a guide for analyzing the advertisements. Then, hand each group an envelope. Have the students work in their groups to analyze the ad or ads contained in their envelope and discuss the questions shown on the Exhibit 4.3 handout. Next, have students create a web diagram based on their analysis of the advertisement and questions. Show them Figure 4.2 as an example. This step should take about fifteen minutes.

Step 3. Discuss the characteristics of persuasive paragraphs and post the students' web diagrams in the classroom.

Exhibit 4.2. Persuading Paragraphs Handout: Entrance Slip.

Name: _____ Date: _____

Directions: Respond to the following questions:

1. What do you think the word "persuade" means?

2. If you want to persuade someone to do something, what strategies do you use? For example, let's say that your curfew on Saturday night is 8 o'clock. How would you convince your parent or guardian to change your curfew to 9 o'clock?

Exhibit 4.3. Persuading Paragraphs Handout:
Directions for Group Exercise Envelopes.

Directions: Examine the advertisement(s) in this envelope.
Discuss and answer the following questions:

1. Identify the product or service being advertised. In other words, what do the creators of the ad(s) want you to buy and/or use?

2. Describe the images that are in the advertisement(s). How are they related to the advertised product(s)?

3. What does the text (writing) say about the product(s)? What do the advertisers want you to know?

4. How is the advertiser trying to convince you that you should try the product or products?

Discovering Organization

Figure 4.2. Persuading Paragraphs Transparency: Web Diagram.

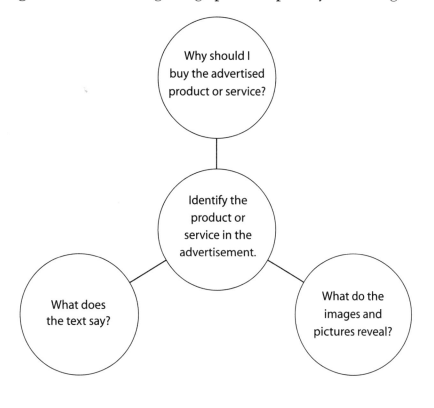

NCTE/IRA Standards

6. Students apply knowledge of language structure, language conventions (e.g., spelling and punctuation), media techniques, figurative language, and genre to create, critique, and discuss print and nonprint texts.

12. Students use spoken, written, and visual language to accomplish their own purposes (e.g., for learning, enjoyment, persuasion, and the exchange of information).

Teaching Writing in the Inclusive Classroom

Beginning-Middle-End

In a nutshell, all writing has a beginning, a middle, and an end. It sounds pretty simple, but student writers need to understand this basic aspect of good writing. This lesson is designed to teach this basic organizational skill. The kinesthetic and group elements of this lesson support a variety of learning styles.

This lesson takes ten to fifteen minutes.

Materials

Gather a week's worth of cartoons from five different series. Make two copies of each set of cartoons. Save one copy as an answer key and cut up the other copy into its individual components. Put the cut-up strips into envelopes. Each cartoon series should be in a different envelope.

Procedure

Step 1. Divide the class into groups of about three to four students. Each group should have one of the prepared envelopes that contain one series of cut-up cartoon strips. Each group should have a different series.

Step 2. Direct the students to put the sections of the cut-up cartoons that are in their envelopes into proper order: beginning, middle, end. Offer these clues to help them sort the pieces:

- Look for transition words, such as "then," "later," "finally," "consequently."
- Pay attention to time of day (morning, afternoon, evening) or season (winter, spring, summer, fall).
- Check the sequence of events in the cartoon.

Step 3. Once the groups have put their cartoons in sequence, have them check their organization of the pieces against the answer key, which shows the original strip in its entirety. The groups of students can then exchange envelopes and organize another series of cartoons for more practice in organizing beginning, middle, and end sequences.

NCTE/IRA Standards

4. Students adjust their use of spoken, written, and visual language (e.g., conventions, style, vocabulary) to communicate effectively with a variety of audiences and for different purposes.

5. Students employ a wide range of strategies as they write and use different writing process elements appropriately to communicate with different audiences for a variety of purposes.

Fitting the Pieces Together

This is another lesson to teach students how to manipulate text and organize it so that it is logical and follows a beginning, middle, end sequence.

This activity takes ten to fifteen minutes.

Materials

In preparation for this lesson, select short stories and cut them into sections. Choose a different story for each group. Keep an extra, intact copy of the stories as an answer key, so the students can check their organization once it is complete. Put a different cut-up story into an envelope for each group.

Procedure

Step 1. Review the elements of story structure and how writing is organized. (Stories have a beginning, middle, and end. Stories contain details that help the reader "see" the story. Authors use transition words.)

Step 2. Divide the students into groups of three to four students and distribute the cut-up story envelopes. Direct the students to arrange the pieces so that they form organized stories.

Step 3. Have the students check their story organization against the answer key. Discuss as a whole group the strategies the students used to organize their stories and how they can relate this exercise to help organize their own writing.

NCTE/IRA Standards

4. Students adjust their use of spoken, written, and visual language (e.g., conventions, style, vocabulary) to communicate effectively with a variety of audiences and for different purposes.

5. Students employ a wide range of strategies as they write and use different writing process elements appropriately to communicate with different audiences for a variety of purposes.

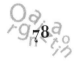

Situation-Problem-Solution

This lesson teaches students sequencing in writing. All pieces of writing present a situation, a problem, and then a solution. By breaking this organizational idea into the smallest increments possible, it has been Katie's experience that students are better able to conceptualize this organizational model.

This lesson takes about ten minutes. The extension activity adds another fifteen minutes.

Materials

Before the lesson, make copies of Exhibit 4.4 for each group. It is helpful to print each group's copy on paper of a different color; this makes it easier to sort the pieces after the lesson. Therefore, depending on how many groups you have, make a set for each group. Put the squares that were cut up from the handout and place them into envelopes.

Procedure

Step 1. Explain to your students that writers often focus on a situation, problem, and solution when they are organizing their ideas. Offer a few examples, such as the following:

Situation	Problem	Solution
I was standing at the bus stop.	When the bus arrived, I realized that I didn't have enough money.	The sweet little old lady smiled and handed me a quarter.
My book report is due tomorrow.	I didn't finish my book.	I stay up late, finish the book, and write my report.
My dog loves to run.	I couldn't keep up with my dog when I took him for a run.	I bought a longer leash and roller skates so I could keep up with my dog.
I ate a huge bean burrito.	It made me sick to my stomach.	I took some antacid.

Step 2. Divide the class into groups (we suggest groups of only two students, if possible). Give each group an envelope that contains the cut-up squares from Handout 1. Direct the students to group the squares into ten different situation-problem-solution sequences.

Step 3. Review the answers with the students and discuss how they organized their sequences. What words or structures offered clues for the sequences?

Extension Activity

Give the students blank squares (see Exhibit 4.5) and ask them to create their own situation-problem-solution sequences. The students can then exchange their sequences and put together the sequences of the other group.

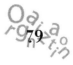

Exhibit 4.4. Situation-Problem-Solution: Handout 1.

Directions: Cut out the individual squares and put into envelopes for each group of students.

Situation	Problem	Solution
I wanted to become a member of the swimming team.	My times weren't fast enough to qualify.	I practiced, improved my times, and qualified the following year.
I ate a huge piece of cake.	My stomach hurt because it was so full.	I took a walk and it made me feel better.
My sister always goes into my room.	My sister messes up my room.	I put a lock on the door to my room.
I wanted to go onto the Internet.	My computer wouldn't start.	I checked the wires and plugged in my computer.
My paper is due on Friday.	I didn't start to write it.	I begged my teacher for an extension until Monday.
I wanted to make chocolate chip cookies.	I didn't have any chocolate chips.	I used cocoa instead and made chocolate cookies.
I entered the store to buy a present for my friend.	I didn't have enough money to buy the present that I wanted to get.	I left the store and bought a different present at a different store.
I love to take vacations.	I couldn't get time off from work.	I took a mini vacation on the weekend.
The grass was overgrown.	My lawn mower was broken.	I borrowed my neighbor's lawn mower and cut the grass.
I love to write.	I never have enough time to write.	I rearranged my schedule so I can now write an hour each day.

Teaching Writing in the Inclusive Classroom

Exhibit 4.5. Situation-Problem-Solution: Handout 2.

Directions: Write a situation, problem, and solution for each sequence set of squares. Once you have written all of your sequences, cut them out and exchange them with another group. After exchanging squares, organize the other group's sequence squares.

Situation	Problem	Solution
Situation	Problem	Solution
Situation	Problem	Solution
Situation	Problem	Solution

NCTE/IRA Standards

4. Students adjust their use of spoken, written, and visual language (e.g., conventions, style, vocabulary) to communicate effectively with a variety of audiences and for different purposes.

5. Students employ a wide range of strategies as they write and use different writing process elements appropriately to communicate with different audiences for a variety of purposes.

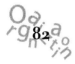

Thesis Statements and Organizing Ideas

Using Dr. Seuss's *Horton Hears a Who,* this lesson was originally developed by Katie's student teacher, Rachel Jarosik.

This lesson can last about thirty minutes or it can be broken into two mini lessons of about fifteen minutes each.

Materials

Get a copy of *Horton Hears a Who* and make copies of the accompanying handouts. Cut Handout 1 (Exhibit 4.6) into strips and place the strips into envelopes, making sure to have enough envelopes for each group of students. We suggest dividing the students into groups of two and making a set for each pair of students.

Procedure

Step 1. Read *Horton Hears a Who* to the class. Afterward, ask them about the ideas and themes raised in the book. One of the major themes is *diversity.*

Step 2. Explain to the students that a thesis statement is a short statement of what you are trying to argue or prove in a piece of writing. Ask the students to write a thesis statement about *Horton Hears a Who.* The following are two possible statements:

In *Horton Hears a Who* Dr. Seuss teaches the importance of respecting diversity.

In *Horton Hears a Who* Dr. Seuss argues that by recognizing commonalities, diverse cultures can bond together.

Here are some examples of poor thesis statements:

Dr. Seuss digs diversity in *Horton Hears a Who.* (This is too broad and uses slang.)

In *Horton Hears a Who* recognizing commonalities and diversities. (This is an incomplete sentence.)

Remind your students that thesis statements must be complete sentences.

Step 3. Once you have discussed thesis statements with the class, discuss the elements of a working outline.

In a working outline, the major points that the writer is discussing should be the major headings.

Minor points and supporting details should be minor headings and subpoints.

When developing their working outlines, tell the students to ask themselves the following questions:

- Are the headings essential to proving my thesis statement?
- Do the minor headings and subpoints contain more specific and detailed information than the major headings?

Step 4. Take time to practice with the working outline. Have students arrange statements into a working outline. Take the copies of the cut-up statements from Handout 1, which you have already placed into envelopes, and give one set (one envelope) to each pair of students. The students should organize the statement strips and then place them on the working outline form shown in Exhibit 4.7.

Step 5. Have the students check their organization of the statement strips against Exhibit 4.8 (the answer key).

Step 6. In a large group, discuss how the students organized their statement strips in the working outline.

Exhibit 4.6. Thesis Statements and Organizing Ideas: Handout 1.

Directions: Cut out these statement strips (shown out of sequence here) and put them into envelopes for each pair of students.

Animals of the Jungle of Nool and the Whos have different characteristics.
Horton promises to protect his friends the Whos, no matter what the jungle animals do.
The animals of the jungle are much bigger than the Whos.
The bird drops the Who clover into a field of clovers.
The Whos face dangers by the animals of the jungle who do not recognize their existence.
Horton hears a noise from a speck of dust.
Horton recognizes the Who culture and builds a relationship based on their commonalities.
The doubting monkeys steal the clover where Horton has placed the Whos.
Horton defends the existence of the Whos to the other animals of the jungle.

Teaching Writing in the Inclusive Classroom

Horton builds a relationship with the Whos based on common characteristics, not differences.
Horton repeatedly says, "A person is a person, no matter how small."
The Whos live in a city as opposed to a jungle.
Horton recognizes that the Who culture exists.
Horton rescues the Who clover from the field.
The animals of the Jungle of Nool recognize that the Whos exist when they shout loud enough for the jungle animals to hear them.

Exhibit 4.7. Thesis Statements and Organizing Ideas: Handout 2.

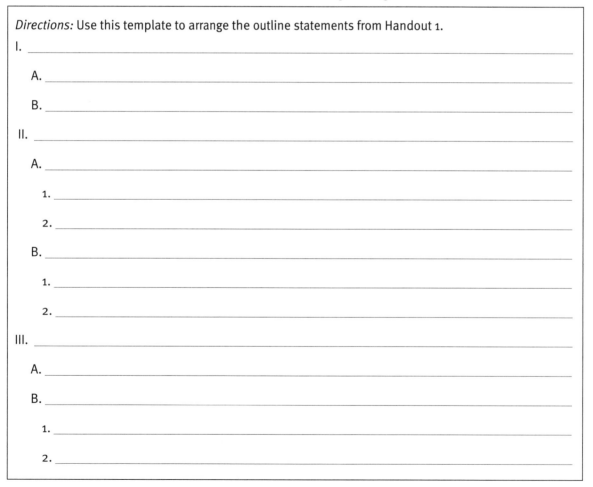

Directions: Use this template to arrange the outline statements from Handout 1.

I. _____

   A. _____

   B. _____

II. _____

   A. _____

      1. _____

      2. _____

   B. _____

      1. _____

      2. _____

III. _____

   A. _____

   B. _____

      1. _____

      2. _____

Copyright © 2007 by John Wiley & Sons, Inc.

Exhibit 4.8. Thesis Statements and Organizing Ideas:
Handout 3: Answer Key.

I. Horton hears a noise from a speck of dust.
    A. Horton recognizes that the Who culture exists.
    B. Horton recognizes the Who culture and builds a relationship based on commonalities.

II. Animals of the Jungle of Nool and the Whos have different characteristics.
    A. Horton repeatedly says, "A person is a person, no matter how small."
        1. The animals of the jungle are much bigger than the Whos.
        2. The Whos live in a city as opposed to a jungle.
    B. Horton builds a relationship with the Whos based on common characteristics, not differences.
        1. The Whos face dangers by the animals of the jungle who do not recognize their existence.
        2. Horton defends the existence of the Whos to the other animals of the jungle.

III. Horton promises to protect his friends the Whos, no matter what the jungle animals do.
    A. The doubting monkeys steal the clover where Horton has placed the Whos.
    B. The bird drops the Who clover into a field of clovers.
        1. Horton rescues the Who clover from the field.
        2. The animals of the Jungle of Nool recognize that the Whos exist when they shout loud enough for the jungle animals to hear them.

NCTE/IRA Standards

5. Students eploy a wide range of strategies as they write and use different writing process elements appropriately to communicate with different audiences for a variety of purposes.

7. Students conduct research on issues and interests by generating ideas and questions, and by posing problems. They gather, evaluate, and synthesize data from a variety of sources (e.g., print and nonprint texts, artifacts, people) to communicate their discoveries in ways that suit their purpose and audience.

12. Students use spoken, written, and visual language to accomplish their own purposes (e.g., for learning, enjoyment, persuasion, and the exchange of information).

Checking It All Out

Editing is one of the most challenging skills for students to learn in the writing process. As a result, Katie developed this checklist for her students to help them develop editing skills for their writing.

This lesson takes about fifteen minutes; it can be longer, depending on the length of the texts that the students are editing.

Materials

Students will need a completed writing assignment that they have not yet handed in. You will also need a piece of your own writing that you would like to share with your students and an overhead projector. Modeling how to use the checklist is an important aspect of this lesson.

Procedure

Step 1. Display your piece of writing on an overhead. Go through the checklist with the students, while editing your own work.

Step 2. After you've modeled your own editing process, explain to the students that they must complete the checklist before the final submission of their work.

Exhibit 4.9. Editor's Checklist.

Name: _____ Date: _____

Project: _____

Directions: Carefully check your writing against this checklist.

☐ My work has an interesting and exciting beginning that draws readers into the story.

☐ There is a defined middle to my work.

☐ My work has an ending or conclusion that satisfies the writing.

☐ I used capitalization rules correctly in my writing.

☐ I used punctuation rules correctly in my writing.

☐ I checked my work for correct spelling.

☐ I checked my work for correct word usage.

☐ I looked for clear sentences in my writing.

☐ I checked all the sentences to make sure they are complete and not run-ons.

☐ I checked to make sure all the paragraphs are formed correctly.

☐ I checked my writing to make sure that it makes sense.

☐ I reread my writing, checking for all kinds of errors.

☐ My work is ready to be submitted to my teacher.

NCTE/IRA Standards

4. Students adjust their use of spoken, written, and visual language (e.g., conventions, style, vocabulary) to communicate effectively with a variety of audiences and for different purposes.

5. Students employ a wide range of strategies as they write and use different writing process elements appropriately to communicate with different audiences for a variety of purposes.

Chapter Five

Learning the Little Stuff

Sentence Structure, Punctuation, Contractions, Descriptive Vocabulary, and More

Many years ago when we entered teaching, literacy educators debated the instructional strategies that would best teach grammar in context. The work of Hillocks (Hillocks, 1986; Hillocks & Shulman, 1999) had established that grammar must be taught in the context of students' writing. To teach grammar through endless drills and worksheets was not effective—students did not transfer their knowledge of grammar to their own writing when it was taken out of context. It's a solid argument that has been further supported by many research studies. Teaching grammar in the context of student writing made sense, but the void in this new instructional approach was a lack of viable models. This is especially critical in classrooms where special education students have been mainstreamed. We will address this later, but first let's look at some of the current thinking about teaching writing and grammar in context.

Several well-known writing teachers offer models and ideas for teaching writing and grammar in context. Two of these gurus are Nancie Atwell (1998) and Constance Weaver (1996). Both have suggested that writing teachers use mini lessons as an instructional strategy for teaching grammar. As new teachers we thought that this made sense, but neither of us had models or lessons in hand when we entered our classrooms.

For the past fifteen years the two of us have created mini lessons for our writing programs. In this chapter we offer some suggestions that are specific to grammar mini lessons. Remember, it is the active nature of mini lessons—the hands-on practice—that promotes retention of the newly introduced skills.

In many ways, teaching grammar consists of some abstract components that are challenging for even the most adept student writer. Yet in our teaching experience, we found it to be particularly critical for special education students. Believe it or not, we borrowed from current math education models that promote manipulatives for abstract concepts to teach grammatical concepts. Like many math problems, grammatical structure can be abstract for the student writer.

As educators, we are of course familiar with Howard Gardner's theory of multiple intelligences (1983, 1984), yet we sometimes found it difficult to integrate kinesthetic experiences in grammar teaching. The lessons that are contained in this chapter rely heavily on the integration/employment of multiple intelligences. These kinds of experiences support *all learners,* not just special education students. However, as we taught the grammar lessons that are contained in this chapter, we soon realized how much they aided our special education students in our mainstreamed classrooms.

Developing Grammar Mini Lessons

Ask Yourself

What do my students already know about grammar? Take a needs assessment of what your students already know and understand about grammar. It is also a great idea to take a needs assessment of the *kinds* of learners in your classroom. These lessons are designed to engage multiple intelligences for all learners.

Scaffold

Although a mini lesson should arise from student needs, you may have to backtrack in order to build up to the grammatical concept that your writers may need. For example, if the students' writing is filled with run-ons and sentence fragments, it's likely that they need a few mini lessons on phrases and clauses before you offer strategies for identifying and revising run-ons and fragments. Similarly, maybe your students need to go back and revisit nouns before they learn when to capitalize proper nouns.

Identify and Practice

If there are specific rules for a grammar issue, identify them with the students' input. Develop a list of very specific criteria and rules and then give them opportunities to practice. Of course, when we say practice we never mean copious

Teaching Writing in the Inclusive Classroom

worksheets. Instead, we mean that the students should be given copious opportunities to apply what they have learned about grammar.

Follow Up

As we already discussed in earlier chapters, the conclusion of the mini lesson should always consider follow-up—that is, what's next. This may mean a follow-up exercise, as shown in some of the mini lessons included here, or another mini lesson entirely, because some of the skills will need to be taught more than once. Many grammatical concepts are challenging for students to grasp. This is why it's necessary to provide ample practice and follow-up. You'll find that most of the lessons we provide in this volume conclude with whole-group discussions. These discussions give students the opportunity to discuss what they already know, what they have learned, and what is still challenging for them. As educators, we know that learners are more likely to retain information and newly learned concepts if they are given opportunities to reflect on what they've learned (Daniels & Bizar, 2005; Hillocks, 1995). In addition to being an important metacognitive strategy, these discussions also serve as an assessment tool for the teacher.

Knowing Nouns and Venturing About Verbs

Knowing Nouns and Venturing About Verbs is an exercise designed to develop students' innate understanding of nouns and verbs. Katie developed this lesson and often uses it to determine what her students already know about grammar, and more specifically, the parts of speech. Definitions such as "A noun is a person, place, or thing" are not very helpful for student writers. Far better is when the students can articulate *how* nouns, verbs, and other parts of speech work in the language. This hands-on lesson actively engages the students as they build on their understanding of nouns.

In this lesson, students articulate their reasons for identifying nouns as nouns. For example, they may develop rules such as the following: *Most nouns can be turned into plurals by adding "s" or "es" at the end. A noun can have "a," "an," or "the" in front of it.* (The latter definition can be a great introduction to articles in addition to determining noun rules.)

Usually, through class discussion, we come up with five or six rules like these by the end of the lesson. Thus, we prompt the students to examine the ways in which language works and how we use it to express ideas. This gives them a far more specific understanding than when they merely regurgitate the familiar definitions. Student writers can tell us a ton about language if we provide them with opportunities to do so, and from there, they can build on their previous knowledge about language.

This activity takes about ten minutes.

Materials

You will need poster paper or large sticky notes, markers, and envelopes. Before you begin, make photocopies of Exhibit 5.1. Cut the words contained in the exhibit into individual strips and put them in envelopes. There should be one envelope for every group of three to five students, and each envelope should include all of the words contained in the exhibit. Write the following directions on the outside of each envelope: *Dump the contents of this envelope onto a desk, and based on what you already know about the parts of speech, divide these words into two separate groups: nouns and verbs.*

Procedure

Step 1. Divide the students into groups of three to five. Give each group one envelope.

Step 2. Direct the students to read and follow the directions on the outside of the envelope.

Step 3. Repeat the directions verbally. Tell students to divide the words into two groups: nouns and verbs.

Step 4. Circulate among the groups and monitor the students' progress. Ask students, "How did you divide the words?" Encourage the students to articulate *why* they divided the words as they did. Ask the students to label each list. The students may develop labels like: nouns and verbs, nonaction words and action words, or things and moving words. All of these are fine, because they will trigger a discussion about what makes a noun a noun and what makes a verb a verb.

Teaching Writing in the Inclusive Classroom

Step 5. Once the students have divided their words, distribute poster paper and markers. Instruct the students to write down the group's reasons for dividing the words as they chose. This should take about five minutes.

Step 6. Conduct a whole-group discussion about the students' lists and create a combined class list that identifies the characteristics of nouns and verbs.

Exhibit 5.1. Knowing Nouns and Venturing About Verbs Handout.

book	birthday cake	answered
walking	ran	flower
computer	music	drove
sings	cutting	oregano
pencil	sandwich	sent
played	growing	paper clip
video game	homework	wrote
cooking	cleaning	box
map	envelope	listening
prepared	painted	refrigerator
studied	compact disk	hears
sports car	questioned	house
leaped	concert	jumped
milkshake		

NCTE/IRA Standard

6. Students apply knowledge of language structure, language conventions (e.g., spelling and punctuation), media techniques, figurative language, and genre to create, critique, and discuss print and nonprint texts.

I'm Just Acting!

I'm Just Acting is an exercise designed to develop students' understanding of subjects and actions in sentence structure. This lesson builds on the students' innate understanding of the parts of speech.

This is a simple activity that takes from five to fifteen minutes.

Materials

You will need index cards or scratch paper.

Procedure

Step 1. Divide your students into two groups.

Step 2. Direct Group 1 to write the name of a person. They can write an actual name, like "Katie" or "Terrence." They can also use a descriptor, like "firefighter" or "rock star." Remind the students that these are the *subjects* for the activity. Ask Group 2 to describe an action on their paper. Some examples might be "jumping" or "think."

Step 3. Collect the cards or papers and put them in two piles. Tell the students that the two piles are titled: "Actor" and "Action."

Step 4. Ask for a volunteer to come up to the front of the classroom and choose a card or paper from each pile. As the actor, this student will perform the action for the class.

Step 5. Conduct a whole-group discussion about the students' two piles of words and create a combined class list that identifies the characteristics of these words.

NCTE/IRA Standards

5. Students employ a wide range of strategies as they write and use different writing process elements appropriately to communicate with different audiences for a variety of purposes.

6. Students apply knowledge of language structure, language conventions (e.g., spelling and punctuation), media techniques, figurative language, and genre to create, critique, and discuss print and nonprint texts.

Postcards from the Past

Postcards from the Past is a mini lesson designed to develop students' understanding of time in their writing. This lesson builds on their innate understanding of verbs in determining time. Verbs are not only action words—they are also time determiners. In this case, they describe past actions.

This activity takes about fifteen to twenty minutes.

Material

You will need postcards with pictures of various tourist destinations, poster paper, and markers.

Procedure

Step 1. Begin a discussion about postcards. Ask the students why people send postcards. What do people write on postcards? Model a postcard that you have written to someone. Then distribute postcards and invite the students to think about the picture on theirs. Ask the students to pretend they've visited the site on the picture and ask them to describe what they did there to a friend at home.

Step 2. Give the students about five minutes to write their postcards.

Step 3. Collect the postcards so you can read some aloud, or read them together in class. Once you have read three or so postcards, ask the students to write down the verbs—or action words—or time determiners. Then read a few more postcards.

Step 4. Ask the students to share their list of verbs and compile a class list. A pattern will form that will be dominated by verbs in the past tense.

Step 5. Conduct a whole-group discussion about past tense verbs and how these words are time determiners.

NCTE/IRA Standards

5. Students employ a wide range of strategies as they write and use different writing process elements appropriately to communicate with different audiences for a variety of purposes.

6. Students apply knowledge of language structure, language conventions (e.g., spelling and punctuation), media techniques, figurative language, and genre to create, critique, and discuss print and nonprint texts.

It's Happening—Right Now!

This is another exercise designed to develop students' understanding of time in their writing. It too builds on the students' innate understanding of verbs in determining time in writing. Again, verbs are not only action words—they are also time determiners. In this case, they describe current events.

This exercise takes about fifteen to twenty minutes.

Materials

You will need paper, pens or pencils, a television, and a video segment from a sporting event.

Procedure

Step 1. Ask your students, "Have you ever noticed that sportscasters on the news often describe the action of the sporting event in the present tense?" Tell your students that you are going to have them view a recent sportscast. Tell them to think about the following as they watch:

How does the sportscaster make you feel as if you are at the event, watching it?

What words stand out as you view and listen to the sporting event?

When does this event take place? Right now? Earlier? Or in the future?

Have them watch the sportscast.

Step 2. Once the students have completed the viewing, discuss the language of the sportscaster and invite the students to identify the verbs, or action words, that stood out. Record the students' responses on a large sheet of paper so they can be displayed in the classroom as a reminder of present tense verbs. Students may come up with words such as *runs, shoots, blocks, delights, scores, makes contact, misses, contacts,* and *rebounds.* These words reveal that the students understand verbs as action words and also as time determiners.

Extension Activities

Invite the students to put the sportscast into another tense—the past or future. How does this affect the time and mood of the sportscast? Conduct a whole-group discussion about past tense verbs and how these words are time determiners.

NCTE/IRA Standards

5. Students employ a wide range of strategies as they write and use different writing process elements appropriately to communicate with different audiences for a variety of purposes.

6. Students apply knowledge of language structure, language conventions (e.g., spelling and punctuation), media techniques, figurative language, and genre to create, critique, and discuss print and nonprint texts.

Teaching Writing in the Inclusive Classroom

Looking into the Future

This is another exercise designed to develop students' understanding of time and action words, or verbs, in their writing. This lesson too builds on the students' innate understanding of verbs in determining time in writing. Verbs are not only action words—they are also time determiners. In this case, they are future tense verbs.

This exercise generally takes from fifteen to twenty minutes.

Materials

You will need to provide copies of horoscopes from such sources as newspapers or magazines. Or assign your students ahead of time to bring these into class.

Procedure

Step 1. Read some sample horoscopes in class and ask the students the following questions: What words indicate that these events will happen in the future? What do these words have in common? What would happen to this horoscope if we put it into the past tense or the present tense?

Step 2. Divide the class into groups of three to four students. Hand out copies of horoscopes, or have students take out those they've brought to class. Direct each student to read one of these horoscopes and identify the verbs it contains that indicate the future.

Step 3. Once each group has compiled a list, have them share their answers with the rest of the class.

NCTE/IRA Standards

5. Students employ a wide range of strategies as they write and use different writing process elements appropriately to communicate with different audiences for a variety of purposes.

6. Students apply knowledge of language structure, language conventions (e.g., spelling and punctuation), media techniques, figurative language, and genre to create, critique, and discuss print and nonprint texts.

Who? What? A World Without Pronouns

This exercise is designed to help students understand the purposes of pronouns in writing. The students will articulate their reasons for using pronouns in writing. Again, this lesson builds on their innate understanding of the parts of speech.

This activity generally takes about ten minutes.

Materials

You will need sheets of paper or large sticky notes, markers, and envelopes containing text samples with some words, including pronouns, missing. Choose samples from literature that your students have read. On the envelopes, write the following directions: *Read the enclosed passage and fill in the blank spaces with words of your choice.*

Procedure

Step 1. Divide the students into groups of three to five.

Step 2. Instruct the students to read and follow the directions on the outside of the envelope.

Step 3. Give the students about five minutes to read the passage and write words in the blank spaces.

Step 4. Once the students have completed the passage, ask them the following questions about the words that they chose to complete the passage: What words did you use? What do these words have in common?

Step 5. Conduct a whole-group discussion about what the students wrote, and create a combined class list that identifies the characteristics of the parts of speech that they used to complete the passage. Put particular emphasis on pronouns.

NCTE/IRA Standard

6. Students apply knowledge of language structure, language conventions (e.g., spelling and punctuation), media techniques, figurative language, and genre to create, critique, and discuss print and nonprint texts.

Dance, FANBOYS, Dance!

Who are the FANBOYS? *For, And, Nor, But, Or, Yet, So.*

Probably one of the most challenging concepts to teach is that of the complete sentence. Students need many opportunities to learn how to avoid run-ons and sentence fragments.

This lesson was adapted from one that Seth D. Watkins, a student in the master of arts in teaching program, created to teach a group of inner-city middle school students about the role conjunctions play in creating a complete sentence; we've included it here with his permission. During an observation of the lesson in action, Katie saw that the students really seemed to develop an understanding of run-ons, fragments, clauses, phrases, and conjunctions. The lesson is interactive, visual, and kinesthetic.

This is a mini lesson in two parts. The first part takes about ten minutes; the second about twenty. The segments may be taught in two separate class periods.

Materials

You will need two sheets of 8½ x 11-inch red construction paper, two sheets of 8½ x 11-inch blue construction paper, ten sheets of 8½ x 11-inch green construction paper, and two sheets of 8½ x 11-inch white construction paper.

Preparation

On the two sheets of red construction paper write a large *P* (for predicate). On the two sheets of blue construction paper write a large *S* (for subject). On the green sheets of construction paper write one word each: *For, Nor, But, Or, Yet, So.* Write *And* on the remaining green sheets. Cut the sheets of white paper in half. Make a large period on one piece and put large commas on the remaining three.

Procedure: Segment 1: Review Parts of the Sentence

Step 1. Review with the students the following parts of speech: subject, predicate, conjunction. The following key (Exhibit 5.2) should be put on the board so students can refer back to it during the activity.

Exhibit 5.2. Parts of Speech: Subject, Predicate, Conjunction.

Term	Definition	Symbol
Subject	Actor (everything to the left of the verb)	S
Predicate	Action (everything to the right of the verb)	P
Sentence	A subject and predicate	S + P
Conjunction	Glue word	conj.
Compound sentence	Two sentences combined with a glue word	(S + P) conj. (S + P)
Compound subject	Two subjects linked with a glue word and a predicate	S conj. (S + P)
Compound predicate	One subject and two predicates linked with a glue word	(S + P) conj. P

Remind the students that when there is a compound sentence, a comma goes before a FANBOY conjunction. When there is a compound predicate or subject, the conjunction does-n't need a comma before it. Color-coded examples on the board help students understand what is going to happen next.

Here are some examples (note that we've used single, double, and dotted underlines rather than colors, which aren't available in this black-and-white volume):

Mr. Watkins jumps.	S + P
Mr. Watkins jumps around the room.	S + P
Mr. Watkins jumps around the room, and he acts silly.	(S + P) conj. (S + P).
Mr. Watkins and the students jump around the room.	S conj. (S + P).
Mr. Watkins jumps around the room and acts silly.	(S + P) conj. P.

As a tool for students to understand whether a word or phrase is a subject or predicate, they can use "That Darned Do" (otherwise known as the "Dummy Do"). If the word or phrase can answer "Who or what did it?" then it is a subject. If the word or phrase can answer "What was done?" then it is a predicate.

Procedure: Segment 2: Putting It into Practice

Step 1. Modeling. Give the students a very simple sentence such as this: "Mr. Watkins jumps." Write the sentence on the board and have them say which part is the subject and which is the predicate. State the subject ("Mr. Watkins," or your name) and point to yourself, then say the predicate ("jumps") and proceed to jump up and down.

Wait for the laughter (and groans) to die down.

Take out one subject and one predicate paper. Show the students how the subject and predicate (S + P) take the structure of the sentence you've just presented. Ask the students what punctuation is needed and hold the papers in proper order for all the students to see. (Blue subject, red predicate, white period.)

Step 2. Students get in the act. Before beginning, set the ground rules of this game, because students are going to make their own sentences. For example: No making anyone in this room or this school a subject. No sex, drugs, or rock and roll as actions (keep it clean).

After taking two volunteers (or two not-so-volunteers) to the front of the class, have them make simple sentences. Whoever has the blue sheet provides the subject and whoever has the red sheet provides the predicate. When a sentence is completed, the student who had the subject takes the predicate sheet and the student who had the predicate sheet picks someone to be the new subject (or someone else volunteers). (You can also have a student hold up the white piece of paper for the period.)

Once students have the simple sentence down pat, you can try having the "subject student" attempt to act out or impersonate the subject and the "predicate student" act out the predicate.

This should only be done three to four times, because most students know how to make a simple sentence.

Step 3. Upping the ante. Ask five students to come to the front of the room. Give two of them subject papers, two of them predicate papers, and the fifth a conjunction paper. Have the students repeat the same activity as in Step 2, but this time creating a compound sentence. The rest of the class is required to make sure that the sentence is grammatically correct by informing you where the proper punctuation goes.

This activity can and should be done a number of times, using additional students to create longer sentences and different kinds of sentences and explore the power of conjunctions in creating meaning.

Using nearly every student in the class, an eighth-grade English class created the following sentence: "The President of the United States choked on his pretzel, but the Secret Service saved him, and people were happy and angry, yet no one knew if the pretzel had salt or didn't." Sentence structure: (S + P), conj. (S +P), conj. (S + P), conj. (S + P) conj. P conj. P.

Extension Activity

Exhibit 5.3 presents a review exercise that can be used to make sure that all students have mastered the concepts covered here. This worksheet is not the teaching tool itself but rather a self-check, so that in the coming days both you and your students will know whether more work will need to be done going over the specific rules of FANBOYS, punctuation, and sentence structure or if the class sufficiently understands the concepts.

Exhibit 5.3. FANBOYS Handout: Additional Practice Worksheet.

Directions: In the following sentences: (1) Circle the FANBOYS. (2) Underline the subject and double-underline the predicate. (3) Put in commas where they are needed.

1. And I attended Marshall Middle School.

2. Huck and Tom went swimming in the river.

3. Jerry said he had a mom but he lied.

4. I wanted to go to the movies but I never made it.

5. So I went home.

6. None of the students got in trouble and the teachers were happy.

7. Neo and Trinity are fictional for they are characters from *The Matrix*.

8. This is not the last question yet some students may wish it were the last.

9. Not everyone in class knows how to use commas so this sentence was written to see if

   you have learned what you need to know and I hope you have.

NCTE/IRA Standards

5. Students employ a wide range of strategies as they write and use different writing process elements appropriately to communicate with different audiences for a variety of purposes.

6. Students apply knowledge of language structure, language conventions (e.g., spelling and punctuation), media techniques, figurative language, and genre to create, critique, and discuss print and nonprint texts.

Crushing Contractions

Crushing Contractions is a kinesthetic lesson that teaches students about the three commonly found English contractions: "have-has" contractions, "not" contractions, and "am-is-are" contractions. It's best to present these as three different groups so that the students can better understand the rules and strategies for each of them.

This activity takes about ten minutes for each contraction group. You can teach each one in a separate mini lesson, or you can teach all of them together in one day as a review.

Segment 1: *Have-Has* Contractions

Materials

You will need index cards, markers of different colors, and tape. You will also need an overhead projector and a transparency made from Exhibit 5.4.

Exhibit 5.4. Crushing Contractions Transparency: Have-Has.

Words	Dropped Letters	Contraction
I have	I + have – ha	I've
you have	you + have – ha	you've
he has	he + has – ha	he's
she has	she + has – ha	she's
it has	it + has – ha	it's
we have	we + have – ha	we've
they have	they + have – ha	they've

1. Create cards that show the following listed words. Make multiple sets so that all students can participate in the activity—one card per student.
2. Use large-size index cards, such as 5 x 7 inches, so students can more easily see the words.
3. Make apostrophe cards that are large enough to cover up the letters that are omitted when contractions are created.

"Have-Has" Contraction Cards

Write the words in this column in one color.	Choose a different color for the words in this column.
I	have
you	have
he	has
she	has
it	has
we	have
they	have

Procedure

Step 1. Discuss the transparency you made from Exhibit 5.4.

Step 2. To create *have-has* contractions, instruct students to "take the laughter" out of the word—that is, remove the HA HA HA's. It works like this example: *I + have – ha* (remember to take the laughter out) = *I've*.

Step 3. Now pass out the cards to the students and have them pair up with one card of each color in each pair so that they can make a contraction with the two words in their possession. Once the students are paired (in the same fashion as the *have-has* contraction list), proceed to the next step.

Step 4. Give the students the index cards with the apostrophes on them. Have them use the apostrophe cards to eliminate the "ha" so that they create a contraction. Ask the students to tape their contraction cards on the chalkboard or to a wall in the classroom.

Segment 2: *Not* Contractions

Materials

You will need index cards, markers of different colors, and tape. You will also need an overhead projector and a transparency made from Exhibit 5.5.

Exhibit 5.5. Crushing Contractions Transparency: Not.

Words	Dropped Letters	Contraction
can not	can + not – no	can't
are not	are + not – o	aren't
do not	do + not – o	don't
does not	does + not – o	doesn't
could not	could + not – o	couldn't
would not	would + not – o	wouldn't
should not	should +not – o	shouldn't
will not	will + not – ill and no + on	won't
have not	have + not – o	haven't
had not	had + not – o	hadn't
has not	has + not – o	hasn't
is not	is + not – o	isn't
was not	was + not – o	wasn't
were not	were + not – o	weren't

1. Create cards that show the following listed words. Make multiple sets so that all students can participate in the activity—one card per student.

Copyright © 2007 by John Wiley & Sons, Inc.

2. Use large-size index cards, such as 5 x 7 inches, so that the students can easily see the words.

3. Make apostrophe cards that are large enough to cover up the letters that are omitted when contractions are created.

"Not" Contractions Cards

Write the words in this column in one color.	Choose a different color for the words in this column.
can	not
are	not
do	not
does	not
could	not
would	not
should	not
will	not
have	not
had	not
has	not
is	not
was	not
were	not

Procedure

Step 1. Explain to students that some contractions are created with the word *not*. Discuss the transparency made from Exhibit 5.5.

Step 2. Explain the following rules: Most *not* contractions are formed when two words are combined by substituting an apostrophe for the "o" in the word *not*. There are two exceptions to this rule: *will not* and *can not*, which become *won't* and *can't*.

Step 3. Now, pass out the cards to the students and have them pair up so they can make a contraction with the two words that they have in their possession.

Step 4. Once the students are paired (in the pairs shown in the list in the *not* contraction list), give them the index cards with apostrophes on them. Have them use the apostrophe cards to eliminate the "o" or other letters so that it creates the contraction. Ask the students to tape their contraction cards on the chalkboard or a wall in the classroom.

Segment 3: *Am-Is-Are* Contractions

Materials

You will need index cards, markers of different colors, and tape. You will also need an overhead projector and a transparency made from Exhibit 5.6.

Exhibit 5.6. Crushing Contractions Transparency: Am-Is-Are.

Words	Dropped Letters	Contraction
I am	I + am – a	I'm
you are	you + are – a	you're
he is	he + is – i	he's
she is	she + is – i	she's
it is	it + is – i	it's
we are	we + are – a	we're
they are	they + are – a	they're

1. Create cards that show the following listed words. Make multiple sets so that all students can participate in the activity—one card per student.
2. Use large-size index cards, such as 5 x 7 inches, so that the students can more easily see the words.
3. Make apostrophe cards that are large enough to cover up the letters that are omitted when contractions are created.

"Am-Is-Are" Contraction Cards

Write the words in this column in one color.	Choose a different color for the words in this column.
I	am
you	are
he	is
she	is
it	is
we	are
they	are

Procedure

Step 1. Discuss the transparency made from Exhibit 5.6. Explain that *am-is-are* contractions are formed by combining the verbs *am, is,* and *are* with the pronouns *I, you, he, she, it, we,* and *they.* In these cases, the "a" or the "i" in the verbs are removed.

Step 2. Pass out the cards to the students and have them pair up so that they can make a contraction with the two words that they have between them.

Step 3. Once the students are paired (with the same words shown in the *am-is-are* contraction list), give the students the index cards with the apostrophes on them. Have them use the apostrophe cards to eliminate the "a" or the "i" so that they create the appropriate contraction. Ask the students to post their contraction cards on the chalkboard or wall in the classroom.

 Teaching Writing in the Inclusive Classroom

NCTE/IRA Standard

6. Students apply knowledge of language structure, language conventions (e.g., spelling and punctuation), media techniques, figurative language, and genre to create, critique, and discuss print and nonprint texts.

Capitalizing Capitalization

In Capitalizing Capitalization students identify the instances where capitalization is needed for proper nouns and create a list of rules for doing so.

This activity takes about ten minutes.

Materials

You will need a blindfold, a large box or bag, and items that can spark discussion about capitalization. Here's a list of possible items:

- Map with a city or location circled

- Newspaper or magazine

- Soup label with the name of the kind of soup (not the brand name) circled

- Soup label with the brand name (not the type of soup) circled

- Book with the title circled

- Spiral notebook

- Compact disc with the artist's name circled

- Stapler

- Compass, with the directions North, South, East, and West capitalized

- DVD

- Picture of a famous person

- CD

- Pencil with the brand name circled

- Notebook with the brand name circled

- Calendar or date book

For fun, label the box "To or Not! That Is the Question."

Procedure

Step 1. Blindfold a student and instruct him or her to remove an item from the box.

Step 2. After retrieving an item, have the student remove the blindfold and determine whether the name of the item should be capitalized. The student must also explain why the item should be capitalized or not.

Step 3. Have another student record the item and the capitalization on chart paper or the chalkboard.

Teaching Writing in the Inclusive Classroom

Step 4. Repeat Steps 1 to 3, with the remaining students taking turns being blindfolded while the observing student records their choices and explanations for why they capitalized the item or not.

NCTE/IRA Standard

6. Students apply knowledge of language structure, language conventions (e.g., spelling and punctuation), media techniques, figurative language, and genre to create, critique, and discuss print and nonprint texts.

Quoting Quotables

Quoting Quotables is an activity designed to develop students' ability to articulate and identify their innate understanding of quotation marks. In small, cooperative groups, the students develop a list of rules and strategies for using quotation marks.

This activity generally takes about fifteen minutes.

Materials

You will need poster paper or large sticky notes, colored markers, and 4 x 6-inch index cards. You will also need a projector and a transparency made from Exhibit 5.7. Before you begin the activity, also cut out the quotation examples from Exhibit 5.8 and glue them onto the index cards.

Procedure

Step 1. Divide the students into groups of three to five.

Step 2. Introduce quotation marks and explain that these punctuation marks indicate the direct words that someone speaks. The open and close quotation marks indicate the beginning and end of a speaker's actual words. In a large group, model the uses of quotation marks and discuss the examples in Exhibit 5.7.

Step 3. Pass out the 4 x 6 index cards with the quotation samples taken from Exhibit 5.8. Ask the students to develop reasons why each example uses quotation marks and have them write down their reasons. As you circulate among the groups, ask the students why and how the quotations are being used in each case.

Step 4. In a large-group discussion, develop a combined list of reasons and strategies for using quotation marks taken from the small-group lists the students developed in Step 3. Use a large sheet of newsprint or poster paper to list the groups' reasons, then display it in the classroom so students will be able to refer to the list when needed.

NCTE/IRA Standard

6. Students apply knowledge of language structure, language conventions (e.g., spelling and punctuation), media techniques, figurative language, and genre to create, critique, and discuss print and nonprint texts.

Exhibit 5.7. Quoting Quotables Transparency.

Quotation example: Biff called the new car "cool" and "bodacious."
Reason for quotation: To highlight key words, phrases, and sentences.

Quotation example: A writer in the school newspaper, *Odyssey,* wrote, "The food in the cafeteria has to improve. Students are turning green in their classes after their lunch period. The food is generally cold and greasy."
Reason for quotation: A direct quote is shown from a written text.

Quotation example: The *Odyssey* writer asked Principal Skinner, "How can the school improve the quality of the cafeteria food?"
The principal replied, "No comment."
Reason for quotation: A direct quote of a statement or question.

Exhibit 5.8. Quoting Quotables: Quotations to Be Cut and Pasted.

Directions: These examples can get you and your students started as they explore the purposes of quotation marks in writing.

"Teenagers today read more paperbacks than ever before," said Mr. Binding.

The rock group's behavior was "outrageously bodacious" as they performed at the arena last night.

Katie Couric, formerly co-anchor of the *Today Show,* asked the secretary of state, "How do you feel about the actions of Congress yesterday?"

The secretary of state replied, "Well, they supported the president and we're very happy about that."

My sense of humor is often described as "silly" and "outrageous."

Bart Simpson's expression "Eat my shorts!" is obnoxious but funny.

My daughter, Ellie, describes her little brother as "Mr. Zoom Zoom," because he frequently runs around the house.

I asked the teacher, "Why do I have to do this assignment?"

The store clerk smiled and said, "Here's your change."

Appropriate Apostrophes

Appropriate Apostrophes creates opportunities for students to identify apostrophe errors and apply the rules for apostrophes. In our experience, apostrophes need to be taught more than once. There is always some confusion about apostrophes, and errors in using this punctuation mark are common.

Here are some reminders about apostrophes that you can share with your students at the beginning of the lesson:

The apostrophe has three functions. It indicates the *possessive case, contractions,* and *plurals of lowercase letters.* (This might seem simple, but it can cause some confusion.)

The possessive case is when something belongs to somebody or something else. Here are some examples of apostrophe use in the possessive case:

The student's book.
The students' books.

When the possessor is single, we indicate possession by using an apostrophe followed by the letter s:

The dog's bark.
My computer's screen.

When the possessors are plural, the apostrophe is placed after the final s:

The students' books.
The workers' paychecks.

When proper names end with the letter s, *the general rule is to add* 's.

James's brother, Ross's land, or Charles's car.

Traditional exceptions to this general rule are *Jesus* and *Moses:*

In Jesus' name and under Moses' leadership.

The apostrophe is never used with possessive pronouns: his, hers, its, ours, yours, theirs. *But it is used with* one: It is best to do one's homework.

Reminder: No apostrophe is required in the plural form of numbers and dates:

In the 1980s.
The crazy eighties.

Teaching Writing in the Inclusive Classroom

In contractions, the apostrophe is used to indicate missing letters. For example:

I am becomes *I'm. He is* becomes *he's. You are* becomes *You're.*
Note the difference between *it's* (contraction for *it is*) and *its* (meaning *belonging to it*).
It's may also be a contraction of *it has.*
Notice that the term *its'* does not exist.

The apostrophe is also used to form the plurals of *lowercase* letters (but *not* capital letters):

Dot your i's and cross your t's.

This activity takes ten to fifteen minutes.

Materials

You will need copies of the signs shown in Exhibit 5.9. You will also need handouts made from Exhibit 5.10, the apostrophe rule sheet.

Procedure

Step 1. Explain to your students that you've collected some signs that you would like to share with them. Display the various signs that contain apostrophes (Exhibit 5.9) and tell your students that you are very confused about what each sign is trying to say because of the punctuation errors, specifically in the use of apostrophes. When Katie teaches this lesson, she makes copies of such signs, adding illustrations, on large paper (11 x 17 inches) and displays them in the classroom. The room becomes a gallery of apostrophe signs. You can also make smaller copies to distribute to the students.

Step 2. Have the students work independently or in pairs. Distribute and discuss the apostrophe rule sheet (Exhibit 5.10) and ask the students to read the different signs and determine what apostrophe rule is creating the confusion. How would they correct the different signs and advertisements? Note that students will see the last signs spelled more than one way. Technically speaking, since the men's room is a room for men (plural), it should have an apostrophe: *men's.* The same goes for the ladies' room. If only one lady used it, it would be the lady's room. A completely wrong example, which can be seen on some rest room doors, is *Ladies's Room.*

NCTE/IRA Standard

6. Students apply knowledge of language structure, language conventions (e.g., spelling and punctuation), media techniques, figurative language, and genre to create, critique, and discuss print and nonprint texts.

Exhibit 5.9. Appropriate Apostrophes.

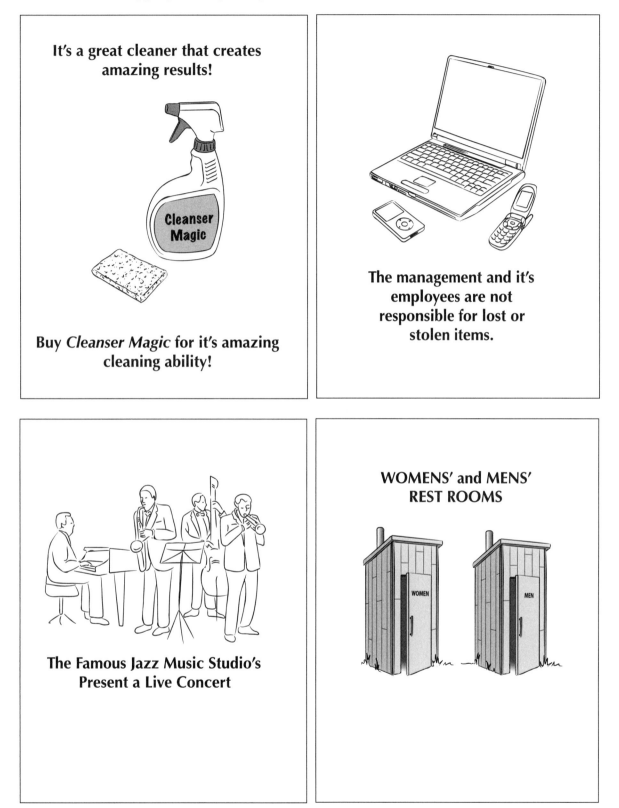

It's a great cleaner that creates amazing results!

Buy *Cleanser Magic* for it's amazing cleaning ability!

The management and it's employees are not responsible for lost or stolen items.

The Famous Jazz Music Studio's Present a Live Concert

WOMENS' and MENS' REST ROOMS

Teaching Writing in the Inclusive Classroom

Exhibit 5.10. Appropriate Apostrophes: Rule Sheet.

The apostrophe has three uses: (1) To form possessives of nouns, (2) to show the omission of letters (contractions), and (3) to indicate certain plurals of lowercase letters. Apostrophes are *not* used for possessive pronouns or for noun plurals, including acronyms.

Rule 1. To form possessives of nouns: To make a possessive, turn the phrase around and make it an "of the" phrase.

The owner of the store = the store's owner
The homework of the students = the students' homework

Remember! No apostrophe is needed if the noun after *of* is a building, an object, or a piece of furniture.

clothes of the doll = doll clothes
room of the school = school room

Now that you know that you need to make a possessive, here are some rules:

1. Add an apostrophe to the singular form of the word (even if it ends in -s): *the dog's bone, Charles's car.*
2. Add an apostrophe to the plural forms that do not end in -s: *children's stories, choir's songs*
3. Add an apostrophe to the end of plural nouns that end in -s: *teachers' lessons, houses' doors*
4. Add an apostrophe to the end of compound words: *my sister-in-law's dress*
5. Add an apostrophe to the last noun to show joint possession of an object: *Roger and Katie's book*

Rule 2. To show omission of letters: Apostrophes are used in *contractions*. A contraction is a word in which one or more letters have been omitted. Why do I need an apostrophe? The apostrophe shows this omission. The apostrophe is used in the place of an omitted letter or several omitted letters: *shouldn't = should not, where's = where is, who's = who is, can't = can not, haven't = have not, it's= it is*

Rule 3. To form plurals of lowercase letters: Apostrophes are used to form plurals of letters that appear in lowercase: *Remember to mind your p's and q's.*

Remember! Apostrophes are *not* used to form plurals of capital letters, symbols, or numbers:

My report card contained all As.
There are a lot of +s.
I love the music from the 1980s.

Defragging Sentence Fragments

This activity is designed to provide practice and application for students to identify and correct sentence fragments. Like apostrophes, sentence fragments and run-ons can be difficult concepts for student writers to grasp. Students need experience with them; they must be taught many times. As students correct their sentences, they will also improve their understanding of a complete sentence structure.

This activity takes about fifteen minutes.

Materials

You will need ruled sheets of paper, a large envelope or other container (such as a cookie jar), one set of fragment slips made by photocopying Exhibit 5.11 and cutting apart the individual phrases, and an overhead transparency made from Exhibit 5.12. You may also want to make copies of Exhibit 5.13; see Step 4.

Exhibit 5.11. Defragging Sentence Fragments: Phrase Slips.

Directions: Cut out each phrase as a separate slip of paper. Put the slips into a container, such as an envelope or a cookie jar, and distribute to the students. Make sure there are enough slips so that each student receives one.

I would like
a large cheese pizza
for dinner
Her little brother loves to play
with different toy trains
almost every day
My favorite music
is often what is played
on the radio
My parents love to tell

Teaching Writing in the Inclusive Classroom

me stories
about their youth
Does anyone
like to eat cheese
with crackers
My favorite cartoon
characters are
usually dogs
The newspaper
was not delivered
last week

Exhibit 5.12. Defragging Sentence Fragments: 1.

Sentence Fragment	What Do I Need to Know?	Complete Sentence
My favorite story in the book	What about the story? Is there a title? What is the story about?	My favorite story in the book is called "My Little Puppy."
Walking to the store	Did something happen when walking to the store? Was there a reason for walking to the store?	Walking to the store, I tripped on a stone.
Wanted to go to an amusement park	Who wanted to go to an amusement park?	I wanted to go to an amusement park.
Thought that looked	Who? What?	I thought that looked delicious.
Very good too	Was something very good too? Or was someone very good too?	My little sister was very good too.

Exhibit 5.13. Defragging Sentence Fragments: 2.

Directions: Write this on a chalkboard or on chart paper, or make copies for all students. Ask the students to fill in the blanks with you.

Fragment	Fragment	Fragment
Created Sentence		

Example

Fragment	Fragment	Fragment
the newspaper	was not delivered	last week
Created Sentence		
Last week, the newspaper was not delivered.		
The newspaper was not delivered last week.		

Procedure

Step 1. Ask your students, "What makes a sentence fragment a sentence fragment?" Using Exhibit 5.12 as a guide, brainstorm with the students as a whole group about the characteristics of sentence fragments. Here are some possible prompts and discussion points:

1. As you look at these examples, ask yourself, What's missing? What don't I know from reading this sentence fragment? How can I add information so that I understand the entire meaning of the possible sentence?

2. Point out that sentence fragments are poor writing because they create confusion for the reader.

Step 2. Discuss with the students the necessities of a complete sentence (refer to Figure 5.1). Point out to the students that the sentence encompasses a subject and a predicate to create a larger ring around these smaller components.

Figure 5.1. What a Sentence Needs.

A Sentence Needs

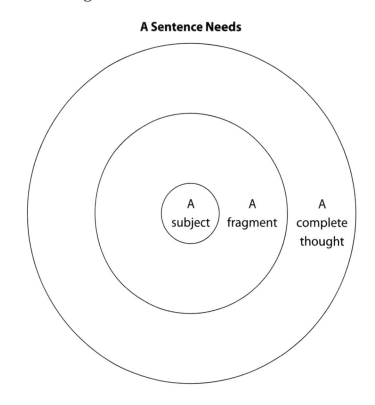

Step 3. Explain the rules for this activity. Each student is to take one slip of paper from your container. Then the students circulate and find another student or students with whom to combine slips of paper to create a complete sentence. Students must combine at least two slips of paper and can combine as many as three slips of paper. They should add punctuation and capitalization to form a complete sentence. When they have a complete sentence, they should stand with the other students with whom they are combining slips and raise their hands.

Step 4. Copy Exhibit 5.13 on the chalkboard or on chart paper, or distribute the copies you have made as handouts. Once all students have created their sentence slips of paper, complete Exhibit 5.13 with the sentences that they created.

NCTE/IRA Standard

6. Students apply knowledge of language structure, language conventions (e.g., spelling and punctuation), media techniques, figurative language, and genre to create, critique, and discuss print and nonprint texts.

Comma Chameleon

Not to sound like a broken record, once again commas have to be taught several times. Like apostrophes and sentence fragments and run-ons, commas are often used incorrectly. Student writers need to learn rules for commas and be given opportunities to play with them so that this punctuation too becomes part of their repertoire. Katie, who developed this lesson, was searching for teaching and learning strategies that incorporate multiple intelligences and different learning styles. It's always challenging to think of grammar lessons that incorporate a variety of strategic learning experiences.

The comma is a useful punctuation device because it separates the structural elements of sentences into manageable segments. It helps students understand the logic and ideas of a sentence since this punctuation separates them into chunks of meaning. This activity provides practice and application of comma rules through several learning experiences. As students correct their sentences, they also apply and practice their understanding of comma rules.

This activity takes about fifteen minutes.

Materials

Make handouts from Exhibits 5.14 and 5.15. If you want to do the extension activity, you will also need paper and markers.

Exhibit 5.14. Comma Chameleon Handout: Identifying Commas.

Name: _____ Date: _____

Directions: Place commas where you think they belong in the following sentences.

1. Katie Roger and Nancy all like to eat chocolate.

2. Katie who is the youngest girl was born in Evanston.

3. Although I have never been to California I have always wanted to visit.

4. The dog growled but let the veterinarian touch him.

5. Colin replied "I would like to play."

6. I love to sing dance and play musical instruments.

Teaching Writing in the Inclusive Classroom

Exhibit 5.15. Comma Chameleon Handout: Comma Rules.

Rule 1. Use a comma before conjunctions *(for, and, nor, but, or, so)* that join the two independent clauses in a compound sentence. *Example:* I love to ride roller coasters, but they make me dizzy.

Rule 2. Use a comma after relatively lengthy introductory phrases or dependent (subordinate) clauses. *Example:* In order to ride roller coasters, I really shouldn't eat right before I go on one.

Rule 3. Use commas to separate items in a series. *Example:* I need pencil, paper, crayons, and markers.

Rule 4. Use commas before and after nonessential elements—parts of the sentence providing information that is not essential to understand its meaning. *Example:* I bought a minivan, which isn't my favorite kind of car, because I drive large groups of people.

Rule 5. Use commas between coordinate adjectives (of equal importance) that modify the same noun. *Example:* The dog's paws were big, brown, and clumsy.

Rule 6. Use commas to separate the elements of dates and places. *Example:* Her daughter was born in Chicago, Illinois.

Rule 7. Use a comma before a direct quotation. *Example:* Katie declared, "That was brilliant!"

Rule 8. Use commas before and after words and phrases like *however, moreover,* and *nevertheless* that serve as interrupters. *Example:* Jim ate the entire container of ice cream. He did not, however, have a stomachache.

Procedure

Step 1. Divide the students into groups of two to three. Explain the origin of the comma as follows: Commas originated from a mark that was made in an actor's script to indicate that a breath or pause should be taken for dramatic effect. The tiny slash mark became commonplace with the invention of the printing press.

Step 2. Distribute the Identifying Commas handout (Exhibit 5.14) and instruct students to take turns reading the sentences aloud. After each sentence is read, discuss and decide where to place commas.

Step 3. Once the students have completed their comma placements, distribute the Comma Rules handout (Exhibit 5.15). Have the students match the rule to each of the sentences in Exhibit 5.14. They may also make changes to their original comma placements.

Step 4. Discuss each sentence in a large group. As you discuss the rules and sentences, your students should reflect on their misconceptions about comma use and compare them with the rules for comma use.

Extension Activity

Have students each create posters with sentences that demonstrate a comma rule. Each poster should contain the comma rule, an example, and a picture that illustrates the rule and example. When they illustrate grammar rules in this way, it facilitates their internalization of the new information. Then display the posters so they serve as a reminder and reinforcement of the rules. This extension activity may be assigned for homework or completed in class.

NCTE/IRA Standard

6. Students apply knowledge of language structure, language conventions (e.g., spelling and punctuation), media techniques, figurative language, and genre to create, critique, and discuss print and nonprint texts.

Prefix Circles

Prefix Circles is a strategy designed to develop students' understanding of prefixes. This is a vocabulary building exercise that develops students' ability to manipulate language, engaging in a challenge that demands logic and word skills. This activity takes about fifteen minutes.

Materials

You will need at least five sheets of poster paper, each one a different color, with one prefix and its definition listed at the top of each. You can select any of those shown in Exhibit 5.16, but make sure that each group has a different prefix.

Procedure

Step 1. Divide the class into groups of three students and give each group a prefix poster paper.

Step 2. Instruct the students to create as many words as they can think of that contain the prefix shown at the top of their paper. Tell them they have one minute to write the words down. For example: *prefix:* dis; *prefix meaning:* opposite, against; *words that begin with the prefix dis:* disagree, disallow, distaste.

Step 3. When one minute has expired, call "Time!" Then instruct the students to leave their prefix poster paper and proceed to the next group. Tell them that they are to add to the prefix list that is now in front of them. Follow this procedure for each group until the students have added words to every list in the class. When the students get to the last couple of lists, Katie lets them look in a dictionary for inspiration.

There may be some words that don't exist in the dictionary. Discuss those words and remind the students that many words are added to the dictionary every year. Writers like Shakespeare invented words all of the time, and one day the students' made-up words might be included in the dictionary. It's also a great idea to display the students' charts in the classroom.

Exhibit 5.16. Common Prefixes.

Prefix	Meaning	Examples
a, an	not, without	anonymous, another
anti	against, opposite	antisocial, antiseptic, antifreeze
audi	to hear	audience, auditory, auditorium
auto	self	automobile, automatic, autograph
bene	good, well	benefactor, beneficial, benevolent, benefit
circu	around	circumnavigate, circumstance, circumference, circulatory
con, com	with, together	convene, compress, contemporary, converge, compact, combine
contra, counter	against, opposite	contradict, counteract, contrary
de	from, down, away	detach, deploy, derange, deodorize, devoid, deflate, degenerate
dei, div	God, god	divinity, divine, deity, divination, deify
demo	people	democracy, demagogue
dia	through, across, between	diameter, diagonal, dialogue, dialect
dis, dys, dif	away, not, negative	dismiss, differ, disallow, disperse, dissuade, disconnect, dysfunction, disrespect, distaste
dyn, dyna	power	dynamic, dynamite, dynamo, dynasty
ecto	outside, external	ectomorph, ectoderm, ectoplasm
equi, equa	equal	equitable, equation, equator
e, ex	out, away, from	emit, expulsion, exhale, exit, express, exceed, explosion
exter, extra	outside of	external, extrinsic, exterior, extraordinary, extracurricular
homo	same	homogenized, homonym, homophone
hyper	over, above	hyperactive, hypersensitive, hyperventilate
hypo	below, less than	hypodermic, hypoglycemia, hypoallergenic
in, im	not	inviolate, innocent, impregnable, impossible
infra	beneath	infrared, infrastructure
inter, intro	between	international, intercept, intermission, interoffice, internal, introvert, introduce
intra	within, into	intravenous
mal	bad, badly	malformation, maladjusted
mega	great, million	megaphone, megabyte
meso	middle	mesoamerica, mesosphere
meta	beyond, change	metaphor, metamorphosis, metabolism

Teaching Writing in the Inclusive Classroom

Prefix	Meaning	Examples
micro	small	microscope, microfiche
mis	bad, badly	misinform, misinterpret, mispronounce, mistake
multi	many	multitude, multiply, multipurpose
neo	new	neoclassic, neophyte
non	not	nonabrasive, nondescript, nonsense
omni	all	omnipotent, omniscient
para	beside	paramedic, paraphrase, parachute
per	through, intensive	permit, perspire, persuade
peri	around	periscope, perimeter
phot	light	photograph, photon
poly	many	polytheist, polygon, polygamy,
port	to carry	porter, portable
re	back, again	report, retract, revise, regain
retro	backwards	retrospect, retroactive
semi	half	semifinal, semiconscious, semiannual, semimonthly, semicircle
sub	under, below	submerge, submarine, substandard
super, supra	above	superior, supernatural, supraoptic
syn	together	synthesis, syndicate
tele	distance, from afar	television, telephone, telegraph
therm, thermo	heat	thermal, thermometer
trans	across	transoceanic, transmit, transport
un	not	uncooked, unharmed
vita	life	vital, vitality, vitamins

NCTE/IRA Standard

6. Students apply knowledge of language structure, language conventions (e.g., spelling and punctuation), media techniques, figurative language, and genre to create, critique, and discuss print and nonprint texts.

Prefix Puzzle

Prefix Puzzle is another strategy to develop students' understanding of prefixes. Once the students organize and connect the puzzle pieces, they can create rules and guidelines for language. The lesson incorporates kinesthetic and visual learning styles. The different colors help the students sort and categorize the pieces.

This activity takes about twenty minutes.

Materials

You will need enough copies of the prefix organization chart (Exhibit 5.17) for each group of students and five different colors of construction paper, one for each of the five different prefix groups, with the puzzle pieces photocopied onto them. For example:

- Group 1: Copy onto blue paper the puzzle pieces with broken words demonstrating the prefix *sub* (sub/way, sub/marine, and so on).

- Group 2: Copy onto red paper the puzzle pieces with broken words demonstrating the prefix *pre* (pre/view, pre/miere).

- Group 3: Copy onto green paper the puzzle pieces with broken words demonstrating the prefix *mis* (mis/take, mis/use).

- Group 4: Copy onto yellow paper the puzzle pieces with broken words demonstrating the prefix *inter* (inter/play, inter/view).

- Group 5: Copy onto brown paper the puzzle pieces with broken words demonstrating the prefix *over* (over/confident, over/indulgent).

Procedure

Step 1. Cut up each sheet so that the puzzle pieces are separated (sub/way, mis/take).

Step 2. Divide the class into groups of three students. Give each group all of the prefix puzzle pieces and a copy of the prefix organization chart. Remember, each prefix group should be on a different color sheet of paper.

Step 3. Instruct the students to put together the puzzle pieces.

Step 4. Once the students have finished assembling the puzzle pieces, have them sort the prefix word pairs into the five color groups.

Step 5. When the students have sorted the puzzle sets by color, they are ready to complete the puzzle organization chart. When that's done, encourage them to create definitions for the prefixes and words on their own; if the students are challenged by this, let them use a dictionary. Katie likes to encourage the students to infer word meanings on their own since this builds on their ability to manipulate language.

Step 6. Once the students have completed the prefix organization chart, they can share what they have discovered about their word pairs.

Exhibit 5.17. Prefix Puzzle Organization Chart.

Puzzle Color	Word	Prefix	Prefix Meaning	Word Meaning	Other Words with Same Prefix
Group 1: Blue					
Group 2: Red					
Group 3: Green					
Group 4: Yellow					
Group 5: Brown					

NCTE/IRA Standard

6. Students apply knowledge of language structure, language conventions (e.g., spelling and punctuation), media techniques, figurative language, and genre to create, critique, and discuss print and nonprint texts.

Bucket o' Words

This is an ongoing strategy that is a great opening activity or closing activity during a class period. The students contribute words that they have encountered in their reading or just have heard and want to learn the meaning. This activity can take anywhere from five to twenty minutes, depending on how many words you and your students want to examine.

Materials

Decorate a large jar or other container and place it at the front of the classroom. Add a side pocket to the container to contain blank Bucket o' Words cards. Katie usually uses 3 x 5-inch index cards cut in half.

Procedure

Step 1. Explain to the students that they should contribute a word to the Bucket o' Words. Several times a week, some words from the bucket will be selected to review.

Step 2. Explain to the students that when they submit a word to the Bucket o' Words, they are to include the following information on the card:

- The word

- The name of the book in which they found it and page number (or description of where they heard the word)

- The sentence in which the word was used

- A dictionary definition

- Their name

Step 3. Select a card from the Bucket o' Words. Have the students try to guess the meaning of the word (the student who contributed the word isn't allowed to guess; that child can be the judge). Once the students guess, read the word in context and give a dictionary definition. The word can be added to a word wall in the classroom or to the students' vocabulary journal or learning log.

NCTE/IRA Standard

6. Students apply knowledge of language structure, language conventions (e.g., spelling and punctuation), media techniques, figurative language, and genre to create, critique, and discuss print and nonprint texts.

Vocabulary Pictures

Vocabulary Pictures is a method for learning new vocabulary through flash cards. Encourage the students to be selective about the words they use; using too many flash cards defeats the purpose.

This activity can take anywhere from five to twenty minutes, depending on how much time the teacher wants to spend on it.

Materials

You'll need 5 x 7-inch index cards or plain paper and markers, crayons, or colored pencils.

Procedure

Model the format for the students. They need to do the following:

- Write the definition of the vocabulary word in the top right corner of the index card.

- Write an antonym for the vocabulary word and draw a red "X" over it in the top left corner of the card.

- Write a sentence that uses the word in context (funny sentences are particularly helpful in learning new vocabulary words) in the lower left corner.

- Draw a picture that illustrates the meaning or concept of the word in the lower right corner.

- Write the word itself in the center.

See Figures 5.2 and 5.3.

Figure 5.2. Vocabulary Pictures: Example 1.

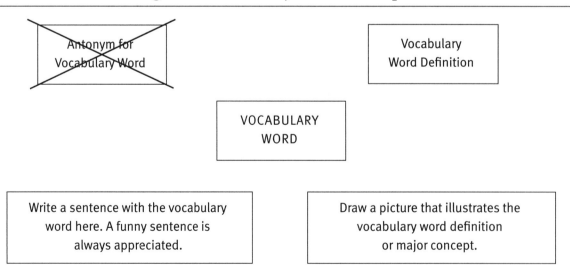

Figure 5.3. Vocabulary Pictures: Example 2.

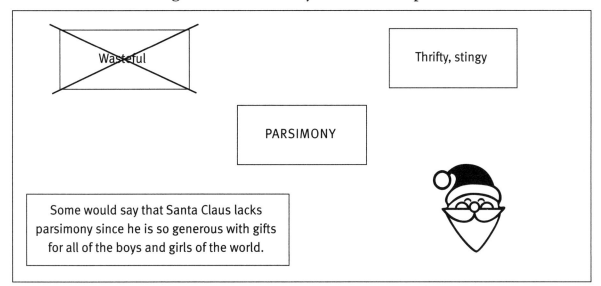

NCTE/IRA Standard

6. Students apply knowledge of language structure, language conventions (e.g., spelling and punctuation), media techniques, figurative language, and genre to create, critique, and discuss print and nonprint texts.

  Teaching Writing in the Inclusive Classroom

It's in the Bag: Adding Descriptive Details

It's in the Bag is designed to help student writers develop and increase their descriptive vocabulary. Students often rely on the same modifiers and rarely stretch their vocabulary unless they are encouraged to do so. This mini lesson will help students enlarge their descriptive vocabulary.

This activity takes ten to fifteen minutes.

Materials

You will need newsprint, pens or markers, brown paper bags, such as lunch bags, and things to fill them with. The contents of each bag should be different. Here are some items that you may use to fill the bags:

Ten to twelve marshmallows

About twenty different metal screws and nuts

Four or five pencil erasers

A small stuffed animal

A pair of knit gloves

A rawhide bone

Paper clips of various shapes and sizes

A paintbrush

A baby pacifier and a small plastic cup

Procedure

Step 1. Gather ordinary objects, such as those suggested in the preceding list, place them into the brown paper bags, and seal them. You'll need to use paper bags because the students have to feel the objects but not be able to see them. The students will rely on kinesthetic input to determine the contents of their bags.

Step 2. Divide the students into groups of two to three. Give each group a bag and strict orders not to open it. Instruct the students to take turns feeling and squeezing their bag and trying to imagine what might be in it. Explain that scientists often work in the same manner: they take what information they can find and make a guess about what is actually in front of them. Sometimes they are right and sometimes they are wrong. What's important is that they are thinking about the items and things that they are studying.

Step 3. Once the students have manipulated their bag for about five minutes, distribute large sheets of newsprint (or standard letter-size) paper and ask them to write down as many words as they can to describe what they have felt in their bag. If the class is having a particularly hard time, the sensory words handout (Exhibit 5.18) can get them started.

Step 4. Once the students have generated and recorded their lists, have them share their lists and add one another's words to their own lists. Keep the bags sealed during the entire lesson, but if the students can't stand the suspense, let them open them and determine if the descriptive words were appropriate for their items.

Exhibit 5.18. Sensory Words Handout.

hear	circular	conical
sharp	see	squared
flat	stubbly	feel
rigid	narrow	sticky
eavesdrop	spherical	flexible
piercing	glimpse	thin
even	lush	caress
quiet	thin	slimy
listen	firm	elastic
jarring	witness	watery
horizontal	smooth	handle
hushed	wide	greasy
snoop	ring-shaped	bendable
razor-sharp	perceive	gummy
vertical	downy	soft
stiff	slender	oily
mutter	globular	plastic
prickly	vision	gooey
crooked	silky	cuddly
gentle	tapered	sweet
whispering	rectangular	metallic
bristly	view	folded
straight	sleek	coarse
round	pointed	sour
shallow	oblong	wooden
barbed	consider	crinkled
diagonal	rough	

NCTE/IRA Standard

6. Students apply knowledge of language structure, language conventions (e.g., spelling and punctuation), media techniques, figurative language, and genre to create, critique, and discuss print and nonprint texts.

Teaching Writing in the Inclusive Classroom

Overusing and Abusing "Very"

Overusing and Abusing "Very" is a mini lesson that Katie developed when she taught tenth-graders. It seemed that every student used the word "very" at least ten times in a paper—the phrase "a lot" (or, as some of Roger's students write, "alot") was also overused. This lesson is another vocabulary stretcher. Students rely on the same modifiers when they have a limited repertoire. In this mini lesson, they enlarge their descriptive vocabulary.

This activity takes about ten to fifteen minutes.

Materials

Photocopy Exhibit 5.19 to make enough handouts to pass to all the students in your class.

Procedure

Step 1. Explain that the word "very" is overused and abused. There are many words that can include the idea of "very."

Step 2. Divide the students into pairs and distribute the handout.

Step 3. Have the students pair as many of the twenty-four expressions and words as they can during about five minutes.

Step 4. To complete the exercise, either regroup the students in teams of four so that they can share and compare their answers or have the groups consult a dictionary.

Exhibit 5.19. Overusing and Abusing "Very" Handout.

Name: _____	Date: _____

Expression Using "Very"	One-Word Equivalent
1. very painful	
2. very stormy	
3. very lonely	
4. very eager	
5. very needy	
6. very indifferent	
7. very wet	

Expression Using "Very"	One-Word Equivalent
8. very dry	
9. very bitter	
10. very firm	
11. very anxious	
12. very ashamed	
13. very critical	
14. very cowardly	
15. very soon	
16. very infrequent	
17. very thin	
18. very powerful	
19. very salty	
20. very clear	
21. very spiteful	
22. very important	
23. very fragrant	
24. very hopeless	

CLUE BOX

arid	apprehensive	briny	zealous
craven	captious	emaciated	doomed
excruciating	potent	obvious	tumultuous
mortified	apathetic	drenched	malicious
imminent	acrid	sporadic	momentous
forlorn	aromatic	destitute	inflexible

Teaching Writing in the Inclusive Classroom

NCTE/IRA Standard

6. Students apply knowledge of language structure, language conventions (e.g., spelling and punctuation), media techniques, figurative language, and genre to create, critique, and discuss print and nonprint texts.

Idiomatic Scavenger Hunt

The Idiomatic Scavenger Hunt gives students an opportunity to manipulate and explore language. The more students are able to play with language, the more comfortable they will become in using language to express their ideas and thoughts in writing.

Student writers need to know about idiomatic expressions because they are a significant part of our language. In addition, idiomatic expressions can teach student writers about the sometimes subtle vagueness of language. Idioms are especially difficult for English language learners (ELL) and special education students because these expressions do not have a literal meaning. Even though exceptional students may not be able to master all of the idiomatic expressions, they too need to have some familiarity so they can understand how to manipulate language.

This activity takes about twenty minutes. The extension activity takes about thirty minutes more, or it can be assigned as homework.

Materials

You will need to photocopy Exhibit 5.20 to make handouts. The thirty-five phrases it lists are just a sampling of the many idiomatic expressions that are commonly used in American English.

In addition, here are two helpful idiom Web sites: http://www.idiomsite.com/ houses an extensive online dictionary for idioms; it includes both the meaning and origin of the idiom. Another online dictionary of idioms and definitions is http://www.usingenglish.com/reference/idioms/. Also helpful is http://www.yourdictionary.com/. Two published references may also be of use: Adam Makkai, Maxine Tull Boatner, and J. E. Gates, *A Dictionary of American Idioms* (Hauppauge, NY: Barron's Educational Series, 1995) and David J. Collis, *101 American English Idioms* (New York: McGraw-Hill, 1987).

Procedure

Step 1. Distribute the handouts and ask students to guess the meaning of the various idiomatic expressions shown.

Step 2. Verify the guess—use any source to discover the actual definition of each expression. Since a dictionary will not have most of them, brainstorm sources for the definitions: the students themselves, Internet Web sites and reference books (see preceding list of sites and works), the teacher, other adults. It is also interesting to trace the origin of some of our more common idiomatic expressions.

Step 3. Ask students to share their answers with the class and discuss how they created a definition for each idiom. How many did they guess correctly?

Extension Activity

Ask the students to create an illustration depicting their favorite idiomatic expression.

Exhibit 5.20. Idiomatic Scavenger Hunt Handout.

Name: _____ Date: _____

Idiom	Meaning Guess	Meaning Actual	Origin
A picture paints a thousand words.			
Apple of my eye			
Back seat driver			
Back to square one			
Bad hair day			
None of your beeswax			
Break a leg.			
Brownie points			
Chip on his shoulder			
Close, but no cigar.			
Cut to the chase.			
Deadline			
Diamond in the rough			
Elvis has left the building.			
Face the music.			
Get out of bed on the wrong side			

Idiom	Meaning Guess	Meaning Actual	Origin
Houston, we have a problem.			
Knock on wood.			
Like a chicken without its head			
Murphy's law			
Nerd			
New kid on the block			
OK			
Over the top			
Pedal to the metal			
Peeping Tom			
Play by ear.			
Put a sock in it.			
Quiz			
Raining cats and dogs			
Sabotage			
Shot in the dark			
Tongue in cheek			
Under the weather			
Wolf in sheep's clothing			

Teaching Writing in the Inclusive Classroom

NCTE/IRA Standards

6. Students apply knowledge of language structure, language conventions (e.g., spelling and punctuation), media techniques, figurative language, and genre to create, critique, and discuss print and nonprint texts.

12. Students use spoken, written, and visual language to accomplish their own purposes (e.g., for learning, enjoyment, persuasion, and the exchange of information).

Chapter Six

Finding Out About Research

Constructing a research paper is one of the most complex and cognitively challenging academic tasks assigned to adolescent writers. In this final chapter, we cover both traditional research papers and I-Search papers. As opposed to traditional research papers, *I-Search papers* incorporate primary source material and personalize the research process.

During her first year of teaching, when she was required by her school to teach the research paper to her eleventh-graders, Katie's students struggled. She taught the research paper exactly the same way in which she had been taught, humbly apologizing to her students. She dug out her college text on how to write a research paper and proceeded to lecture them. She relayed the familiar adages: "Choose a topic that interests you!" "Use 4 x 6 index cards for notes and 3 x 5 cards for your bibliography!"

Katie's students were frustrated, and so was she. The truth came crashing down when she observed Darius, one of her struggling students, in the library. As he copied sources down, she realized that he was plagiarizing—a capital offense among most English teachers. This wasn't anything she didn't know already about Darius and his classmates. She decided to ask him what he was doing. He responded that he was taking notes. The fact was, he really didn't know

how to synthesize information. It was then that Katie realized that this was the root of the problem when it came to teaching the research paper. She had given her students many requirements but few opportunities for them to practice and synthesize the skills they were learning as they constructed their papers.

Over the next ten years, Katie developed as many kinesthetic and hands-on lessons as she could to provide opportunities for her students to practice the skills that they were learning in meaningful ways. The mini lessons offered in this chapter are the fruits of that labor. They are intended to help students synthesize all of the new information and skills that are required for research projects.

Developing Research Skill Mini Lessons

- *Keep it simple.* It's critical to get the concept for the research mini lesson down to the bare components. This makes it easier for the students to synthesize the new skills that they are learning.

- *Use hands-on activities.* Using hands-on activities is a must in research mini lessons. The more the students practice their new skills, the less they will have to think about them when it comes time for them to write their actual papers. As a teacher, you want your students to have experience with the new skills so that they become part of their skill set as writers. Writing is an individual experience; it provides students with needed accommodations to develop proficiency, voice, and in this particular case, research skills.

- *Chunk ideas.* Build the lessons so that the skills being taught are complementary. In other words, group the lessons by skill. For example, in teaching students how to take notes effectively, teach some content reading strategies, then paraphrasing, and then actual note taking.

- *Practice.* Once again, the more your students practice a skill, the more likely the strategy will become part of their writing repertoire. Even if you think they have mastered paraphrasing, for example, revisit the skill again about a week after you first teach it.

Noting Notes

Teaching student writers the art of paraphrasing and taking notes can be challenging. This activity is designed to help students pull key information from their research sources.

This activity takes about fifteen to twenty minutes.

Materials

You will need lined paper and highlighters of different colors. You will also need copies of two selected texts. Choose texts that are appropriate for the reading level of the students in your class. The selections may be from a piece of literature or a nonfiction piece on science, history, or other subject. For this exercise, it may be better to select a text that is relatively easy for the students to read. You will also need a projector. Make a transparency from Figure 6.1 and make handouts from Exhibit 6.1.

After selecting two different text passages, put copies of one of the texts in an envelope along with markers in two different colors, a copy of the handout, and the lined paper. Prepare enough envelopes for each group in your class, including three to five students in each group.

Figure 6.1. Noting Notes Transparency.

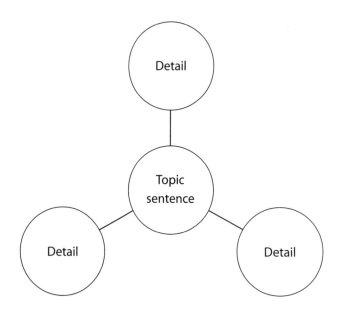

Exhibit 6.1. Noting Notes Handout.

Directions: Now that you know how to identify the topic sentence and important details in a text, it's time to practice this skill with your small group.

Steps	*Check This Box When Your Group Has Completed This Step*
Read the enclosed passage with your group.	☐
Identify the topic sentence of the passage.	☐
Highlight the topic sentence with one of the highlighters.	☐
As a group, identify the *three most important details* in the passage.	☐
Use another highlighter to highlight these details.	☐
List the topic sentence and the details that you selected on the accompanying diagram.	☐
Great job!	

Procedure

Step 1. Distribute copies of the first text to your students. Read it together in large group.

Step 2. Ask the students to identify the topic sentence in the text and then highlight it. Once they have identified the topic sentence, instruct them to identify the three most important details in the passage. The students should highlight these with a different colored highlighter pen.

Step 3. Discuss and brainstorm the details of the passage as a whole group. It's especially useful to write the topic sentence and details on the chalkboard as a Venn diagram. Show the transparency you made from Figure 6.1.

Step 4. Give each group an envelope that contains the second piece of literature or nonfiction passage, highlighter pens in two different colors, and the lined paper. As you did during the large group, have them read and identify the topic sentence and the details, as explained in Exhibit 6.1.

NCTE/IRA Standard

7. Students conduct research on issues and interests by generating ideas and questions, and by posing problems. They gather, evaluate, and synthesize data from a variety of sources (e.g., print and nonprint texts, artifacts, people) to communicate their discoveries in ways that suit their purpose and audience.

Building Focused Thesis Statements

Building a focused thesis statement is another challenging activity for research paper writers. This mini lesson breaks the thesis statement down into chunks that students can comprehend.

This activity generally takes fifteen to twenty minutes.

Materials

You will need 4 x 6-inch index cards for all students, a piece of large paper, and tape.

Procedure

Step 1. Explain to your students that you will discuss the elements of a thesis statement. Display Exhibit 6.2 as you discuss and model thesis statements.

Exhibit 6.2. Building Focused Thesis Statements: Transparency 1.

Thesis statements help writers focus their research papers. A thesis statement contains:
  A subject
  A verb
  A key term that can be divided into constituent parts (see the following example)

Example: The school parking lot needs three major improvements.
  Subject: the school parking lot
  Verb: needs
  Key term: improvements

Identify the subject, verb, and key term in the following thesis statements:

  American society today embraces many different lifestyles.

  Reading books can help people escape from reality in different ways, such as triggering imagination, through visualizing settings, or by relating to characters, among others.

Step 2. Distribute the 4 x 6-inch index cards and instruct the students to complete this practice exercise. The first step in developing the thesis statement is modeled, and the students should be prompted to develop their thesis statements. For example, write the following on the chalkboard. Explain that the students have to fill in a verb to create a complete sentence.

Subject: The poetry of Langston Hughes

Emerging thought (becomes the key term): Musical styles

Image list: Blues, jazz, spirituals

Thesis statement: Ask students to create a one-sentence thesis statement on an index card. For example:

The poetry of Langston Hughes was influenced by musical styles such as blues, jazz, and spirituals.

Step 3. After the students have created their statements, ask them to tape the statements on a wall or chalkboard and invite them to read their classmates' statements.

Step 4. Divide the students into groups. Now that students have identified the parts of a thesis statement and practiced the steps in writing one, use Exhibit 6.3 as a model to guide them through the process of creating their own thesis statements. After each group has completed its statement, again invite them to tape their thesis statements on the chalkboard or classroom wall. The students should read each other's thesis statements. This activity provides the students with the opportunity to further share and discuss the elements of a thesis statement.

Exhibit 6.3. Building Focused Thesis Statements: Transparency 2.

Directions: Choose one of the following subjects. Develop an emerging thought, an image list, and a thesis statement for the subject you choose. Be sure to create a complete sentence by including a verb.

Possible subjects: Shakespeare, Maya Angelou, Stephen King

Chosen subject: _____

Emerging thought (becomes the key term): _____

Image list: _____

Thesis statement: _____

_____

NCTE/IRA Standard

7. Students conduct research on issues and interests by generating ideas and questions, and by posing problems. They gather, evaluate, and synthesize data from a variety of sources (e.g., print and nonprint texts, artifacts, people) to communicate their discoveries in ways that suit their purpose and audience.

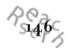

Teaching Writing in the Inclusive Classroom

Working Out a Working Outline

This hands-on exercise is designed to teach students how to organize and categorize information. The exercise actively engages students in developing a working outline for their research paper.

This activity should take fifteen to twenty minutes.

Materials

You will need index cards, large paper, tape, and four to five envelopes (one per group).

Before you begin, copy the outline shown in Exhibit 6.4 on the chalkboard or on a large sheet of butcher block paper.

Exhibit 6.4. Working Out a Working Outline Handout.

Make enough copies of the Exhibit 6.4 handout to give one copy to each group of two to three students. Make them big so that students can place their index cards in the appropriate place on the outline form. Also make copies of Exhibit 6.5, cut apart the sentences, and tape them onto the index cards. Place one set of index cards and one copy of Exhibit 6.4 in

an envelope for each group of students. On the outside of the envelope, write these instructions: *Organize these headings as needed on the provided outline.*

Exhibit 6.5. Working Out a Working Outline Strips.

Sleep deprivation has been linked to a number of health problems.

Sleep deprivation also contributes to poor personal health.

The *Times* also blames falling asleep at the wheel for 6,500 U.S. traffic deaths each year.

The typical adult needs eight hours of sleep to function effectively during the day.

Second, it increases the risk of heart diseases.

The same study showed that 20 percent of people get fewer than six hours of sleep a night.

Most Americans do not get the sleep they need on a regular basis.

The statistics linking sleep deprivation to traffic accidents and deaths are alarming.

Yet most Americans consistently get fewer than eight hours of sleep a night.

First, it weakens the immune system.

Sleep deprivation is the leading cause of traffic accidents and deaths.

It has been reported that sleep deprivation is one of the most pervasive health problems in the U.S.

Sleep deprivation is a major cause of traffic accidents and death.

Several studies show that over half of people get fewer than seven hours of sleep a night.

Third, it contributes to gastrointestinal illness.

It has been reported that drowsiness causes 200,000 auto accidents each year.

You may notice that the directions are brief. There's a reason for that. We have found that it is better to give students fewer directions as they develop their individual skills and critical thinking to resolve the writing problem that is presented. In this case, it's outlines. Every writer organizes and outlines in different ways. For example, Roger loves to use mind maps. This drives Katie nuts, and she uses linear outlines. Of course, Roger hates that organizational method. In the spirit of this book, we don't give directions that rescue kids. Make them figure out a solution; they can do it. By allowing students to experiment and figure out solutions on their own, they are developing their individual and unique skill set as writers.

Procedure

Step 1. Discuss with students the outline format shown in Exhibit 6.4. Describe and define the difference between major points, minor points, and tertiary points.

Step 2. Divide the class into groups of two to three students each. Instruct the students to read the directions on their envelope and organize the headings into the big outline format shown in Exhibit 6.4. It's best that the students organize the headings in their groups; then they can tape them onto the big outline.

Step 3. Discuss and make any revisions that may be necessary for this working outline.

NCTE/IRA Standard

7. Students conduct research on issues and interests by generating ideas and questions, and by posing problems. They gather, evaluate, and synthesize data from a variety of sources (e.g., print and nonprint texts, artifacts, people) to communicate their discoveries in ways that suit their purpose and audience.

Developing I-Search Research Papers

One of the difficulties students have with formal research papers is the emotional detachment of the format. Standard research papers are written using discipline-specific language, which is particularly dull and unattractive for students learning to conduct and document research for the first time. In addition, with most research papers, students simply read, then synthesize and rehash what they have read in the body of their papers. No time is spent engaged with primary sources or materials. In fact, instructors rarely encourage using primary sources, and sometimes don't even mention doing so.

Unlike research papers, I-Search papers place the student in the center of the inquiry process. First proposed by Ken Macrorie (1988) in *The I-Search Paper*, this format guides students through inquiry-based projects, personalizing their research process and writing by allowing them to choose a topic that interests them (thus, "I-Search"). I-Searching is constructivist practice at its best. This personalized process allows students to focus on the important task of learning how to conduct a research project and how to document their findings.

Also unlike with research papers, when conducting an I-Search students are required to speak with experts in the field rather than simply read articles written by authorities or third parties. I-Searchers cannot help but become engaged with primary source material—it is a part of the underlying concept of the I-Search to engage one-on-one with real people. When conducting an I-Search, students are encouraged to engage in serious inquiry, answering authentic questions about a content area of interest.

In addition, the I-search paper is written in the first person in a narrative style and allows students to document their findings and the path they took to obtain the information. They are, in effect, telling the story of their investigation, what prompted them to think about this question, what they read to help inform their knowledge of the problem, whom they spoke with and how that helped them better understand the subject, and finally, what it is that they learned about their particular inquiry question.

Here are some guidelines to consider when evaluating the varied audiences for the I-Search paper.

- *Special needs students, ESL students, and middle school students:* These students do not need to typewrite or word-process their papers. They need to cite sources, but do not need to adhere to a specific reference format.

- *High school students:* These students should typewrite their papers and follow Modern Language Association (MLA) guidelines to format them. They should write their I-Search papers in standard English, using clear, concise language. Their papers should be error-free.

The following mini lessons will help you teach your students how to plan, organize, research, and write an I-Search paper. None should take more than fifteen minutes to review with students. The worksheets are, then, useful as scaffolding for students as they engage in their I-Search.

Brainstorming I-Search Topics

An I-Search topic must be directly related to the content of the course and also be one that the student is interested in learning more about. Thus, the first requirement is that there be an interest in a topic.

Make photocopies of Exhibit 6.6, or create your own version of it and print copies to hand out to your students. Have your students use these charts to explore several topics that might prove fertile ground for an I-Search paper.

Exhibit 6.6. Looking at Potential Topics.

Potential topic 1: _____

This interests me because:

Potential topic 2: _____

This interests me because:

Narrowing Down the I-Search Topic

Once each student has chosen a few topics, all should bring their ideas to class—or to their group, if the students are working in groups—and explain to the other students how they became interested in their topics.

After this discussion, have the students write down the advantages and disadvantages of all their potential topics. For example, does the subject still seem interesting now that they have discussed it with their classmates? Once they list all this information, the choice will be easy for them to make. Provide enough "T" charts (Exhibit 6.7) for each student to account for each topic he wishes to explore. We suggest limiting potential topics to no fewer than two and no more than six or the project may seem overwhelming.

Exhibit 6.7. The "T" Chart.

Topic 1	Topic 2
Advantages:	Advantages:
Disadvantages:	Disadvantages:

Developing a Search Plan

Once they identify and narrow down a topic, students need to create a search plan (Exhibit 6.8). There are four phases in developing a plan. Students need to:

1. Identify existing knowledge.

2. Identify potential resources.

3. Identify potential experts.

4. Determine what they still need to learn.

Exhibit 6.8. Developing a Search Plan.

My topic is _____

I already know. . . .

I want to learn. . . .

Now break down the items listed into three main sections:

Big question: _____

Minor question 1: _____

Minor question 2: _____

Minor question 3: _____

Identifying Potential Resources

After breaking down the questions, students must identify potential resources. The following charts (Exhibits 6.9 and 6.10) will help them do so.

Students will need to find experts or authorities who know about the topic they are interested in. Remind your students that experts are persons who know a lot about something. They need not hold an official position or be of a certain age. A student's best friend may be the best authority on, say, skiing in your area.

Before they interview people who know a lot about their topic, students will need to think about the best way to approach these experts. Recommend to the students that they learn something about the topic prior to approaching an expert in the field.

When speaking with the experts, students will need to ask the experts to refer books, magazine, journals, and so on that might be useful research tools for the subject matter they are researching. They will also need to decide which resources they want to explore first. For example, do they want to interview an expert first or do a literature review first?

Students need to consult both primary sources (people who can talk to them about what they're doing or about objects and events they observe on their own) and secondary sources (books, magazines, newspapers, or people who tell you about what others have done).

Exhibit 6.9. Primary Sources.

Name of Potential Expert	Field of Interest	Reasons Why This Source Will Be Helpful

Exhibit 6.10. Secondary Sources.

Source Type (Book, Magazine or Journal, Encyclopedia, Other Compilations)	Title	Author	Reasons Why This Source Will Be Helpful

Teaching Writing in the Inclusive Classroom

Gathering Information, Integrating Information, and Self-Evaluation

The last three phases in the I-Search process are to gather and integrate information and to self-evaluate. At this point students are used to the scaffolding worksheets that help guide them through the I-Search process. These additional worksheets (Exhibits 6.11, 6.12, and 6.13) may be given to students with or without explanation. We suggest that if you introduce these worksheets in class you do so in the form of mini lessons. Each worksheet is designed to stand alone as a support for students as they continue to I-Search.

Exhibit 6.11. Gathering Information.

Type of Source	Name of Expert/Author	Field of Interest	Information I Learned from This Source

Exhibit 6.12. Integrating Information.

Topic Questions		Sources					
		Expert 1	*Expert 2*	*Magazine/ Journal 1*	*Magazine/ Journal 2*	*Book 1*	*Book 2*
	Big question						
	Minor question 1						New sources from reading
	Minor question 2						
	Minor question 3						
	New questions						
	Identify conflicts between sources						
	Reconcile conflicts between sources						
	Conclusions						

Teaching Writing in the Inclusive Classroom

Exhibit 6.13. Evaluation Checklist for the I-Search Project.

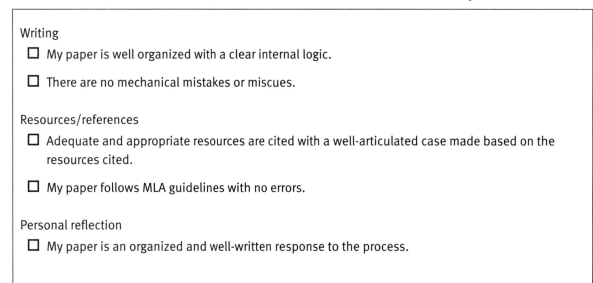

Writing

☐ My paper is well organized with a clear internal logic.

☐ There are no mechanical mistakes or miscues.

Resources/references

☐ Adequate and appropriate resources are cited with a well-articulated case made based on the resources cited.

☐ My paper follows MLA guidelines with no errors.

Personal reflection

☐ My paper is an organized and well-written response to the process.

Appendix: National Council of Teachers of English and International Reading Association (NCTE/IRA) Standards for the English Language Arts

1. Students read a wide range of print and nonprint texts to build an understanding of texts, of themselves, and of the cultures of the United States and the world; to acquire new information; to respond to the needs and demands of society and the workplace; and for personal fulfillment. Among these texts are fiction and nonfiction, classic and contemporary works.
2. Students read a wide range of literature from many periods in many genres to build an understanding of the many dimensions (e.g., philosophical, ethical, aesthetic) of human experience.
3. Students apply a wide range of strategies to comprehend, interpret, evaluate, and appreciate texts. They draw on their prior experience, their interactions with other readers and writers, their knowledge of word meaning and of other texts, their word identification strategies, and their understanding of textual features (e.g., sound-letter correspondence, sentence structure, context, graphics).
4. Students adjust their use of spoken, written, and visual language (e.g., conventions, style, vocabulary) to communicate effectively with a variety of audiences and for different purposes.

5. Students employ a wide range of strategies as they write and use different writing process elements appropriately to communicate with different audiences for a variety of purposes.

6. Students apply knowledge of language structure, language conventions (e.g., spelling and punctuation), media techniques, figurative language, and genre to create, critique, and discuss print and nonprint texts.

7. Students conduct research on issues and interests by generating ideas and questions, and by posing problems. They gather, evaluate, and synthesize data from a variety of sources (e.g., print and nonprint texts, artifacts, people) to communicate their discoveries in ways that suit their purpose and audience.

8. Students use a variety of technological and information resources (e.g., libraries, databases, computer networks, video) to gather and synthesize information and to create and communicate knowledge.

9. Students develop an understanding of and respect for diversity in language use, patterns, and dialects across cultures, ethnic groups, geographic regions, and social roles.

10. Students whose first language is not English make use of their first language to develop competency in the English language arts and to develop understanding of content across the curriculum.

11. Students participate as knowledgeable, reflective, creative, and critical members of a variety of literacy communities.

12. Students use spoken, written, and visual language to accomplish their own purposes (e.g., for learning, enjoyment, persuasion, and the exchange of information).

Appendix A.1. NCTE/IRA Standards Met in Lessons and Activities.

Chapter	Strategy/Mini Lesson	Standards Met
2	Alien Encounter	4, 5, 11, 12
5	Appropriate Apostrophes	6
2	Archaeologist	4, 5, 11, 12
2	Basic Description	4, 5, 11, 12
4	Beginning-Middle-End	4, 5
2	Blueberry	4, 5, 6, 11, 12
5	Bucket o' Words	6
6	Building Focused Thesis Statements	7
5	Capitalizing Capitalization	6
4	Checking It All Out	4, 5
5	Comma Chameleon	6
5	Crushing Contractions	6

Chapter	Strategy/Mini Lesson	Standards Met
5	Dance, FANBOYS, Dance!	5, 6
5	Defragging Sentence Fragments	6
4	Don't Spill the Topics	5
4	Fitting the Pieces Together	4, 5
2	Frame	4, 5, 11, 12
2	Friday Essay	3, 4, 5, 11, 12
2	Hall Walk	4, 5, 11, 12
5	Idiomatic Scavenger Hunt	6, 12
5	I'm Just Acting!	5, 6
5	It's Happening—Right Now!	5, 6
5	It's in the Bag: Adding Descriptive Details	6
5	Knowing Nouns and Venturing About Verbs	6
2	Lists of Ten	12
5	Looking into the Future	5, 6
6	Noting Notes	7
5	Overusing and Abusing "Very"	6
4	Paragraph Jigsaw	5
4	Persuading Paragraphs	6, 12
2	Picture Writing	4, 5, 11, 12
5	Postcards from the Past	5, 6
5	Prefix Circles	6
5	Prefix Puzzle	6
5	Quoting Quotables	6
2	Reporter	1, 3, 4, 5, 6, 7, 8, 11, 12
2	Rich Description	4, 5, 11, 12
2	Round Robin Theme Exchange	4, 5, 11, 12
4	Situation-Problem-Solution	4, 5
2	Sight, Smell, Taste-Touch, Sound (SST-TS)	4, 5, 11, 12
4	Sweet Organization	5
4	Thesis Statements and Organizing Ideas	5, 7, 12
2	Transactional Writing	4, 11, 12
2	Visualizing	4, 5, 6, 11, 12
5	Vocabulary Pictures	6
5	Who? What? A World Without Pronouns	6
6	Working Out a Working Outline	7
2	Writing Directions	3, 4, 5, 11, 12

References

Applebee, A. N. (1996). *Curriculum as conversation: Transforming traditions of teaching and learning.* Chicago: University of Chicago Press.

Atwell, N. (1987). *In the middle: Writing, reading, and learning with adolescents.* Portsmouth, NH: Boynton/Cook.

Atwell, N. (1989). *In the middle: New understandings about writing, reading, and learning.* Portsmouth, NH: Heinemann.

Atwell, N. (1998). *In the middle: New understandings about writing, reading, and learning* (2nd ed.). Portsmouth, NH: Heinemann.

Bloom, H. (1987). *The closing of the American mind: How higher education has failed democracy and impoverished the souls of today's students.* New York: Simon & Schuster.

Bradbury, R. (2005). *A sound of thunder and other stories.* New York: Harper Perennial.

Brodkin, K. (1998). *How Jews become white folks & what that says about race in America.* New Brunswick, NJ: Rutgers University Press.

Calkins, L. M. (1994). *The art of teaching writing* (rev. ed.). Portsmouth, NH: Heinemann.

Cochran-Smith, M., & Lytle, S. L. (1993). *Inside outside: Teacher research and knowledge.* New York: Teachers College Press.

Csikszentmihalyi, M. (1990). *Flow: The psychology of optimal experience.* New York: HarperCollins.

Daniels, H., & Bizar, M. (2005). *Teaching the best practice way: Methods that matter, K–12.* Portland, ME: Stenhouse.

Daniels, H., & Zemelman, S. (1985). *A writing project.* Portsmouth, NH: Heinemann.

Derrida, J. (1999). *The monolingualism of the other: Or, the prosthesis of origin.* (P. Mensah, Trans.) Stanford, CA: Stanford University Press.

Derrida, J. (2002). Faith and knowledge: The two sources of "religion" and the limits of reason alone (S. Weber, Trans.). In G. Anidjar (Ed.), *Acts of religion* (pp. 42–101). New York: Routledge.

D'Souza, D. (1991). *Illiberal education: The politics of race and sex on campus.* New York: Vintage Books.

DuBois, W.E.B. (1989). *The souls of black folks.* New York: Penguin Books. (Originally published 1903.)

Emig, J. (1977, May). Writing as a mode of learning. *College Composition and Communication, 28,* 122.

Fish, S. (1999). *The trouble with principle.* Cambridge, MA: Harvard University Press.

Flower, L., & Hayes, J. R. (1997). A cognitive process theory of writing. In J. V. Villanueva (Ed.), *Cross-talk in comp theory: A reader.* Urbana, IL: National Council of Teachers of English.

Gardner, H. (1983). *Frames of mind.* New York: Basic Books.

Gardner, H. (1984). The seven frames of mind. *Psychology Today, 18*(6), 21–26.

Geuder, P., Harvey, L., & Loyd, D. (Eds.). (1974). *They really taught us how to write.* Urbana, IL: National Council of Teachers of English.

Hillocks, G. (1986). *Research on written composition: New directions for teaching.* Urbana, IL: National Conference on Research in English.

Hillocks, G. (1995). *Teaching writing as reflective practice.* New York: Teachers College Press.

Hillocks, G., & Shulman, L. (1999). *Ways of thinking, ways of teaching.* New York: Teachers College Press.

Hirsch, E. D. (1987). *Cultural literacy: What every American needs to know.* Boston: Houghton Mifflin.

Illinois Learning Standards. (1997). Springfield: Illinois State Board of Education.

Kohn, A. (1999, November). *The deadly effects of "tougher standards": Challenging high-stakes testing and other impediments to learning.* Paper presented at the annual meeting of the National Council of Teachers of English, Denver.

Macrorie, K. (1988). *The I-Search paper.* Rochelle Park, NJ: Hayden Book Company.

Marzano, R. J., & Kendall, J. S. (1998). *Awash in a sea of standards.* Aurora, CO: Mid-Continent Regional Educational Laboratory.

Metz, M. H. (1990). Real school: A universal drama amid disparate experience. In D. Mitchell & M. E. Goertz (Eds.), *Educational politics for the new century: The twentieth anniversary yearbook of the Politics of Education Association* (pp. 75–91). Philadelphia: Falmer Press.

Murray, D. A. (1991, February). All writing is autobiography. *College Composition and Communication,* n.p.

Murray, D. A. (1997). Teach writing as a process not product. In J. V. Villanueva (Ed.), *Cross-talk in comp theory: A reader.* Urbana, IL: National Council of Teachers of English.

Newmann, F. M., Byrk, A. S., & Nagaoka, J. K. (2001). *Authentic intellectual work and standardized tests: Conflict or coexistence* (Special report series). Chicago: Consortium on Chicago School Research.

Newmann, F. M., Marks, H. M., & Gamoran, A. (1995a). *Authentic pedagogy: Standards that boost student performance* (Issue Report No. 8). Madison, WI: Center on Organization and Restructuring of Schools.

Newmann, F. M., Secada, W. G., & Wehlage, G. G. (1995b). *A guide to authentic instruction and assessment: Vision, standards and scoring.* Madison: Wisconsin Center for Education Research.

Newmann, F. M., & Wehlage, G. G. (1993). *Standards of authentic instruction* (Issue Report No. 4). Madison, WI: Center on Organization and Restructuring of Schools.

Passman, R. (2001, December). *The TIP Writing Project: Developing a Writing Program in Two West Texas Rural School Districts.* Paper presented at the annual meeting of the National Reading Conference, San Antonio.

Passman, R. (2003). It's about time! Lengthen student writing. *Academic Exchange Quarterly, 7*(3), 279–282.

Passman, R. (2004, January). *Engaging teachers—engaging students: Focused reflection and student engaged classroom practice.* Paper presented at the Hawaii International Conference on Education, Honolulu.

Perl, S. (1979). The composing processes of unskilled college writers. *Research in the Teaching of English, 13*(4), 317–336.

Ravitch, D., & Finn, C. E., Jr. (1987). *What do our 17-year-olds know? A report on the first national assessment of history and literature.* New York: HarperCollins.

Ryle, G. (1949). *The concept of mind.* Chicago: University of Chicago Press.

Schlesinger, A. M., Jr. (1998). *The disuniting of America: Reflections on a multicultural society* (rev. ed.). New York: Norton.

Schön, D. (1982). *The reflective practitioner: How professionals think in action.* New York: Basic Books.

Street, B. V. (1995). *Social literacies: Critical approaches to literacy development, ethnography and education.* London: Longman Group.

Tuchman, B. (1978). *A distant mirror: The calamitous fourteenth century.* New York: Random House.

Weaver, C. (1996). *Teaching grammar in context.* Portsmouth, NH: Boynton/Cook.

Index

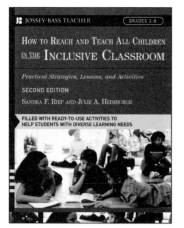

How to Reach and Teach All Children in the Inclusive Classroom
Practical Strategies, Lessons, and Activities
2nd Edition

Sandra F. Rief and Julie Heimburge

Paper   ISBN: 0-7879-8154-0
www.josseybass.com

"This best-practice toolkit for reaching and teaching all students—including those at risk—is practical, easy to use, and highly effective."
   —Greg Greicius, senior vice president for education,
      Turnaround for Children, New York City

This thoroughly updated edition of the best-selling book gives all classroom teachers, special educators, and administrators an arsenal of adaptable and ready-to-use strategies, lessons, and activities. *How to Reach and Teach All Children in the Inclusive Classroom* is a comprehensive resource that helps teachers reach students in grades 3–8 with varied learning styles, ability levels, skills, and behaviors. Topics include how to:

- Effectively differentiate instruction

- Make accommodations and modifications for students based on their learning styles, abilities, and behaviors

- Engage reluctant readers and writers

- Motivate all students to be successful mathematicians

- Increase communication and collaboration between home and school

- Build students' organization, time management, and study skills

- Implement positive behavioral supports and interventions

- Create classroom and schoolwide programs designed to enhance students' resiliency and self-esteem

Sandra Rief (San Diego, CA) is an award-winning educator with over two decades of teaching experience. Specializing in instructional and behavioral strategies for meeting the needs of children with learning, attention, and behavioral challenges, Sandra works as a consultant with the New York City school system and is a faculty member of the ADHD project of the National Initiative for Children's Healthcare Quality (NICHQ).

Julie Heimburge (San Diego, CA) has taught at the elementary level in the San Diego Unified School District for the past 25 years. As a mentor teacher, she has been involved with curriculum writing, staff development, demonstration lessons, and in-service training. Her workshops focus on developmental learning, thematic teaching, language arts, and multiple intelligences.

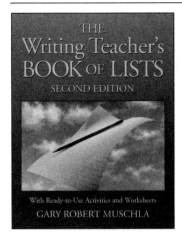

The Writing Teacher's Book of Lists
Ready-to-Use Activities and Worksheets
2nd Edition

Gary Robert Muschla

Paper   ISBN: 0-7879-7080-8
www.josseybass.com

This is the second edition of the unique information source and timesaver for English and language arts teachers. *The Writing Teacher's Book of Lists* features 90 useful lists for developing instructional materials and planning lessons that help elementary, middle, and secondary students improve their writing skills, word usage, and vocabulary.

- **Lists and Activities for Special Words and Word Groups:** Contains the information students need on topics such as synonyms, antonyms, hard-to-spell words, easily confused words, and words associated with time.

- **Lists and Activities for Nonfiction Writing:** Aids students in their understanding of nonfiction topics including advertising, ecology, education, government and politics, newspapers and magazines, sciences, and travel.

- **Lists and Activities for Fiction Writing:** Helps students grasp concepts of fiction and contains words related to various genres including adventure and romance, science fiction and fantasy, and westerns.

- **Lists and Activities for Writing Style:** Offers ways to improve students' writing skills including information on alliteration, clichés, figures of speech, overblown phrases, and transitional words and phrases.

- **Rules, CheckLists, and Activities for Student Writers:** Helps students learn the rules of capitalization, punctuation, and spelling.

- **Special Lists for Student Writers:** Includes lists on a variety of topics such as finding ideas for writing, common writing mistakes, manuscript preparation, markets for student writers, ways to improve scores on writing tests, and Web sites for student writers.

- **Special Lists for Teachers:** Contains information about creating a classroom atmosphere conducive to writing, ways to publish the writing of students, tips for conducting writing conferences with students, and a self-appraisal for writing teachers.

Gary Robert Muschla, B.A., M.A.T., taught reading and writing for more than 25 years at Appleby School in Spotswood, New Jersey. He is the author of several practical resources for teachers, including *Writing Workshop Survival Kit, English Teacher's Great Books Activities Kit, Reading Workshop Survival Kit,* and three books of Ready-to-Use Reading Proficiency Lessons and Activities for the 4th, 8th, and 10th grade levels, all published by Jossey-Bass.

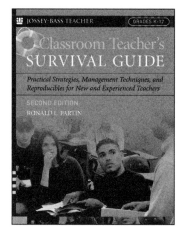

Classroom Teacher's Survival Guide
Practical Strategies, Management Techniques, and Reproducibles for New and Experienced Teachers
2nd Edition

Ronald L. Partin

Paper   ISBN: 0-7879-7253-3
www.josseybass.com

"I use the Survival Guide throughout the year as a reference tool and give it as a practical gift to my student teachers—they love it!"
   —Elizabeth Eddy, National Board Certified Teacher, Westerville South High School

Designed for both the new and experienced teacher, this fully updated second edition of the best-selling *Classroom Teacher's Survival Guide* offers a practical source of ready-to-use tips and strategies for solving the everyday problems teachers face while organizing and managing a classroom.

Here is a sampling of the topics and reproducibles you'll find in each section:

- **Create a Supportive Learning Environment:** The First Day of School . . . Humor in the Classroom . . . Thirty Hot Tips for Managing Classroom Behavior

- **Creating Successful Lessons:** Lesson Plans . . . Twenty Tips for Closing a Lesson . . . Putting More Pizzazz in Your Presentation . . . Homework That Helps

- **Alternatives to Lectures:** Twenty-Two Tips for Asking Effective Questions . . . Journal Keeping . . . Field Trips . . . Videotaping

- **Building a Learning Community:** Twenty-Four Hot Tips for Working with Other Teachers . . . Guidelines for Collaborative Teams

- **In Search of Educational Excellence:** Twenty-Two Tips for Becoming an Effective Teacher . . . Why Teachers Fail

- **Effective Use of School Time:** The Erosion of School Time . . . Block Scheduling . . . Eleven Tips on Minimizing Classroom Interruptions

- **Helpful Teaching Resources:** The Internet as a Learning Resource . . . Tips on Getting Started on the Internet . . . Computer Software for Improving Teacher Productivity

Ronald L. Partin, Ph.D., holds a doctorate in educational psychology and counseling and has more than thirty-five years of experience as an educator, scholar, counselor, consultant, and presenter. Partin is the author of *The Social Studies Teachers' Book of Lists, 2nd Edition* from Jossey-Bass.

Library of Congress Cataloging-in-Publication Data

Supportive care of children with cancer: current therapy and
   guidelines from the Children's Cancer Group / edited by Arthur R.
   Ablin. — 2nd ed.
      p. cm.
Includes bibliographical references and index.
ISBN 0-8018-5726-0 (hc : alk. paper). — ISBN 0-8018-5727-9 (pbk. alk. paper)
     1. Tumors in children—Adjuvant treatment. 2. Tumors in children
  —Treatment—Complications—Treatment. 3. Tumors in children—
  Psychological aspects. I. Ablin, Arthur. II. Children's Cancer Group.
    [DNLM: 1. Neoplasms—therapy. 2. Neoplasms—in infancy &
  childhood. QZ 266 S9592 1997]
  RC281.C4S94 1997
  618.92 ' 99406—dc21
  DNLM/DLC
  for Library of Congress   97-26952
                                      CIP